Certification Exam Review for the Pharmacy Technician

WITHDRAWN

Certification Exam Review for the Pharmacy Technician

THIRD EDITION

Mike Johnston, CPhT

PEARSON

Boston   Columbus   Indianapolis   New York   San Francisco   Hoboken
Amsterdam   Cape Town   Dubai   London   Madrid   Milan   Munich   Paris   Montreal   Toronto
Delhi   Mexico City   São Paulo   Sydney   Hong Kong   Seoul   Singapore   Taipei   Tokyo

Publisher: Julie Levin Alexander
Publisher's Assistant: Sarah Henrich
Product Manager: Marlene Pratt
Program Manager: Faye Gemmellaro
Program Management, Team Lead: Melissa Bashe
Project Management, Team Lead: Cindy Zonneveld
Project Manager: Yagnesh Jani
Editorial Assistant: Lauren Bonilla
Marketing Manager: Brittany Hammond
Senior Marketing Coordinator: Alicia Wozniak

Marketing Specialist: Michael Sirinides
Full-Service Project Management: George Jacob, Integra
Senior Operations Specialist: Mary Ann Gloriande
Media Project Manager: Lorena Cerisano
Creative Director: Andrea Nix
Art Director: Diane Ernsberger
Cover Image: diplomedia/shutterstock
Composition: Integra
Printing and Binding: Edwards Brothers Malloy
Cover Printer: Edwards Brothers Malloy

Credits and acknowledgments for material borrowed from other sources and reproduced, with permission, in this textbook appear on the appropriate page within the text.

Library of Congress Cataloging-in-Publication Data
Johnston, Mike (Pharmacy technician), author.
   Certification exam review for the pharmacy technician/Mike Johnston.—Third edition.
      p. ; cm.
   Preceded by Certification exam review for the pharmacy technician/Mike Johnston ... [et al.].
2nd ed. c2011.
   Includes index.
   ISBN 978-0-13-405644-9—ISBN 0-13-405644-2
   I. Title.
   [DNLM: 1. Pharmacy—Examination Questions.   2. Certification—Examination Questions.
3. Pharmacists' Aides. QV 18.2]
   RS122.95
   615'.1076—dc23
                                                                  2014048545

10 9 8 7 6 5 4 3 2 1

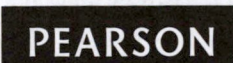

ISBN 10:   0-13-405644-2
ISBN 13: 978-0-13-405644-9

Dedication

Harry F. Banks once said, "For employee success, loyalty and integrity are equally important as ability," which explains why I view my staff to be so successful.

Each and every member of my team, although unique and individual, consistently demonstrates unshakable loyalty, integrity, and incredible ability. There is no doubt that I am blessed to work with such amazing individuals. To each member of my team—this book is dedicated to you.

—Mike Johnston

Brief Contents

Contents

Preface

Certification Exam Review for the Pharmacy Technician is a core title in Pearson Education's pharmacy technician educational list of books. This text has been developed and designed to ensure greater success for the pharmacy technician student.

About the Book
More than 525,000 individuals have become nationally certified pharmacy technicians in the United States. Many states now require national certification to practice, and becoming certified makes sense as more are looking to adopt such regulations. Achieving recognized credentials will increase both your salary and your career opportunities.

Weighted Content
The key advantage of this book is that the text content is weighted according to the national certification exam. The PTCB, the certifying board, clearly defines the percentage of content covered by the exam, yet other "review books" cover the content equally—making them, in essence, training manuals. This book has one fundamental purpose: to aid you in successfully passing the PTCB national certification exam on the first attempt. This text has removed all of the "fluff" and focuses on presenting you with the specific information and concepts you need to master to pass the exam. It is that simple.

Practice Exams
To ensure your success, we have included five complete certification practice exams. Each exam has 90 multiple-choice questions, weighted according to PTCB content guidelines, and should be completed within 3 hours—providing a true replica of the certification exam process.

The answers for each practice exam are provided at the back of the manual and include the rationale for each answer for the first practice exam—again, all to ensure your success!

New to the Edition
In addition to enhancing and updating the original content, we have added:

Nine all-new chapters to match the new exam blueprint:

- Pharmacology for Technicians
- Pharmacy Law and Regulations
- Sterile and Non-sterile Compounding
- Medication Safety
- Pharmacy Quality Assurance
- Medication Order Entry and Fill Process
- Pharmacy Inventory Management
- Pharmacy Billing and Reimbursement
- Pharmacy Information Systems Usage and Applications

About the Author

Mike Johnston, CPhT   Mike is known internationally as a respected author and speaker in the field of pharmacy. He published his first book, *Rx for Success—A Career Enhancement Guide for Pharmacy Technicians*, in 2002.

In 1999, Mike founded the NPTA in Houston, Texas, and led the association from 3 members to more than 20,000 in less than 2 years. Today, as executive director of the National Pharmacy Technician Association and publisher of *Today's Technician* magazine, he spends the majority of his time meeting with and speaking to employers, manufacturers, association leaders, and elected officials on issues related to pharmacy technicians.

About the NPTA

The NPTA, the National Pharmacy Technician Association, is the world's largest professional organization established specifically for pharmacy technicians. The association is dedicated to advancing the value of pharmacy technicians and the vital roles they play in pharmaceutical care. In a society of countless associations, we believe it takes much more than a mission statement to meet the professional needs and provide the needed leadership for the pharmacy technician profession—it takes actions and results.

The organization is composed of pharmacy technicians practicing in a variety of practice settings, such as retail, independent, hospital, mail-order, home care, long-term care, nuclear, military, correctional facility, formal education, training, management, and sales. The NPTA is a reflection of this diverse profession and provides unparalleled support and resources to members.

The NPTA is the foundation of the pharmacy technician profession. We have an unprecedented past, a strong presence, and a promising future. We are dedicated to improving our profession while remaining focused on our members.

For more information on the NPTA:
Call 888-247-8700
Visit www.pharmacytechnician.org

Acknowledgments

This book has been both an exhilarating and an exhausting project. To say that it is the result of a collaborative team effort would be a gross understatement.

Sandy—your revisions to this third edition have made this a better and stronger book. I appreciate your dedication to this project.

Mark—thank you for believing in my initial vision and concept for this project, which was anything but traditional. I will always remember the day we spent in New York City talking about cover concepts and the like at coffee shops and art galleries. More important, I am honored to have gotten to know you, Alex, and now little Sophie—and I consider each of you friends.

Julie—thank you for taking risks (plural) on this project, compared with standard policies and procedures. In the end, your support and belief in this project have allowed a truly innovative product to be published.

Robin—your commitment to this project, to exceeding all expectations, and to developing the best training series for pharmacy technicians available has been amazing. You are a wonderful, gifted individual—but most important, I am thankful to call you a friend.

Most important, I wish to thank my family. The past several years have been difficult and trying, but the strength, love, and support that you've given me have always pulled me through. Thank you.

Reviewers

George W. Strothmann Jr., CPhT, RPhT
Program Director, Pharmacy Technician

Sanford-Brown College Fort Lauderdale
Fort Lauderdale, FL

Michelle C. McCranie, AAS, CPhT, CMA (AAMA)
Medical Assisting Instructor
Ogeechee Technical College
Statesboro, GA

Shelby Newberry, CPhT
Pharmacy Technician Program Director
Vatterott College of Kansas City
Kansas City, MO

Jayson K. Parshall, BAS CPhT, RPhT
Pharmacy Technician Program Chair
Sanford-Brown College
Jacksonville, FL

Laura S. Skinner
Program Director of Pharmacy Technology
Wayne Community College
Goldsboro, NC

Pilar Perez-Jackson, PRS, CPhT, RPhT
Pharmacy Technician Program Director
Sanford-Brown Institute
Iselin, NJ

Shelby Newberry, MCPhT
Pharmacy Program Director
Vatterott College of Kansas City
Kansas City, MO

Paula Silver, B.S Biology, PharmD
Medical Assisting Faculty
ECPI University
Newport News, VA

Bobbi J. Steelman, B.S.ED, M.A.ED, CPhT
Pharmacy Technician Program Director
Daymar College
Bowling Green, Kentucky

Getting Certified

LEARNING OBJECTIVES

Learning objectives for this chapter will include:

- Definition and explanation of what a pharmacy technician is.
- Professional credentialing available to the pharmacy technician.
- Explanation of national certification and the two exams offered.
- Categories of questions and the format for both exams.
- Costs associated with both the exams as well as when they are offered.
- Professional difference between the pharmacist and the pharmacy technician.
- Benefits of pharmacy technician certification.
- Areas of competency covered by both exams.
- Requirements of updating the exam details, such as expiration, cost, and continuing education credits.

Starting at the Beginning

Each and every story, process, explanation, rule, or regulation has a beginning. This is no less true for the field of pharmacy, and of course, the pharmacy technician. In order to understand where we are going, we need to understand where we have been. So, as is the case with most things, we need to start from the beginning.

The practice of pharmacy has had such undeniable influence on civilization and the creation of society, as we know it today that it even has roots in Greek mythology. As the Greek myth goes, Asclepius, the god of medicine or god of the "healing heart," allocated the task of compounding his remedies to his apothecary, Hyiela. So, in this recording of Greek mythology, Hyiela is essentially the world's first pharmacist.

A more reliable account of the history of pharmacy can be traced back to as far as 4000 B.C., when the people of Sumeria, what would be known today as Iraq, compounded medications from plants native to the region. Licorice, opium, and mustard were just a few of the common ingredients used to compound cures for illnesses. The Sumerians are the first recorded civilization that sought to separate treating a disease from diagnosing a disease, which in today's society is the duty associated with a pharmacist and a physician. Additionally, evidence exists which proves that the Sumerians were the first civilization to employ written prescription. Proof of these early prescriptions still exists today, dating back to as far as 2700 B.C.

In Ancient Egypt, the Pastophor was considered a position of great importance or status. Pastophors were those permitted to compound or prepare medications. Borrowing from the Sumerians, the Ancient Egyptians sought to create distinct markers between those that diagnosed disease and those that created the treatments for the disease. The Ebers Papyrus dated 1500 B.C. proved the existence of the Egyptians' pharmaceutical exploration. The Ebers Papyrus, the oldest known medical papyrus or recorded paper, verifies the Egyptians' compounding of infusions, ointments, lozenges, suppositories, lotions, enemas, and pills—an unbelievable documentation of more than 875 prescriptions and 700 drugs.

Throughout the years the practice of pharmacy progressed. According to the Royal Pharmaceutical Society, based in London, England, the first record of medications was sold for profit in 1345 in London. The term *pharmacist* was first attached to the profession in 1834, when it was published in *The Last Days of Pompeii,* a novel written by the Victorian period author, Edward Bulwer-Lytton. However, the word "pharmacy" has been used in print for an even longer period of time. *The Knight's Tale,* written by Geoffrey Chaucer, defines the act of preparing medication from plants as "farmacies of herbs."

When English colonists sought refuge in the New World, so did the practice of pharmacy or apothecary, the common name of the time. As the practice of pharmacy grew, so did the need for regulation. Edward Parrish, considered by some to be the pioneer of pharmacy ethics, was an American pharmacist that fought for national standardization of pharmacy practice. In 1850 and 1860, Parrish was a member of the committee established to make practice changes to the U.S. pharmacopeia as well as an established member of the American Pharmaceutical Association, now known as the American Pharmacists Association (APhA). Through his efforts to create an environment of standardization and safety in the field of pharmacy, Parrish and his colleagues helped to lay the groundwork for legislation and regulation that affects us even today.

Other significant events related to the practice of pharmacy include the following:

- 1820—The first **U.S. Pharmacopeia** was established in Washington, DC. It is the first compilation of standards for drugs in the United States.
- 1848—**Drug Importation Act** was passed. The Act was passed in order to control the amount of altered drug entering the United States from overseas.
- 1902—**Biologics Control Act** was passed. Quality controls for purity and safety were established for serums and vaccines used to prevent and treat disease in humans.
- 1906—President Theodore Roosevelt passed the first **Food and Drug Act.** Under the original Act, the interstate trade of foods, drinks, and drugs was regulated to prevent being misbranded or contaminated.
- 1914—**The Harrison Narcotic Act** was passed. Mandated record keeping was required for narcotics by pharmacists and physicians as well as prescriptions for narcotics that were filled beyond the allowable limits.
- 1937—One hundred and seven people, of which the majority were children, were killed when diethylene glycol, a poisonous solvent, was found in Elixir of Sulfanilamide. Sulfanilamide had been used to treat streptococcal infection, but it was available only in tablet or powder form. Owing to patient demand, liquid form was created, but it was never tested for purity and safety before being introduced to the public.
- 1938—**The Federal Food, Drug, and Cosmetic Act** was enacted by the Congress primarily as a result of the 1937 Elixir of Sulfanilamide incident. The new act was a revamping of the original 1906 Food and Drug Act passed during Theodore Roosevelt's presidency. Some of the key points under the new act included the following:
  - Greater control for cosmetics and other therapeutic devices.
  - New documentation and regulation requirement for new drugs, before they are marketed to the U.S. consumers.
  - Changes concerning intend to defraud with drug misbranding.
- **Amendments under the Federal Food, Drug, and Cosmetic Act of 1938**
  - 1941—**Insulin Amendment** required FDA testing and certification of insulin safety and purity before it was released to the public.

- 1945—**Penicillin Amendment** required FDA testing and certification of penicillin safety and purity before it was released to the public. The Amendment would later grow to include all antibiotics in the U.S. market. However, in 1983 it was found that regulation was no longer needed, and the Amendment was eliminated.

- 1951—**Durham–Humphreys Amendment** allowed separation of drugs that may be used safely with little to no medical supervision and those that require medical supervision in order to be safe. Consequentially, the terms *over the counter* and *prescription* were created. The Amendment lays down that a licensed physician will have to provide a written prescription for those drugs that are labeled as prescription medications. Additionally, the Amendment decided which prescription medications and refills could be authorized from a licensed physician to a pharmacist over the phone.

It is undeniable that the Federal Food, Drug, and Cosmetic Act of 1938 and its subsequent amendments have played a very significant role in the field of pharmacy. While it may seem that pharmacy's past has very little to do with the field of pharmacy today or with the career of the pharmacy technician, this is far from the truth. Philosopher and novelist George Santayana has aptly said, "Those who do not remember the past are condemned to repeat it." In the field of pharmacy, remembering our past helps us improve upon the future of the patients we serve. Pharmacy manufacturers, pharmacists, and pharmacy technicians are all responsible for the safety of the patient. In order to ensure safety for the patient, the field of pharmacy must always undergo progressive change, of which the pharmacy technician must constitute an integral part.

Now that we have understood how the field of pharmacy established, we need to understand the role of pharmacy technician. If you visit State Boards of Pharmacy Web sites, you will find that a pharmacy technician is defined as "An individual who is responsible in a pharmacy to provide technical services that do not require professional judgment regarding preparing and distributing drugs and who works under the direct supervision of and is responsible to a pharmacist." Today's pharmacy technician, however, plays a much more significant role than just being the pharmacist's assistant. Today's pharmacy technicians require training and education in order to keep pace with the changes bound to take place in the field of pharmacy.

While the definition of a pharmacy technician states that there be no "professional judgment" made by the pharmacy technician concerning the preparing and distribution of drugs, there is still a specific level of skill, training, and education required by the pharmacy technician in order to provide safe and effective experience for the patient. Essential to securing the value of the pharmacy technician's skill level, along with training and education, is national certification.

Pharmacy technicians can be found working in any number of pharmacy settings, but two most common settings are ambulatory pharmacies and institutional pharmacies. Ambulatory pharmacies are more commonly referred to as retail or community pharmacies. This type of pharmacy setting would include not only large retail pharmacies such as Walgreens or Rite-Aide, but also small single-proprietor pharmacies. Mail order, home health care, and clinic pharmacies are also labeled as ambulatory pharmacies.

Institutional pharmacies, on the other hand, are typically housed within a hospital or other health-care facility. The purpose of an institutional pharmacy is to provide pharmacy services for the patients of the hospital or health-care facility. This is also referred to as inpatient services. While the majority of institutional pharmacies will provide care as inpatient services, some institutional pharmacies will also provide care as an outpatient services. Institutional pharmacies that provide outpatient services generally provide this service as a convenience to the patient. Patients that utilize the services of an institutional pharmacy's outpatient services are typically patients that are being discharged from the facility's emergency department, same-day surgery, or inpatient services. However, institutional pharmacies may also provide outpatient services to the facility's clinics, such as an oncology or pain clinic. Long-term care, assisted-living facilities, as well as retirement homes may also be classified as institutional pharmacies.

When trying to distinguish an ambulatory pharmacy from an institutional pharmacy, a good rule of thumb is that if patients travel to the pharmacy or the pharmacy travels to the patient, it is an ambulatory pharmacy. If the patients and the pharmacy are housed in the same facility, it is an institutional pharmacy. Of course, you must also keep in mind that some institutions provide outpatient services for their patient as well.

Pharmacy technicians are health-care professionals, and as health-care professionals they are expected to possess, not only a certain level of skill, education, and training, but also professionalism and integrity. Professionalism and integrity go hand in hand; one cannot truly possess one without the other. On a daily basis, pharmacy technicians process confidential patient information. Patient demographics, medical histories, insurance information, and payment information are all available to the pharmacy technician at the touch of a button. Confidentiality of patient information is imperative whenever pharmacy services are provided to a patient. The Health Insurance Portability and Accountability Act of 1996 (HIPAA) speaks directly of the issue of patient information and privacy. Violation of HIPAA regulations can lead to suspension of licensure, immediate dismissal, or even prison sentence. HIPAA is taken quite seriously in the medical community and should be respected as such.

A pharmacy technician must always work under the direct supervision of a licensed, registered pharmacist. There is absolutely no exception to this rule. The pharmacist is a licensed professional with years of training specifically in the field of pharmacy. If an error is made, the liability ultimately falls on the pharmacist. However, a pharmacy technician may be accountable for errors that are made out of negligence or omission. Pharmacy is a profession that thrives on the trust of the public as well as other health-care professionals. Once the trust is broken, it is very difficult to regain the same trust; using sound judgment and caution is mandatory within the profession of pharmacy.

The profession of pharmacy is one of the most respected career fields today. In the December 2013 Gallup poll, pharmacists ranked second only to nurses when the general public was asked to rank professions according to honesty and integrity. Pharmacy technicians should maintain the same demeanor as their pharmacist counterparts. A technician that is not willing to put the patient first while abiding by the rules and regulations set by state and federal agencies should probably rethink about his or her career path.

Evidence shows that the practice of pharmacy has roots as far back as the Ancient Egyptians and even Greek mythology. Fortunately, the profession has evolved remarkably and continues to evolve with changing generations of pharmacists and pharmacy technicians. Pharmacy technicians update themselves with changes in pharmacy processes. Pharmacy technicians have gone from ringing up prescriptions, to compounding intravenous solutions, to medication reconciliation duties, and even to supervising the work of other pharmacy technicians. Change is imminent and necessary for growth. The pharmacy technician is an excellent example of change within the profession of pharmacy.

Today, pharmacy technicians are finding themselves completing tasks once reserved for pharmacists. The changing tide of patient care is moving toward a more clinic-based aspect. Recent laws and regulations require the pharmacist to counsel patients on their medication as well as collaborate with physician on medication therapies. The result of this change is evident. More and more duties that were once tasked to the pharmacist are being handed over to the pharmacy technician. It is for this reason that training, education, and national certification for the pharmacy technician is so fundamental.

A great number of pharmacy technicians employed today may have received training through programs offered by their employers. On-the-job training today is not as prevalent as it was in past decades, and it can still be an effective way to train the pharmacy technician, but its reach can be short, and the pharmacy technician learn little to nothing about theory or background surrounding pharmacy. Today's technicians require more than a simple "instruct and do" training. In order to provide the patient with the best, safest care, the pharmacy technician must attain both training and education.

Pharmacy technician education has become more widespread. Pharmacy technicians may receive education through a number of sources. Accredited technical schools, health systems, professional organizations, and community colleges offer education and training programs for the pharmacy technician. Upon completion of one of these programs, the pharmacy technician receives a certificate of completion, program diploma, or an Associates of Applied Science (AAS) in Pharmacy Technology depending on the chosen program.

Every pharmacy technician program will vary slightly from any other program, but some of the basic courses that a prospective student can expect to take include the following:

- Introduction to Pharmacy Technology
- Pharmacy Calculations
- Pharmacy Operations
- Pharmacology for Pharmacy Technicians
- Pharmacy Laws and Ethics
- Computer Applications in Pharmacy
- Sterile Products
- Inter-professional Relationships in Pharmacy

As previously stated, courses will vary depending upon the program, but most will be similar to those previously mentioned. In addition to course work, students will most likely be required to complete an internship with a local retail and institutional pharmacy. Some programs may require the student to take a specialized internship, such as sterile IV or chemotherapy compounding.

Pharmacy technician students who choose a program that offers an Associates of Applied Science (AAS) in Pharmacy Technology will be required to complete all of the same courses as the certificate or diploma programs, but will be required to complete courses in the following subjects as well:

- English
- Biology
- Advanced Mathematics, such as College Algebra
- Chemistry
  - General and Organic
- Humanities
- Social Sciences
- Communications

An AAS in Pharmacy Technology will take longer than a certificate or diploma program, but may also provide the pharmacy technician student greater career potential. Pharmacy technician supervisor and pharmacy technician educator are just a few career paths that may be available to pharmacy technicians with AAS in Pharmacy Technology.

Whenever a potential student is contemplating a career as a pharmacy technician, there are things that need to be taken into consideration. One of the first questions a potential pharmacy technician should ask is, "Why do I want to become a pharmacy technician?" Knowing why you want to become a pharmacy technician will not only motivate you but also prepare you. Chances are that if students understand their reasons for becoming a pharmacy technician, they will be more eager to overcome any challenges that may come their way. Pharmacy technician students that are not motivated and do not fully understand why they want to become a pharmacy technician, or simply feel that the career path is just a "means to an end," will most likely not perform well as a student or as a pharmacy technician. Students with this mind-set should rethink their career path.

Once a potential pharmacy technician student decides to take this career path, he or she should explore training programs. If several pharmacy technician programs are offered within a community, the pharmacy technician student should evaluate each program and decide which one best fits his or her needs. When evaluating a program, a student should check for the following points:

- Verify the program accreditation—Legitimate programs will be accredited by either the Accreditation Council on Pharmacy Education (ACPE) or the American Society of Health System Pharmacist (ASHP).
- Evaluate the program courses—If the program does not offer courses in pharmacy calculations, pharmacology, pharmacy ethics, and professionalism or pharmacy law, it may be time to explore other programs. Courses such as those previously mentioned help the pharmacy technicians to not only build a solid knowledge basis, but also develop a greater understanding of the profession as a whole.
- Check if national certification is a program goal—Many employers require national certification as a condition of employment. Additionally, many state boards of pharmacy also require national certification, before a technician is permitted to be employed by a retail or institutional pharmacy.
- Check if the program offers career development—Pharmacy technician programs should be able to assist pharmacy technician graduates with development of their career. It should help them in understanding how to write an effective resume and cover letter as well as successfully navigating the interview process.

Pharmacy technician programs that are fully accredited offer a solid learning experience for the students and provide future employers with employees that are well educated and have a complete understanding of the practice of pharmacy. Programs that offer career planning and development bring pharmacy technicians and future employers together.

Learning About National Certification

National certification—what exactly does it mean and why is it so important to the career of a pharmacy technician? These are two very appropriate questions that will be discussed and answered in the next few paragraphs. National certification has become the standard for the pharmacy technician. Currently, there are only six state boards of pharmacy that do not require national certification in order to practice as a pharmacy technician. As previously addressed, the move toward pharmacy technicians that have better training and more education is not just a trend, but also a need, and national certification fits this criteria.

The Merriam Webster dictionary defines certification as *the act of making something official: official approval to do something professionally and legally.* In other words, certification is the recognition of a person's professional or technical skills and abilities. Certification is not the only term attached to the profession; but registration and licensing are also valid; however, there is a distinct difference between the three.

- **Registration**—*the act or process of placing names on an official list*
- **Licensing**—*permission is granted by a government entity for an individual to perform an activity. Specific criteria must be met before licensing can occur, which is a means of protecting the public*
- **Certification**—*the act of making something official: official approval to do something professionally and legally*

So, while each one of these terms has its own specific meaning, they all have to do with official recognition of a particular act or skill. Two more terms that may be associated with any one of the three previously mentioned terms are *credentialing* and *accreditation*. Credentialing is the act of granting formal recognition of professional or technical competency, whereas accreditation typically refers to an institution that has met a specific set of standards set by an agency and has received that agency's seal of approval. For example, The Any City Hospital strives to meet certain criteria in order to receive the Joint Commission's Gold Seal of Approval. Receiving Joint Commission's Gold Seal of Approval allows the hospital's patients and the public the security of knowing the hospital has met certain standards in order to provide the safest experience possible.

For the intent and purposes of this text, we will be focusing on certification of the pharmacy technician. Certification, as we previously explored, is official recognition, typically by a nongovernmental agency, that an individual has met a specified level of competency in order to perform a particular task or tasks. A pharmacy technician can obtain national certification through one of the two means—either through an exam given by the Pharmacy Technician Certification Board (PTCB) or through an exam given by the National HealthCareer Association, known as the Exam for Certification of Pharmacy Technician (ExCPT). It is important to recognize that successful completion of either of these exams gives the pharmacy technician national certification, which is recognized throughout the United States, and can become an invaluable career tool.

Differences Between the Two Exams

In 1995, several professional pharmacy organizations recognized a need for the standardization of the knowledge and skills required to become a competent pharmacy technician. The American Pharmacists Association (APhA), the Illinois Council of Health-System Pharmacist (ICHP), the Michigan Pharmacist Association (MPA), and the American Society of Health System Pharmacist (ASHP) came together with one single goal in mind—to create a nationally recognized exam that would help to standardize and identify the skill and knowledge of the pharmacy technician. The outcome of the meeting was the formation of the Pharmacy Technician Certification Board (PTCB).

Since it first started administering the exam in 1995, PTCB has nationally certified more than half a million pharmacy technicians. The Pharmacy Technician Certification Exam (PTCE) was the first accredited exam available for pharmacy technicians seeking national certification. The PTCE is offered continuously throughout the year at various testing sites nationwide. To take the exam candidates can apply online at the PTCB Web site http://www.ptcb.org. Once the application has been approved by PTCB, the candidate will have 90 days to take the exam at their chosen testing center. A list of testing centers is made available once the candidate's application has been approved.

The PTCE is proctored and administered by Pearson Vue. Once candidates have received application approval, they may schedule the exam through the Pearson Vue Web site http://pearsonvue.org or by phone at (866) 902-0593. A pharmacy technician that requires special accommodation due to a chronic illness, disability, or travel issues is required to take permission from PTCB before a special accommodation can be made. PTCB complies with the Americans with Disabilities Act of 1990 (ADA), but requires candidates to complete the "Special Accommodations" request form. The form is available on the PTCB Web site http://www.ptcb.org/docs/get-certified/accommodations-form. Once approval is granted, candidates can call Pearson Vue at (800) 466-0450.

Canceling and/or rescheduling of the exam are handled through Pearson Vue. Candidates may cancel or reschedule their exam as long as the request to cancel or reschedule is initiated no less than one business day prior to the exam. All applicable fees of candidates that fail to arrive at their scheduled time or are more than 30 minutes late for the exam will be forfeited. Candidates that still wish to obtain the certification will be required to re-apply for the exam and pay all applicable exam fees.

Candidates must be able to present a valid, nonexpired, government-issued photo ID on the day of the exam. Candidates who are not able to present the required ID will not be permitted to take the exam. Valid forms of identification include the following:

- Government-issued passport with photo ID
- State-issued driver's license or permit
- Official photo ID issued by a state or federal agency
- Permanent Resident Card (Green Card)
- U.S. Department of Homeland Security-issued Employment Authorization Card
- Immigrant and nonimmigrant visas issued by the United States.

Names of candidates on IDs must match with their names on their PTCB accounts. Candidates that cannot provide a valid ID will need to re-apply for the exam and pay all applicable exam fees.

Candidates that are unable to complete the exam within the 90-day window or need to withdraw from the exam may do so by logging onto their PTCB account; however, an administration fee of $25.00 will be deducted from their application refund. All application fees of candidates that fail to take the exam before the 90-day window expires or fail to withdraw within the allowable time period will be forfeited. Candidates wishing to obtain certification at a later date will be required to re-apply and pay all applicable exam fees.

Sometimes there are extenuating circumstances that may not allow a candidate to take the exam on their scheduled testing date. Candidates that miss their scheduled testing date or the 90-day exam window due to emergency circumstances may petition PTCB for an emergency withdrawal. Candidates must provide PTCB with an Emergency Withdrawal form available at http://www.ptcb.org/docs/default-source/get-certified/emgergency-withdrawal-form, as well as documentation to support the need for an emergency withdrawal. Situations that may be considered for an emergency withdrawal include the following:

- Death of a family member
- Serious illness or injury
- Hospitalization
- Court appearance
- Other extenuating circumstances

PTCB and its Board will have the final approval on all emergency withdrawals. Emergency withdrawals that do not have supporting documentation will not be considered.

Certification as a pharmacy technician will be granted only under the following conditions set forth by PTCB:

- Have a high school diploma or equivalent such as a G.E.D. or foreign diploma
- Provide PTCB with full disclosure of all criminal and State Board of Pharmacy registration and licensing action
- Comply with all PTCB certification policies as they apply to the candidate
- A passing score on the Pharmacy Technician Certification Exam (PTCE)

PTCE candidates are held to strict Code of Conduct. A full disclosure of PTCB's Code of Conduct is available on the PTCB Web site http://www.ptcb.org/resources/code-of-conduct. Candidates that violate PTCB certification policies or Code of Conduct, or are in violation of State Board of Pharmacy registration or licensing regulations will not be eligible to apply for exam certification. Candidates are also cautioned that past, current, or pending criminal conduct will be grounds for ineligibility. PTCB reserves the right to request background checks or future verification of candidates at their discretion.

The exam consists of 90 questions, 80 scored and 10 unscored. The certified pharmacy technician candidate will have 110 minutes to take the exam. The PTCE is a weighted exam, which means that some questions will hold more points or value than others, and the final score will be based on the number of questions answered correctly. The PTCB exam is entirely computer based and graded as an immediate "pass" or "fail" once the candidate has completed the exam. In order to receive certification, candidates must obtain a score of no less than 1400 points out of a possible 1600.

Candidates can take up to four attempts to pass the exam. A candidate not able to qualify in the first attempt must wait for a period of no less than 60 days before taking the second attempt. After the first and second attempts are exhausted, a candidate must wait for a period of no less than six months before retaking the exam for the third and final time. Candidates should note that the cost of each attempt of the exam is $129.00. Candidates are encouraged to check with their employers regarding the reimbursement of exam fees, as many employers will pay for certification as an employment benefit.

As previously mentioned, questions on the exam are weighted or carry more point value than others. Questions on the exam are based on surveyed information received from pharmacy technicians across the country. The PTCB exam covers the following areas as they relate to the pharmacy technician:

- **Pharmacology for the Pharmacy Technician**
  - Brand and generic names
  - Therapeutic equivalents
  - Drug interactions
    - Drug–disease
    - Drug–drug
    - Drug–dietary supplement
    - Drug–OTC
    - Drug–nutrient
    - Drug–laboratory
  - Drug doses, strengths, forms, physical appearance, route of administration, and duration of therapy
  - Common and severe adverse side effects, allergies, and therapeutic contraindications associated with medications
  - Dosage and indication legends, OTC medications, and herbal and dietary supplements
- **Pharmacy Laws and Regulations**
  - Storage, handling, and disposal of hazardous substances and waste
    - Material Safety Data Sheets (MSDS)
  - Hazardous substances exposure, prevention, and treatment
    - Eye wash stations
    - Hazardous drug and chemotherapy spill kits
    - Personnel Protective Equipment (PPE)
  - Drug Enforcement Agency (DEA) Regulations
    - Regulations for controlled substance transfer
    - Documentation for controlled substances
      - Ordering
      - Returning
      - Loss/theft
      - Destruction
    - How to verify a prescriber's DEA number

- Documentation and retention of prescriptions
  - Basic record-keeping criteria
  - Length of time prescriptions must remain on file
- Requirements for dispensing restricted drug programs
  - Processing requirements
    - Thalidomide
    - Isotretinoin
    - Clozapine
- Professional requirements and expectations concerning patient information
  - Health Information Portability and Accountability Act
    - Confidentiality of patient information
  - Security and integrity of patient data
    - Backing up and archiving data
- Omnibus Budget Reconciliation Act of 1990 (OBRA '90)
  - Specific requirements of pharmacist–patient consultation
- Food and Drug Administration (FDA) recall classification
  - Requirements of each recall class
- Standards for infection control as set by OSHA, USP<797>, and USP<795>
  - Hand washing
  - Clean room standards
  - Laminar airflow requirements
  - Cleaning of equipment in a pharmacy
    - Counting trays, countertops, balances, other instruments of measure
- The Joint Commission and the State Board of Pharmacy
  - Record-keeping requirements
    - Repackaged drug products
    - Recalled drug products
    - Supplies
  - Professional responsibilities and standards
    - Role of the pharmacist
    - Role of the pharmacy technician
    - Role of other pharmacy personnel
  - State and federal laws and regulations
    - Understanding their interactions
    - Understanding authoritative priority
  - Facilitative requirements of a pharmacy
    - Equipment and supplies
    - Dimensions and space
    - Reference materials
    - Storage of prescription files
    - Public health and cleanliness factors
- **Sterile and Nonsterile Compounding**
  - Infection control measures
    - Personal protective equipment
    - Hand washing recommendations
      - Centers for Disease and Control and Prevention (CDC)
      - World Health Organization (WHO)

- **Medication Safety**
  - Preventing errors during data entry
    - Correct patient, correct medication order or prescription
  - Patient medication precautions and directions
    - Patient package inserts
    - Medication-specific information requirements
    - Auxiliary labels
    - Special precautions
  - Recognizing patients and medication therapies that require pharmacist intervention
    - Recommendations for OTC medications
    - Therapeutic substitutions
    - Misuse of medication
    - Missed dose
    - Drug Utilization Review (DUR)
      - What is a DUR
      - Issues addresses with DUR
    - Adverse Drug Events (ADE)
      - What is an adverse drug event
      - Reporting and adverse drug event
    - Look alike/sound alike medications
      - Recommendations from the Institute for Safe Medication Practices (ISMP)
    - High-alert and high-risk medications
      - ISMP recommendations
        - In an ambulatory or community pharmacy
        - In an institutional or acute care pharmacy
    - Approaches for safe patient medication practices
      - Tall man, short man letter
      - Separation of inventory
        - Hazardous drug
        - Chemotherapy agents
      - Leading and trailing zeros
      - Use of abbreviations
        - Error-prone abbreviations
        - Approved abbreviations
- **Pharmacy Quality Assurance**
  - Quality assurance measures for medications and inventory control
    - National Drug Code (NDC)
      - Identification
    - Drug bar coding
    - Data entry
  - Infection control guidelines
    - Documentation
    - Procedure recommendations
    - Personnel Protective Equipment
    - Safety measures during needle recapping

- Risk management guidelines and regulations
  - Recommendation for prevention of medication errors
- Appropriate use of communication
  - Use of proper channels and chain of command
  - Problem solving
  - Follow-up and resolution
    - Drug recalls and shortages
- Productivity, efficiency, and customer satisfaction measures
- **Medication Order Entry and Fill Process**
  - Order entry
  - Interpreting and receiving patient data for entry
  - Dose calculation requirements
  - Physician order and prescription fill procedures
    - Correct drug for the correct patient
    - Special handling
    - Measurements
      - Counting
      - Liquid measure
    - Final check of product
  - Patient label requirements
    - Patient-specific information
    - Auxiliary and warning labels
    - Expiration dating
    - Refill requirements
    - Prescriber information
  - Prescription and order packaging
    - Types of containers
      - Syringes
      - Bags
      - Glass
      - PVC
    - Child-resistant packaging
      - Regulations
    - Light-resistant packaging
  - Dispensing procedures
    - Prescription and order
      - Validation
      - Documentation
      - Distribution
- **Pharmacy Inventory Management**
  - Function and application of NDC number
    - Lot numbers and expiration dates
  - Formulary or approved/preferred product list
  - Ordering and receiving inventory stock
    - Par levels
    - Rotation of stock

- Drug Storage Requirements
  - Room-temperature medications
  - Refrigerated medications
  - Freezer medications
- Removal of medications from inventory
  - Recalls
  - Returns
  - Outdates
  - Reverse distribution
- **Pharmacy Billing and Reimbursement**
  - Prescription plans and reimbursement
    - Health Maintenance Organizations (HMO)
    - Preferred Provider Organizations (PPO)
    - Centers for Medicare and Medicaid Services (CMS)
    - Private plans
  - Solving third-party payer issues
    - Prior authorizations
    - Rejected claims
    - Plan limitations
  - Payment from third-party payers
    - Medication assistance programs
    - Coupons
    - Self-pay
    - Pharmacy Benefits Management (PBM)
  - Health-care reimbursement systems
    - Home health
    - Long-term care
    - Home infusion
  - Coordination of patient pharmacy benefits and plans
- **Pharmacy Information System Usage and Applications**
  - Pharmacy-related computer applications for documenting the dispensing of prescriptions or medication orders
    - Electronic Medical Records (EMR)
    - Patient compliance
    - Patient risk factors
      - Alcohol use
      - Drug allergies
      - Side effects
    - Database, pharmacy computer applications, and documentation management
      - User access
      - Drug database
      - Interface
      - Inventory report
      - Usage reports
      - Override reports
      - Diversion reports

The Pharmacy Technician Certification Board (PTCB) made extensive updates to its exam in November 2013. The categories listed above provide a complete listing of those revisions. Along with a blueprint of the exam, PTCB also provides percent of content based upon the exam knowledge categories. A review of exam content, as per PTCB's Knowledge Domains and Areas, is provided below.

- Pharmacology for Pharmacy Technicians   13.75% of exam content
- Pharmacy Laws and Regulations   12.50% of exam content
- Sterile and Nonsterile Compounding   8.75% of exam content
- Medication Safety   12.50% of exam content
- Pharmacy Quality Assurance   7.50% of exam content
- Medication Order Entry and Fill Process   17.50 % of exam content
- Pharmacy Inventory Management   8.75% of exam content
- Pharmacy Billing and Reimbursement   8.75% of exam content
- Pharmacy Information Systems   10.00% of exam content

Pharmacy technicians preparing to take the PTCE should have a well-rounded knowledge base as it pertains to the practice of pharmacy. Pharmacy technicians should use PTCB's Knowledge Domains and Areas as a study guideline, but should be cautioned not to overlook an exam area based upon the projected percentage of content. Pharmacy technicians participating in the PTCE should also remember that while not directly referenced in PTCB's Knowledge Domains and Areas, the use of pharmacy calculations plays a significant role in the exam.

Candidates that successfully pass the PTCE will be awarded the title of Certified Pharmacy Technician, or CPhT. PTCB-certified pharmacy technicians are required to renew their certification biannually. As part of the renewal process, the CPhT must pay a biannual fee of $40.00 and complete not less than 20 hours of continuing education (CE) credits during the 2-year period prior to their renewal date.

Qualified CE credits must be accredited by the Accreditation Council for Pharmacy Education (ACPE) and should meet all of the following requirements:

- No less than 1 credit hour of pharmacy law
- No less than 1 credit hour concerning patient medication safety measures
- CE credit must pertain specifically to the field of pharmacy and the pharmacy technician and may cover any of the following subjects:
  - Distribution of medication
  - Inventory control measures
  - Mathematics
    - Pharmacy weights and measures
    - Pharmacy calculations
  - Biology
  - Pharmaceutical science
  - Pharmacy law
  - Pharmacology/drug therapy
  - Roles and duties of the pharmacy technician
  - Patient medication safety measures

CPhTs that are applying for certification reinstatement must follow the same requirements under the renewal process with the following exceptions:

- No less than 2 CE credits dealing in pharmacy law
- No less than 1 CE credit dealing with patient medication safety measures

Renewal and reinstatement candidates are permitted to apply not more than 15 hours of applicable college credits toward the minimum required 20 CE credits as long as the course was completed prior to the renewal or within the reinstatement period and the candidate received a passing grade of "C" or better. Candidates for renewal and reinstatement may also apply not more than 10 CE credits from in-services completed prior to the renewal or reinstatement period.

The Examination for Certification of Pharmacy Technician

The Examination for Certification of Pharmacy Technician (ExCPT) is the second recognized examination for national certification for pharmacy technicians. While ExCPT is fully accredited, it is the lesser known of the two pharmacy technician certification exams. Certification applicants should check with their state's board of pharmacy or mandating employer before applying for ExCPT. Although ExCPT is fully accredited and nationally recognized, some employers and state boards of pharmacy only accept certification through the PTCE.

ExCPT, which was originally administered by the Institute for the Certification of Pharmacy Technicians (ICPT), is now administered by the National HealthCareer Association (NHA). The exam consists of 120 multiple-choice questions, 100 questions are scored for the test, and 20 questions are pretested for future exam questions. Like PTCE, ExCPT is completely computerized. Results of the exam are given to the candidates on the day of the exam.

The cost of the exam, which is offered 310 days a year at a cost of $105.00, may be taken at PSI/LaserGrade Testing Centers across the United States. Application for ExCPT may be completed online at the NHA Web site http://www.nhanow.com/pharmacy-technician.aspx. Once application for the exam has been verified, the candidate may register for the test by calling PSI/LaserGrade at (800) 211-2754. A complete listing of PSI/LaserGrade Testing Centers may be found by logging onto http://www.candidate.psiexam.com.

As is the case with PTCE, ExCPT candidates will need to meet eligibility requirements for taking examination. Basic eligibility requirements include the following:

- At least 18 years of age
- High school graduate or completed G.E.D. or foreign diploma equivalent
- Have completed a pharmacy technician training program or have at least 12 months of experience in the field of pharmacy within the last 36 months
- Have no felony drug charges

Candidates should log onto the NHA Web site http://nahanow.com/pharmacy-technician.aspx to read the full disclosure on exam eligibility before applying to the exam.

Candidates are required to provide proof of identification on the day of the exam. Only a government-issued photo ID is acceptable. ID requirements are similar to those of the PTCE. Acceptable forms of ID include

- Valid passport
- State-issued driver's license
- US Armed Forces photo ID
- Non-driver's ID issued by a state department of motor vehicles

The candidate's ID must have his or her clear and decipherable photo as well as his or her name. The name on the candidate's ID must match with the name on the exam registration form. In case the name does not match, further proof of identification in the form of a certified or notarized document need to be produced, such as a marriage license or divorce decree. If a candidate's address is different from his or her chosen form of ID, a current utility bill must be provided to prove residency.

Candidates should be aware that books, cell phones, calculators, pagers, scanners, cameras, or PDAs are not permitted in the exam centers. A secure area will be provided for candidates to store their personal belongings during the exam. Coincidentally, these same rules apply to the PTCE as well. Candidates with further questions concerning personal items should refer to their chosen exam's Web site.

Candidates for the ExCPT must arrive at their scheduled exam time. If candidates cannot keep with their scheduled exam time, they must notify PSI/LaserGrade no less than 24 hours before their exam time. Candidates that fail to notify PSI/LaserGrade within the stipulated time or fail to keep their scheduled exam time will not be refunded any exam fees. If the candidates decide that they would like to obtain certification, they must re-apply for examination and pay the required examination fee.

There are certain cases where a candidate may need to make special exam accommodations due to a disability or other extenuating circumstances. The NHA fully complies with the ADA and will provide special accommodations for those candidates that warrant them. Candidates will need to submit an Accommodations Request form, available on NHA Web site http://www.nhanow.com/forms.aspx. Candidates must also provide full documentation supporting their disability or extenuating circumstance.

NHA will allow reasonable accommodations for those candidates with special needs, but will only do so as long as the accommodations continue to create an equal balance with other candidates. There will be no accommodations provided that place any candidate at an unfair or unequal balance with other candidates. Additionally, any special accommodations that come as an added expense to NHA will need to be paid for by the candidate. Please note that NHA will also not make special accommodations for those that do not speak English, nor will translation dictionaries be permitted in the exam centers.

Candidates will have 2 hours and 10 minutes to answer 120 multiple-choice questions, 100 that are scored and 20 that are pretested and reviewed for future examinations. As previously mentioned, the exam is proctored by PSI/LaserGrade, which is a fully accredited, computer-based testing organization with more than 500 exam centers across the United States, Canada, and overseas. PSI/LaserGrade has central headquarters in Burbank, California, and Vancouver, Washington. Further information regarding PSI/LaserGrade can be found on their Web site http://candidate.psiexam.com.

ExCPT focuses on testing the pharmacy technician on three key areas: Regulation and Technician Duties, Drugs and Drug Products, and the Dispensing Process. Taking up 52% of the test questions, the Dispensing Process is the largest knowledge area. Regulation and Technician Duties and Drugs and Drug Products are split almost evenly at 25% and 23%, respectively. A more detailed offering of exam material is given here.

Regulations and Technician Duties

- General outline of technician duties
  - Role of the pharmacist and technician
  - Duties the pharmacy technician may and may not perform
  - Security within a pharmacy
  - Pharmacy workflow
  - Inventory control
- Controlled substances
  - Controlled substance schedules
  - Refill requirements and prescription transfers
  - Handling Schedule V sales
  - DEA numbers
  - The Controlled Substance Act
- Other laws and regulations
  - Health Insurance Portability and Accountability Act (HIPAA)
  - Laws concerning brand–generic substitutions
  - Child-resistant packing requirements

- Government agencies
  - Drug Enforcement Agency (DEA)
  - State Board of Pharmacy
  - Food and Drug Administration (FDA)
- OTC packaging requirements
- Manufacturer drug label requirements

Drugs and Drug Therapy

- Drug classifications
  - National Drug Code (NDC)
  - Dosage forms and routes of administration
  - OTC products
  - Major drug classifications
- Drugs most frequently prescribed
  - Brand–generic name
  - Pharmacology as well as drug class
  - Drug indications
  - Adverse drug events
    - Interactions
    - Reactions
    - Contraindications

Dispensing Process

- Required prescription information
  - Patient demographics
  - Prescription directions
  - Commonly used and approved prescription abbreviations
  - Prescriptions via the fax and phone
  - Refills
- Preparing and dispensing prescriptions
  - Avoiding errors
  - Entering prescriptions into the computer
  - Proper labeling
  - Packing and storing of prescriptions
  - Managing care prescriptions
  - Documentation and patient records
  - Verifying prescription before it goes to the patient
- Calculations
  - Calculations during compounding
  - Dosage and administration times for sterile IV compounds
  - Pricing, markup, and inventory control
  - Patient dosing calculations
  - Pharmacy-based conversions and units of measure
  - Prescription ingredients
- Sterile products, unit dose, and repackaging
  - Drug dispensing systems used in hospitals and nursing homes
  - Repacking medications
  - Aseptic technique and laminar flow workstations

- Special precautions for chemotherapy
- Sterile IV products
- Compounding and labeling of sterile IV products
- Routes of administration for parenteral products

A more extensive detailing of the ExCPT blueprint of exam areas is available online at http://nhanow.com/libraries/pdf/excpt_candidate_handbook.sflb.ashx. Once again, candidates are encouraged to review the ExCPT blueprint and guide prior to applying for the exam in order to obtain a full understanding of the exam's requirements and content.

Candidates that receive a passing grade on the ExCPT will be eligible for the title of Certified Pharmacy Technician, or CPhT. Like PTCB certification, successful ExCPT examinees will be required to apply for recertification on a biannual basis. NHA also requires recertification candidates to complete not less than 20 hours of continuing education hours or credits before completing the recertification process. Continuing education credits must be completed within the 2-year period prior to recertification and include not less than 1-hour dealing in pharmacy law.

Continuing education credits must be pharmacy based and pertain to duties and areas specific to the pharmacy technician. One hour of CE must be completed in pharmacy law or else the candidate's application for recertification will be rejected. Other suggested CE topics include the following:

- Preparing sterile IV compounds
- Pharmacy calculations
- Pharmacy inventory control
- Drug therapies and management
- Pharmacy operations
- Professional communication
- Interacting with patients

Please note that NHA clearly states on their Web site that they reserve the right to reject any CEs determined not to be pertinent to the practice of pharmacy or the duties of a pharmacy technician.

A maximum of 10 credit hours in employer-provided training or projects will be accepted toward the mandated 20 CE credits as long as the training or project pertains to the practice of pharmacy and helps to further establish and advance the knowledge base of the CPhT. Training and projects must be completed under the supervision of a licensed, registered pharmacist, and the CPhT must obtain the supervising pharmacist sign and complete the ExCPT Continuing Education form, which is available at the NHA Web site http://nha.com/pharmacy-technician/recertification.aspx.

College course in subjects directly related to the practice of pharmacy, such as mathematics, life sciences (biology and microbiology), or pharmaceutical sciences (organic and inorganic chemistry), will also be considered toward completion of the mandated CEs. Candidates may apply up to 15 CE credits from college course taken within the 2-year window prior to the candidate's recertification period. Candidates using college course toward CE completion must provide a college transcript as the Certification of Participation.

Candidates must complete the NHA ExCPT Recertification Application Form available on the NHA Web site http://nhanow.com/pharmacy-technician/recertification.aspx, provide the accompanying $40.00 recertification fee, and have completed all mandated CEs, in order to be considered for recertification. Recertification candidates have four options available for filing their application with NHA:

- Online at http://nhanow.com/pharmacy-technician/recertification.aspx
- Fax at (913) 661-6214

- Regular postal mail—NHA, 11161 Overbrook Road, Leawood, KS, 66211
- Email continuingeducation@nhanow.com

Recertification candidates have a 90-day window to apply for recertification. Once the 90-day window is over, a pharmacy technician will lose the title of Certified Pharmacy Technician. If this is the case, the pharmacy technician may apply for reinstatement with NHA; however, the reinstatement cannot be completed if the request is made after more than 12 months from the date of the pharmacy technician's original recertification date.

What is the Advantage to Certification?

No matter which test pharmacy technician choses to take, the PTCB or the NHA certification exam, one thing is certain, the pharmacy technician will be able to clearly establish their knowledge and skills as a pharmacy professional. Both exams are fully accredited by national accrediting bodies, and both exams successfully test the skills, knowledge, and training of the pharmacy technician.

The requirement for national certification of the pharmacy technician has grown by leaps and bounds over the past two decades. Most employers require certification as a term of employment, and all but six State Boards of Pharmacy. There is a greater push toward a nationalized standard for the pharmacy technician, and certification plays a central role.

Professional pharmacy organizations such as American Society of Health System Pharmacist (ASHP), American Pharmacist Association (APhA), Pharmacy Technician Educators Council (PTEC), American Association of Pharmacy Technicians (AAPT), and the National Pharmacy Technician Association (NPTA) are strong proponents for the standardization of pharmacy technician education and certification.

Pharmacy technicians that seek national certification may receive higher wages, have greater opportunity for career advancement, or be placed in or authoritative positions, such as pharmacy technician supervisor. The career advantages associated with national certification are undoubtedly growing with the profession.

The role of the pharmacy technician is to assist the pharmacist. As laws governing the practice of pharmacy continue to change, specifically the expansion of clinical roles for the pharmacist, so do the duties of the pharmacy technician. Although the pharmacist always has the final check, most dispensing and compounding duties have fallen on the pharmacy technician. Keeping this in mind, a pharmacy technician who has achieved national certification bring an added value of trust and assurance to the practice of pharmacy. Their skills and knowledge have been tested, and this, along with experience, becomes invaluable.

In the reality of it, the question of whether or not to become certified should be a passing thought. National certification for the pharmacy technician is no longer a question, but rather just another step in the career advancement and professional advancement of the pharmacy technician.

CHAPTER REVIEW QUESTIONS

1. Ebers Papyrus, which is believed to date back as far as 1500 B.C., is one of the most substantial pieces of evidence proving the existence of pharmaceutical practices by the Ancient Egyptians. The scroll contains documentation of more than _____ prescriptions and _____ drugs.
   a. 500/250
   b. 800/70
   c. 900/850
   d. 875/700

2. The only two nationally recognized exams for pharmacy technicians are _____ and _____.
   a. ASHP/PTCB
   b. ExCPT/ASHP
   c. PTCE/ExCPT
   d. NPTA/PTCE

3. The _____ was passed in _____ as a result of the 1937 Elixir of Sulfanilamide incident.
   a. Pure Food and Drug Act/1922
   b. Harris/Humphreys Amendment/1934
   c. Federal Food, Drug, and Cosmetic Act/1938
   d. Medication Safety Act /1906

4. The 1951 Durham–Humphreys Amendment creates distinction between _____ and _____.
   a. Generic/brand name drugs
   b. Prescription medication/non-prescription medication
   c. Physician's orders/pharmacist consultation
   d. Pharmacist/pharmacy technician

5. The two most common pharmacy practice settings for the pharmacy technician are _____ and _____ pharmacies.
   a. Ambulatory/institutional
   b. Community/retail
   c. Hospital/institutional
   d. Insurance companies/community

6. Pharmacy technicians must always work under the supervision of a _____.
   a. Licensed physician
   b. Licensed, registered pharmacist
   c. Pharmacy supervisor
   d. State Board of Pharmacy

7. According to a 2013 Gallup poll, _____ is one of the most trusted professions in the United States.
   a. Health care
   b. Pharmacy
   c. Administration
   d. Information technology

8. _____ by definition is the act of making something official.
   a. Registration
   b. Licensing
   c. Certification
   d. Qualifying

9. PTCB offers the _____ and NHA offer _____ the exam.
   a. ExCPT/PTCE
   b. Certification/registration
   c. Registration/licensure
   d. PTCE/ExCPT

10. In order to pass the PTCE the exam, a candidate must obtain a score of at least _____ out of 1600 in order to become certified.
    a. 1000
    b. 1400
    c. 1200
    d. 1300

Pharmacology for the Pharmacy Technician

LEARNING OBJECTIVES

Learning objectives for this chapter will include:

- Definition and explanation of the term *pharmacology* and any associated terminology.
- Reasons why pharmacology is important to the pharmacy technician.
- Providing a base knowledge of pharmacology.
- Explanation of how absorption, distribution, metabolism, and elimination play specific roles in pharmacology.
- Explanation of routes of administration and duration of medication therapies.
- Explanation of medication dosage forms and appearance.
- Providing a brief synopsis of drug classifications.
- Examining common drug interactions, allergies, and side effects.
- Understanding brand and generic names as well as therapeutic equivalence.

When attempting a definition for the term *pharmacology*, we need to look at the origin of the word. *Phar.ma.col.o.gy*, it is easy enough to pronounce, and if broken down, easy to understand. Pharmacology in its simplest of meanings is the study of how drugs work and react within an active living system, primarily human beings. Toxicology, which is the study of poisonous drugs and their effects on the body, and therapeutics, the study of treatments and cures for disease, are also significant to the science of pharmacology.

As one might guess, pharmacology plays a central role in the practice of pharmacy. Pharmacist and pharmacy technician become educated in pharmacology in order to provide the patient with the best treatment option available and to better understand the mechanisms, and chemical and physical properties, of the drugs they are dispensing. A pharmacist's knowledge of pharmacology is indispensable when consultation is needed for patient drug therapies or treatment plans, and while it is important for the pharmacy technician to be educated in pharmacology, he or she will not apply knowledge in the same way as the pharmacist.

Pharmacy technicians are never permitted to dispense information concerning medications to anyone. Not only is it against federal and state pharmacy laws, but unprofessional as well. Although the pharmacy technician is a valid and central part of the pharmacy profession, the fact remains that he or she simply does not have the same in-depth educational background of a pharmacist.

So the question arises, "Why do pharmacy technicians need to know pharmacology?" Even though the pharmacy technicians are prohibited from consultation or giving advice or information about medications, it does not mean they shouldn't have a working knowledge of the medications they help to dispense. A pharmacy technician with a well-informed background in pharmacology may help to alert the pharmacists to potential reactions, duplication of therapies, or dosing that is inconsistent with a patient's weight, age group, or demographic. Possessing the knowledge to safeguard against any one of these contradictions will protect patients from medication errors, or possibly even save a life. So, pharmacology is a major part of the training and education needed for pharmacy technicians.

Four Central Stages: Learning About Pharmacokinetics

In order for medications to work as they should, they need to be moved or transported throughout the body's systems. Pharmacokinetics is the study of how this process is completed. Pharmacokinetics is the branch of pharmacy dealing with how medications are transported through the body's systems. There are four central stages or phases associated with pharmacokinetics: absorption, distribution, metabolism, and elimination. The phrases "onset of action," "peak effort," and "duration of action" will also be referred to with the four central stages of pharmacokinetics.

The phrase "onset of action" is simply the amount of time a drug needs before it starts to work within the body. For example, when you have an ache or pain, you may take a class of drugs known as analgesics, such as acetaminophen. You do not feel instantaneous relief from your pain after you take the drug, but after a period of time, typically less than an hour, you could have received some if not complete relief from your pain. The drug needs time to be absorbed by the body's system and bloodstream in order to be successful in controlling the pain.

On the other hand, "peak effort" refers to the time in which the drug is working at its best or giving the patient the greatest benefit. Peak effort depends greatly on how a drug is distributed or moved through the body to the circulatory system. Once the drug has been distributed successfully to its intended site of action, it begins to perform in its most beneficial stage.

Finally, there is "duration of action." Duration of action can be explained easily. It is the period of time from which the drug begins working to the period of time in which it stops working. Duration of action is the accumulation of efforts associated with the four central stages of pharmacokinetics: absorption, distribution, metabolism, and elimination.

There are several ways in which medications can enter the body. The way a medication enters the body or its "route of administration" plays a large role in how it is absorbed into the body. Absorption is the process that medications undergo in order to enter into the bloodstream. There are a number of factors that might hinder absorption.

- **The medication form:** Tablets and capsules take longer to "break down" and enter the bloodstream compared to an intravenous (IV) medication that is injected directly to the vein.
- **Medication taken with or without food:** Some medications should not be taken with food because they can greatly affect the absorption of the drug. For example, penicillin-based antibiotics, like ampicillin, should be taken with an empty stomach. Conversely, some medications need to be taken with a full stomach because they may be absorbed too quickly on an empty stomach. HIV medications like ritonavir and saquinavir are two examples of medications that need to be taken on a full stomach.
- **Patients' disease state:** Patients with underlying medical conditions, such as liver or kidney damage and/or failure, may see a decrease in drug absorption because the organ used to "filter" the drug into the blood stream cannot or is not working up to its capacity.
- **Patient compliance:** This may not be seen as an issue that can affect absorption, but patients who are noncompliant or inconsistent in taking their recommended drug therapies will not have the same drug absorption rates as patients who are compliant and consistently take recommended drug therapy.

These are just a few issues that may delay the absorption of a drug. It shows just one more example of how valuable pharmacy intervention is to the success of a patient's well-being and safety. Although it will be the pharmacist who provides clinical intervention, the pharmacy technician is often the patient's first line of contact. Pharmacy technicians with a base knowledge of pharmacology will be able to recognize patients who may need more direct patient-to-pharmacist consultations.

Medications taken orally (by mouth), which include tablets, capsules, elixirs, suspensions, and solutions, are the most common form of medication administration. Oral medications come with various "release mechanisms" or ways the medication is released into the bloodstream. Some example include the following:

- **Time—Released or Delayed Release:** Medication is released slowly into the bloodstream over a specified period of time. Administration of time-released oral medications not only allows the patient to receive the medication in a consistent manner, but may also allow them the luxury of once-daily administration. This is particularly important when patient compliance is of concern or when a patient is taking several medications as part of their daily regimen.

- **Immediate or Quick Release:** Medication is released into the patient's bloodstream over a short period of time, typically 30 minutes or less. Immediate or quick release medications allow the patient to receive the benefits of the medication at a much faster pace than time release. Morphine IR is a good example of this, as the patients most likely receive relief from their pain in less than 30 minutes.

- **Sublingual and Buccal:** Sublingual mediations are administered underneath the tongue as relief needs to be immediate. Nitroglycerin tablets are given underneath the tongue or sublingually because the patients need immediate relief from chest pain. Buccal medications are also administered by mouth but need to be placed between the cheek and gums. Buccal, as well as sublingual, medications should never be chewed or swallowed whole, but rather left to dissolve at their place of administration.

Intravenous administration is done via the veins and arteries of the body and is one of the fastest routes of administration. Subcutaneous medications are injected into the body just beneath the first, epidermis layer of the skin. Insulin is a good example of a medication that is given subcutaneously. When a medication, such as an antibiotic, needs to be administered into a muscle, its route of administration is known as intramuscular. However, antibiotics, like Rocephin, are given intramuscularly, rather than intravenously, because a patient's veins or arteries cannot to handle the strain of IV administration.

Transdermal administration of medications is, as it sounds, transportation of medication through the dermis or skin. Transdermal administration is still a fairly new process of administration, but as new medications are brought to the market, more and more are being offered transdermally. Transdermal administration is completed through the use of a time-released patch that the patient wears on a specific area of the body's skin. Transdermal patches are typically applied on a patient's upper arm, chest, or back; however, manufacturer instructions should be read by the patient or caregiver, before application, as recommendations vary.

Topical medications are applied directly to the surface of the skin or mucus membranes. Ointments, creams, lotions, foams, powders, shampoos, and some solutions are all considered to be topical medications. However, ophthalmic, otic, and nasal preparations are also considered to be topical medications because they involve immediate release through a mucosal membrane or area of the skin.

Rectal medications are administered primarily as either a suppository or as an enema. Rectal medications are given to the patient through the rectum where the medication is released into the vessels of the bloodstream. Rectal medications are often times given to small children or to those who may be unable to swallow the oral form of the medication. Medications that reduce fever, such as acetaminophen, and medications that provide relief from nausea and vomiting, such as promethazine, are common examples of rectal medications. Enemas are most often given to soften stool or stimulate bowel production. Enemas intended for use as a laxative may be saline or mineral oil based, and some may contain other active ingredients such as bisacodyl.

Inhalations are medications that are inhaled into the lungs or nasal passages. Quick relief is essential to patients suffering from respiratory illnesses, such as asthma and COPD. Inhalation medications for respiratory illnesses are manufactured as aerosolized or powdered medications that can be delivered directly to the lungs and the blood vessels of the lungs. Inhalers, such as albuterol, provide the patient with almost instantaneous relief, opening up the passage ways of the lungs and allowing them to breath much more freely.

Nasal inhalations come in the form of a spray that the patient can spray into the nasal passages and inhale into the mucus membranes. As with respiratory inhalations, relief is almost immediate as the medication is delivered directly to the blood vessels of the nasal passages. Allergy relief medications, such as Flovent, are the most common nasal medications, but flu vaccines and medications used to fight osteoporosis, such as calcitonin, are also available as nasal sprays. It is believed that in the near future insulin will be available as a nasal spray as well, eliminating the need for daily injections required by those who suffer from diabetes.

Another route of administration is vaginal administration. Medications that are administered vaginally need to have direct absorption in to the vagina or vaginal lining. Suppositories are the most common form of vaginal administration, but tablets, creams, ointments, and gels may also be used. A good example of a drug commonly used for vaginal administration would be miconazole nitrate or as it is more readily known and marketed, Monistat. Miconazole nitrate or Monistat is an antifungal used to treat fungal or yeast infection. It is available as a vaginal cream and tablet.

Distribution forms the second stage of pharmacokinetics. Distribution is the transportation of the medication into the bloodstream and further across cell membranes and barriers where it finally begins its onset of action and eventually performs at its "peak efficiency."

Distribution is key to the performance of a drug. If the drug is unable to reach its intended site of reaction, the patient will receive little or no benefit. The drug is eventually eliminated from the body and efforts to control the patient's pain or symptoms become a useless event. Each pharmacokinetic stage builds off from its previous stage. Distribution cannot happen without absorption, and metabolism cannot take place without distribution, which leads us to the third stage or pharmacokinetics, metabolism.

Everyone has heard the term *metabolism* tossed about at one time or another. Metabolism in literal terms is the chemical process the body uses to break down substances within the body. When we talk about metabolism in regard to diet, it means food is converted into energy and used within the body. When we talk about metabolism in regard to pharmaceuticals, it means a drug is broken down in the body after it has been distributed thorough the body's bloodstream.

Most medications, but not all, are metabolized through the kidneys or the liver. It is for this reason a patient's kidneys and liver functions become a concern when some medications need to be administered. A patient who has kidneys that do not function with full efficiency or a liver that is compromised by a disease, such as cirrhosis of the liver, will not be able to properly break down the medication. The end result leaves the patient with little or no benefit from the drug and, in some cases, may cause more damage to the already compromised organ. Without the ability to metabolize medications, the medication will never be able to reach its peak efficiency.

The final stage of pharmacokinetics, elimination, may seem like it needs little explanation, but as with the relationship between metabolism and distribution, elimination cannot be processed without metabolism. Elimination is the way or method a medication leaves the body. In order for a drug to be efficiently removed from the body, it must be broken down, and as we have already discussed, this process most often takes place within the kidneys and, sometimes, the liver. During the elimination stage, the kidneys continue their work by eliminating or flushing the drug from the body's system after it has completed peak efficiency and "duration of time."

Once again, poorly functioning kidneys can have a tremendous effect on a body's overall functions. Kidneys that are unable to eliminate medications from the body's system lead to a build-up of toxic levels of the medication, putting the patient at further risk and causing irreversible harm to an already compromised system.

It is for this reason certain drugs, such as a group of IV antibiotics known as aminoglycosides, require regular blood draws to check for metabolism and elimination. Gentamicin, amikacin, tobramycin, and kanamycin are just a few of the drugs listed under the antibiotic sub-classification of aminoglycoside. When a patient is prescribed a therapy involving an aminoglycoside, the physician or sometimes the clinical pharmacist will order a daily blood draw known as a "peak and trough." A "peak and trough" is actually two separate blood draws. The "peak" is typically drawn half hour after a patient has received the aminoglycoside antibiotic and the "trough" is typically drawn half hour before the patient's next scheduled dose of the aminoglycoside antibiotic.

When the clinical pharmacist receives the "peak" and "trough" values for the patient, they are able to ascertain if the patient is receiving too little or too much of the drug. The tests also alert the clinical pharmacist to any drug elimination issues the patient may potentially be experiencing. Based upon the findings of the "peak" and "trough," the clinical pharmacist makes a recommendation to increase, decrease, or sustain the patient's current drug dose and regimen.

The Name Behind the Name: Generic Versus Brand Names

Having a base understanding of pharmacokinetics is mandatory for a pharmacy technician, merely because it is the process that pharmacology is built upon. Medications are created by incorporating chemical compounds, and it is from these chemical compounds that medications derive their generic and brand names. When a new drug is created, it receives a chemical name. A chemical name of a drug is based upon the chemical structure of the drug and is usually referred to as the drug's scientific name. The drug's chemical name or scientific name will rarely be used while marketing the drug to the general population. For example, the chemical name for Prilosec (omeprazole), a common Proton Pump Inhibitor (PPI) used to treat peptic ulcers and gastrointestinal reflux, is **di-5-methoxy-2- [[(4-methoxy-3, 5-dimethyl-2-pyridinyl) methyl] sulfinyl]-1H-benzimidazole magnesium**. Most of us could not even begin to pronounce this jumble of chemical compounds, let alone understand what they mean. So, for that reason, drug companies market medications under a generic name and a brand name.

Generic Versus Brand: What Makes Them Different? What Makes Them the Same?

The Food and Drug Administration (FDA) is responsible for assuring that the medications produced and marketed to the citizens of the United States are safe and effective. It is a very long and arduous process for a new drug to make it from the research laboratory to FDA approval, and onto the general public. In fact, it takes a pharmaceutical researcher an average of 12 years and 350 million dollars just to make it to the FDA approval stage.

Pharmaceutical manufacturers hold the patent on a new drug for a period of 20 years from the date the patent is filed with the FDA. Once the patent expires, other pharmaceutical manufacturers can seek approval from the FDA to manufacture a generic version of the drug. This process also may last for several years before the generic drug is approved for the consumer.

Brand name drugs are drugs that have a trade name as established by the manufacturer and hold a patent that is proprietory to the drug manufacturer's trade name. For example, Advil is a brand name for ibuprofen, and ibuprofen is the generic name. Additionally, there may be several brand names for a generic drug. Keeping with the example of the generic drug ibuprofen, Motrin, Advil, and PediCare Fever are all brand names whose main ingredient is ibuprofen. So while the brand or trade name is proprietory, several manufacturers may produce the drug as long as they hold a patent for that particular trade name.

According to the World Health Organization (WHO), a generic drug is defined as "a pharmaceutical product usually intended to be interchangeable with an innovator product that is manufactured without a license from the innovator company and marketed after the expiry date of the patent or other exclusive rights." In other words, a generic drug is the bioequivalent of the brand name drug but is being manufactured and marketed from a pharmaceutical company other than the original patent holder.

Generic drugs, per FDA regulations, must contain the same active ingredient, strength, dosage form, and route of administration as the brand name drug. The FDA has established that a generic drug must be the bioequivalent of the brand drug; however, the FDA does allow for variance with the inactive ingredients of the generic drug.

Bioequivalent simply means the generic drug must have exactly the same active ingredients as the brand name drug, as well as perform exactly the same action as the brand name drug. The inactive ingredient in a drug compound refers to the ingredients in the drug that have no physiological effect within the drug compound. For example, dyes, preservatives, flavorings, and binding material are all examples of inactive ingredients. They may serve a specific purpose within the drug compound, but if they were removed from the compound, it would not diminish the effects of the drug.

Which One to Dispense, Brand or Generic?

There is no doubt that generic drugs save the consumer hundreds of thousands of dollars each year, but when is it appropriate to dispense a generic drug versus a brand name drug? Does the consumer have any say as to whether their prescription is filled with a brand or generic drug? As we have already seen, a generic drug, per FDA-mandated regulations, must provide the consumer with exactly the same bioequivalent as its brand name counterpart. Additionally, the generic drug must have the same strength, dosage form, and route of administration, and perform just as the brand name. The only variance or difference between the brand and generic is the presence of inactive ingredients, such as dyes and binders.

When a prescription is written for a patient, the physician must write out the name of the drug to be dispensed, the strength of the drug, the dosage form of the drug, the drug quantity, the instructions, and of course, the physician's signature, but there is one more item if written on the prescription which will dictate whether or not it will be filled with a brand name drug or a generic drug.

If the physician writes the words "Brand Name Necessary" or "Fill with Brand Name Only," the prescription must be filled with the brand name drug. Additionally, the physician must reference the brand name drug on the prescription. However, if the physician does not make specific reference to the brand name, the prescription may be filled with the generic equivalent. In fact, every state has regulations regarding the substitution of generic drugs.

Each state varies on how it handles the substitution of generic drugs, so it is always best to check with your state's board of pharmacy in order to obtain a clear understanding of brand to generic substitution requirements. Most states go by either a "positive" formulary or a "negative" formulary to determine if a generic drug may be substituted for a brand name drug. States that go by a "positive" formulary substitution list brand name drugs that may be substituted for generics, and states that go by a "negative" formulary substitution list brand name drugs that may not be substituted. There are also states that use neither a "positive" nor "negative" formulary, but allow the pharmacist to substitute based upon the generic drug match for bioequivalence. States that allow generic substitution require pharmacies to post notice to the consumer that generic substitution will be used when applicable unless the physician mandates brand name only.

Patients may request that a generic substitution be made or that the brand name be filled, but some insurance plans may not allow payment for the brand name drug, leaving the patient responsible for any cost beyond their typical co-pay. Once again, if uncertainty arises about a state's brand–generic drug substitution laws, the state board of pharmacy is the best source for reference.

Drug Classifications

Drug classifications are an important part in understanding pharmacology. There are thousands of prescriptions and OTC drugs available to consumers in the United States, and more reaching the market everyday. Drug classification is a way of organizing drugs within a specific group or class. Drugs that fall under the same classification will have similar chemical structure, work much the same way as other drugs in that class, as well as treat similar disease states. For example, Prozac is a drug that is often prescribed to treat depression; however, Zoloft is also a drug prescribed to treat depression. Collectively, these two drugs fall under the drug classification known as antidepressants.

The following table lists some of the most common drug classifications. It is important to note that some drugs may fall under more than one classification because the drug has been approved from the FDA to treat more than one disease state or symptom.

DRUG CLASSIFICATION	DRUG ACTION	EXAMPLES OF DRUG WITHIN CLASSIFICATION
Anesthetic	Induces loss of sensation with or without consciousness	propofol, thiopental, sevoflurane, desflurane, etomidate
Antibiotic	Prevents or destroys the microorganisms that produce infection within the body	penicillin, amoxicillin, doxycycline, cephalexin, erythromycin, ciprofloxacin
Antifungal	Prevents or destroys the growth of fungi within the body	amphotericin B, fluconazole, ketoconazole, iraconazole, voriconazole
Antihistamine	Blocks histamine produced by the body that may help to induce allergic reaction	fexofenadine, loratadine, diphenhydramine, chlorpheniramine, certirizine,
Antipruritic	Helps to reduce itching	hydroxyzine, hydrocortisone, diphenhydramine
Analgesic	Relieves pain	acetaminophen, ibuprofen, morphine, hydrocodone
Antipyretic	Relieves fever	acetaminophen, ibuprofen aspirin
Non-Steroidal Anti-Inflammatory (NSAID)	Reduce swelling and pain	ibuprofen, aspirin, ketoprofen, naproxen
Antiarrhythmic	Stabilizes cardiac arrhythmia	amiodorone, atenolol, betaxolol, bisoprodol
Anticholinergic	Blocks the neurotransmitter acetylcholine, reducing impulses to the parasympathetic nerve	atropine, Scopolamine, acetylcholine, tolterodine

(Continued)

DRUG CLASSIFICATION	DRUG ACTION	EXAMPLES OF DRUG WITHIN CLASSIFICATION
Anticoagulant	Prevents the clotting of the blood	warfarin, heparin, enoxaparin rivaroxaban, dalterparin
Antihypertensive	Lowers blood pressure	lisinopril, metoprolol HCTZ, clonidine, atenolol
Beta Blockers	Blocks action of beta-receptors allowing decrease in rate and flow of heart contraction and blood pressure	propranolol, pindolol, nadolol, atenolol, metoprolol
Thrombolytic Agents	Dissolves blood clots	antistreplase, reteplase, streptokinase, Activase, tenecteplase
Vasoconstrictor	Decreases the flow of blood to the heart by constricting or narrowing the blood vessels	phenylephrine, oxymetazoline, pseudo-ephrine, EPINEPHrine, ePHEDrine, caffeine, cocaine
Angiotensin-Converting Enzyme (ACE) Inhibitor	Causes the dilation of blood vessel and increases blood flow to the heart	lisinopril, captopril, enalapril, ramipril, losartan
Calcium Channel Blockers	Decreases the flow of calcium to the cells of the heart and blood vessels, allowing more oxygenated blood to reach the heart so it may work more efficiently	amlodipine, nifedipine, verapamil, diltiazem
Diuretic	Increases the production of urine	Furosemide, bumetanide, torsemide, chlorothiazide, metolazone, spironolactone, acetazolamide
Statins	Decreases cholesterol in the blood and in turn increases blood flow	pravastatin, rosuvastatin, simvastatin, atorvastatin, fluvastatin, lovastatin
Anti-Diabetics	Treats and reduces the effects of diabetes mellitus	Insulin, metformin, tolazamide, glimepride, glipizide
Antiemetic	Prevents or controls nausea and vomiting	ondansetron, metoclopramide, promethazine, prochlorperazine
Antineoplastic	Treats the cells that cause cancer	doxorubicin, methotrexate, gemcitabine, bleomycin, cisplatin
Benzodiazepine	Treats and reduces the effects of anxiety and panic disorders	diazepam, oxazepam, clorazepate, lorazepam, clonazepam,
Anti-Psychotic	Manages disorders associated with psychosis, such as schizophrenia and bipolar disorder	aripiprazole, chlorpromazine, olanzapine, quetiapine, risperidone, ziprasidone
Proton Pump Inhibitors (PPI)	Treats the effects of gastrointestinal reflux and stomach ulcers by greatly reducing the production of gastric acid	pantoprazole, lansoprazole, omeprazole, esomeprazole, rabeprazole
Histamine-2 Receptor Antagonist	Blocks histamine receptors and decreases gastric acid associated with peptic ulcers	ranitidine, famotidine, cimetidine
Antidiarrheal	Lessens and controls the effects of diarrhea	loperimide, diphenoxylate/atropine, paregoric, bismuth subsalicylate, sodium bicarbonate oral
Laxative	Treats constipation and softens the stool	docusate sodium, bisacodyl, methylcellu-lose, psyllium, polycarbophil, polyethylene glycol 3350, magnesium hydroxide
Stimulant	Temporarily increases physiological function, commonly used to treat and control the symptoms of Attention Deficit Disorder Hyperactivity (ADHD)	methylphenidate, amphetamine/dextroamphetamine, dextroamphetamine, atomoxetine, caffeine

DRUG CLASSIFICATION	DRUG ACTION	EXAMPLES OF DRUG WITHIN CLASSIFICATION
Contraceptives	Drugs or devices used to prevent pregnancy	desogestrel/ethinyl/estradiol ethynodiol/ethinyl/estradiol levonorgestrel/ethinyl/estradiol norethindrone
Vitamins and Nutritional Supplements	Helps supplement organic substances found in the body and needed for normal metabolic function	retinol, thiamine, riboflavin, ascorbic acid, ergocalciferol, cholecalciferol, phytonadine, potassium, phosphate salts
Bronchodilators	Dilates bronchi and bronchioles and increases airflow	Albuterol, theophylline, beclamethasone, salmeterol, tiotropium, formoterol, ipratropium
Vaccines and Toxoids	Prevents or treats a specific disease state, such as smallpox or rabies	hepatitis B vaccine, human papillomavirus vaccine, influenza vaccine, polio virus vaccine, rabies vaccine, rotavirus

Side Effects, Adverse Reactions, and Allergies

As drug therapies have become beneficial in the battle to prevent and cure diseases, they do not come without the potential for harm. Side effects, adverse reactions, and allergies are all very real possibilities when a patient begins a new drug therapy or has been taking a particular drug therapy for an extended period of time. While the terms *side effects, adverse reactions,* and *allergies* can sometimes be grouped into one, each term truly has its own specific meaning.

Understanding the definition and specifics of each term will allow the pharmacy technician to understand more clearly how significant these terms are within the practice of pharmacy. Understanding how these terms should be used when speaking about patient drug therapies will allow the pharmacy technician to alert a pharmacist to any potential issues, and keep the patients safe from harm.

Side effects are the unwanted effects that may occur when taking a particular drug therapy. While the majority of drug side effects are usually mild and harmless, there are some instances when the side effects are quite substantial and possibly detrimental to the patient. For example, diphenhydramine, a drug used to combat allergies, may cause the patient to become sleepy or have a dry mouth. Side effects such as those experienced with diphenhydramine are more of a nuisance than harmful; they are unwanted, but they aren't typically going to harm the patient.

A more aggressive and alarming example of a side effect is of the drug warfarin. Warfarin is an anticoagulant used to reduce the risk of blood clots. Patients on warfarin therapy, especially those over the age of 75 and those who have had long-term use, are at an increased risk for severe bleeding, severe bruising, and numbness and tingling in the body. Patients on warfarin must have periodic blood test to keep their clotting factors in check and are given certain dietary restrictions, such as avoiding consuming dark, leafy, green vegetables.

Side effects like those potentially seen in patients on warfarin therapy are still considered unwanted and, although if monitored, will most likely not cause harm to the patient; they do put the patient at greater risk than some other drug side effects may. As stated earlier, patient monitoring is essential when there is the potential for serious side effects. Pharmacy technicians that recognize drugs with harmful side effects, like warfarin, can help to keep the pharmacists informed when patients alert them about their concerns.

It can sometimes be difficult to comprehend the difference between a drug side effect and a drug adverse reaction. Neither event is a wanted reaction from the drug, but the key difference is that an adverse reaction, unlike a side effect, significantly places the patient in harm's way. Adverse reactions may cause harm to the patients from the onset of use or over a nonspecific period of time. Drug manufacturers must report any known adverse reactions to the FDA's MedWatch Web site. MedWatch, established by the FDA in 1993, is another way of safeguarding the public from medications that are at a greater risk for causing harm. The process is completely voluntary for health professionals, with the exception of vaccine events, but is greatly encouraged by the FDA as well as most health-care institutions and providers. Pharmacy technicians and pharmacy technician students are urged to learn about the MedWatch system. Information about MedWatch is available at http://www.accessdata.fda.gov/scripts/ MedWatchLearn/.

Allergies are a vital piece of a patient's medication history and profile. Patient allergies will alert the pharmacy technician and the pharmacist to drugs that may have the potential for causing harm to the patient. A patient may have an allergic reaction to a drug the first time he or she uses the drug or even after he or she has taken the drug multiple times. Allergic reactions are hypersensitive reactions brought on by the ingestion of an unknown element into the body's system or for our purposes, a drug. Allergic reactions to a drug might include hives or rashes, swelling of the face or extremities, or swelling of the tongue and throat. These types of allergic reactions are known as anaphylactic reactions, and in case of swelling of the tongue and throat, they may become life threatening.

Penicillin falls under the classification of antibiotic and is further categorized under the sub-classification of beta-lactam antibiotics, with beta-lactam referring to the chemical structure of the drug. Having an allergic reaction to penicillin is not uncommon. What the pharmacy technician must recognize is that the patient will also have the potential for allergic reaction to other beta-lactam antibiotics as well, such as amoxicillin and ampicillin. If while verifying a patient's drug allergies, the pharmacy technician discovers an allergy, such as penicillin, the pharmacy technician should inquire further to ascertain what type of reaction the patient has had to penicillin. If the patient had any of the reactions previously discussed, then the patient has a true allergic reaction to the penicillin and will most likely have a reaction to other medications within that class. If the patient states that they had a reaction such as nausea, vomiting, or diarrhea, then the patient experienced a drug side effect and not an allergic reaction.

Pharmacy technicians should always be certain that the pharmacist is aware of any allergic reactions a patient may have had to a medication, including those that might be considered a side effect and not an allergic reaction. It will be the best judgment of the pharmacist that determines whether or not the reaction was a side effect or an allergic reaction. If the pharmacist feels the patient had an allergic reaction, he or she will interview the patient for further verification and follow up by consulting the patient's physician. Anaphylactic reactions, such as those potentially seen with a penicillin allergy, can be life threatening and should be highlighted on a patient medication history or profile. Pharmacy technicians that are aware of the risk will be able to alert the pharmacist to potential danger and, once again, keep the patient from harm.

Legend, Over-the-Counter, and Supplements: Defining and Understanding the Terms

As we have already discovered, the FDA plays a very significant part in the practice of pharmacy. Regulations set forth by the FDA help to assure the patient is receiving medication produced under strict quality and safety assured guidelines. In 1938, Congress passed the Food, Drug and Cosmetic Act (FDCA). Spurred by the deaths of more than 100 deaths, most of them children, from an untested, unregulated drug, it would be a huge step forward for the safety of the patient. Although the law required the drug be proven safe, before being marketed to U.S. consumers, there was still an issue with medications that required medical supervision in order to be considered safe for the patient. So, in 1951, after much debate, Congress amended the FDCA and passed the Durham–Humphrey Amendment.

The Durham–Humphrey Amendment of 1951 provided an extra layer of protection for the patients by creating two separate categories of drugs, legend drugs and over-the-counter (OTC) drugs. Under the amendment, any drug that was considered to have insufficient instruction and therefore needed more medical supervision in order to be safely consumed would be labeled as a legend drug.

Legend drug would require a written prescription from a licensed physician before being acquired by the patient. Additionally, all legend drugs would be mandated to state on their manufacturer packaging, "Caution: Federal law prohibits dispensing without a prescription." However, in 1997, manufacturers were permitted to print the words, "*Rx Only*" on their packing, simplifying legend-labeling requirements.

The pharmacist would also be required to place a label on the medication clearly stating the physician's instructions for the drug. For example, "Take one capsule twice a day." Prescription or legend drugs must be kept behind the pharmacy counter, away from patient's reach, at all times. Prescriptions obtained outside these guidelines are considered to be illegal and punishable under state and federal law.

The Durham–Humphrey's Amendment also provided regulation concerning the number of refills for legend or prescription medications as well as the allowance of oral or verbal prescription orders.

OTC drugs are considered safe for the public to consume with little to no medical supervision. OTC drugs can be acquired without a written prescription from the patient's physician and, therefore, not required to be kept behind the pharmacy counter. The one exception to this rule involves the sale of pseudoephedrine and products containing pseudoephedrine.

The USA Patriot Act of 2006, signed into law by President George W. Bush, included a provision known as the Combat Methamphetamine Epidemic Act of 2005. A small part of the Act requires that all sales of pseudoephedrine products be completed behind the pharmacy counter, even though the drug is considered to be an OTC or non-prescription drug. Further details of the Act will be covered in the chapter, "Pharmacy Laws and Regulations."

Herbal and dietary supplements make up a large part of the OTC products marketed to U.S. consumers. It is for this reason that President Bill Clinton signed into action the Dietary Supplement Health and Education Act of 1994 (DSHEA). As with other FDA regulations, DSHEA was created out of a concern for the safety of the U.S. consumer. The Act, which was an amendment to the FDCA of 1938, spelled out the definition of a dietary supplement as well as product safety and claims.

DSHEA defines a dietary supplement as "a product intended to supplement the diet that bears or contains one or more of the following dietary ingredients:

1. A vitamin
2. A mineral
3. An herb or other botanical
4. An amino acid
5. A dietary supplement used by man to supplement the diet by increasing total dietary intake
6. A concentrate, metabolite, constitute, extract or combination of any ingredient described"

While dietary supplements, such as those listed earlier, may prove useful to a patient's overall well-being, caution should be observed when taking them with prescription medications. There are several valid examples that prove this point, and since the safety and well-being of the patient should be the first concern in the practice of pharmacy, pharmacy technicians that are able to identify potential risk factors and alert the pharmacist may very well prevent an adverse event.

A prime example of such risk exists with the herb ginkgo biloba. Extract made from the leaves of the ginkgo biloba plant are thought to help in retaining memory by increasing blood flow to the brain. It is often given to patients that have been diagnosed with Alzheimer's disease or other forms of dementia because it has been found that patients with these types of diagnoses have a significant decrease in blood flow to the brain, explaining at least part of the reason for memory loss.

While conclusive studies on the link between ginkgo biloba and memory are still inconclusive, precautions remain a major concern, especially for patients on a regimen that might include anticoagulants. Since ginkgo biloba has been proven to increase blood flow, patients taking such drugs as warfarin, aspirin, ibuprofen, or any other medication used to slow clotting of the blood should steer clear of taking it. Ginkgo biloba has also been proven to interact with benzodiazepines, such as alprazolam, as well as antidepressants, such as fluoxetine.

St. John's Wort is another herbal supplement that has gotten a lot of attention over the last several years. St. John's Wort is thought to help with the effects of depression, as well as the symptoms associated with menopause and premenstrual syndrome. However, just as with ginkgo biloba, precautions should be observed when St. John's Wort is taken with certain prescription medications.

Citaloprim, escitaloprim, and paroxetine are just a few commonly prescribed antidepressants that are known to interact with St. John's Wort. The antihistamines loratadine, cetirizine, and fexofenadine have also been proven to interact with St. Johns's Wort. So, it is clear that precaution must be taken when herbal supplements are taken along side prescription medications.

Pharmacy technicians should always obtain as much information about a patient's medication history as possible, especially if the patient is new to the pharmacy. Pharmacy technician must learn to ask the patients about all medications and supplements that they might be taking in order to give the pharmacist a complete view of a patient's medication history and current regime. Not only will this allow the pharmacist to assist the patient further, but also possibly prevent potential drug interactions, duplication of therapy, or a fatal drug allergy from happening, or causing harm to the patient.

CHAPTER REVIEW QUESTIONS

1. _____ is the study of how drugs work and react within a living system, primarily human beings.
   a. Pharmacology
   b. Kinetics
   c. Toxicology
   d. Distribution

2. _____ is the branch of pharmacy of how drugs are transported through the body's system.
   a. Toxicology
   b. Pharmacology
   c. Pharmacokinetics
   d. Absorption

3. The four central stages involved in pharmacokinetics are _____, _____, _____, and _____.
   a. Elimination, metabolism, structure, and absorption
   b. Absorption, distribution, metabolism, and elimination
   c. Metabolism, structure, elimination, and distribution
   d. Distribution, elimination, absorption, and structure

4. The chemical name of a drug is based upon a drug's _____.
   a. Chemical structure
   b. Indication
   c. Form
   d. Route of administration

5. In order for a prescription to be filled with a brand name drug the prescription must contain the words, _____.
   a. Generic only
   b. Brand necessary or fill with brand name only
   c. Chemical name only
   d. Doctors orders

6. According to FDA regulations, a generic drug must be the _____ equivalent of the brand name drug.
   a. Price
   b. Chemical
   c. Genetic
   d. Daily

7. _____ are a class of drug used to treat the symptoms associated with nausea and vomiting.
   a. Anticonvulsive
   b. Antiulcer
   c. Antiemetic
   d. Anticholesterol

8. _____ are a class of heart medications.
   a. Angiotensin-converting enzyme (ACE) inhibitor
   b. Antihypertension
   c. Anticholesterol
   d. Antibiotics

9. _____ are the classification of drugs used to control cholesterol in the blood and increase blood flow.
   a. Antibiotics
   b. NSAIDS
   c. Statins
   d. Beta Blockers

10. The drug classification known as _____ help to decrease the symptoms associated with of anxiety and panic disorders.
    a. NSAIDS
    c. Benzodiazepines
    c. Antibiotics
    d. Calcium channel blockers

3 Pharmacy Laws and Regulations

Learning objectives for this chapter will include:

- Description of pharmacy laws that affect everyday pharmacy practice.

- Explanation of the intent of pharmacy laws.

- Description of major pieces of federal pharmacy legislation and explanation of how they affect the practice of pharmacy.

- Stating the intent of the Poison Prevention and Packaging Act (PPPA) and listing exceptions to it.

- Definition of theories of ethical reasoning.

- Explanation of the importance of law and ethics in the pharmacy practice.

- Comparison of the difference between lawful and ethical behavior.

An Introduction to Pharmacy Law

Laws are an important part of everyday life. If you drive a car you obey the law by not going over the permissible speed limit or by fastening your seat belt. You pay taxes to local, state, and federal agencies because it is the law. In some professions, such as of a pharmacist, you must complete specific educational requirements and be licensed and registered with the state you wish to practice in, before you can proceed further with your chosen career. We often have "laws" for our home lives, even though these are more commonly referred to as rules.

Laws are created by positions of authority in a community, state, or country and are typically created in order to protect the citizens of the community, state, or country. Unfortunately, laws are generally put in place after there has been an event or situation that has endangered the public. The practice of pharmacy has several examples of laws and regulations that were enacted after tragedies struck. Take, for example, the case of "Mrs. Winslow's Soothing Syrup."

"Mrs. Winslow's Soothing Syrup" was a product that was first marketed to the public in 1849. The product, created by a midwife, Charlotte Winslow, was advertised to sooth crying infants that suffered from teething pain. The product, main ingredient of which was 65 mg of morphine sulfate, went largely unregulated. Since the package labeling did not fully divulge the syrup's ingredients, many parents would overdose their crying infants with morphine, which would eventually lead to the infant's death.

Once the deaths of infants from "Mrs. Winslow's Soothing Syrup" became known to the public, there was an outcry from parents and professionals alike, demanding the federal government to enforce regulations on such acts of deception and quackery. The result was the passing of the 1906 federal regulation known as the Pure Food and Drug Act. The purpose of the new law was to prohibit interstate commerce of misbranded or adulterated food and drugs in the United States. False claims used to advertise the drug failed to hold up in court as "misbranding." Additionally, the act did not grant any legal authority to any governmental agency to ban or recall any drugs that might potentially be unsafe. Rather than put a false label on a drug, the manufacturer could just leave off the label and not list all the ingredients, which, coincidentally, was the case for "Mrs. Winslow's Soothing Syrup."

In 1910, the *New York Times* ran an article declaring the dangers of "Mrs. Winslow's Soothing Syrup," and in 1911 the American Medical Association (AMA) christened the concoction as a "baby killer." Sadly, prior to the Pure Food and Drug Act of 1906, remedies like Mrs. Winslow's were not uncommon, many with the same disastrous results. While the 1906 Pure Food and Drug Act was not as effective as had been hoped, it did pave the way for later amendments and regulations that would be successful in protecting the public.

Federal Authorities

There are two Federal authorities, which are key players in the development of laws pertaining to pharmacy, the Drug Enforcement Agency (DEA) and the Food and Drug Administration (FDA). Both these entities have produced regulations that have not only improved safety for U.S. consumers, but have also improved the outcome of health care.

The DEA was born under the Nixon administration in July 1973. The sole purpose for the formation of the DEA, which resides under the administration of the Department of Justice, was to extinguish an ever-growing drug issue in the United States. In 1970, Congress enacted Title II of the Comprehensive Abuse Prevention and Control Act or as it has come to be known today, the Controlled Substance Act. The DEA is a federal agency and is responsible for carrying out the statutes of the Controlled Substance Act.

Formerly known as the Bureau of Narcotics and Dangerous Drugs (BNDD), the DEA was the Nixon administration's response to two international treaties: the 1961 Single Convention on Narcotic Drugs and the 1971 Convention on Psychotropic Substances. These two conventions set about to establish classifications for controlled substances. The formation of the DEA, a branch of the Federal Bureau of Investigation (FBI) under the authoritative power of the Department of Justice (DOJ), as well as the enactment of the Controlled Substance Act completed this task.

Starting out with a task force of just under 1500 agents and a budget of 75 million dollars, the DEA has grown to be a formidable force in the war against illicit drugs, now boosting a staff of 5000 special agents and a 2.2 billion budget. Throughout the history of the DEA, amendments to the Controlled Substance Act have called for more stringent regulations of controlled substances and in most recent years a crackdown on the illegal trade of opioid drugs, such as OxyContin and hydrocodone. The street value of these drugs on the illegal drug market continues to rise, causing unwanted pains for the DEA and the pharmacy community.

The FDA is the other half of the Federal authority, which is a guiding principle behind putting into force legislation and statutes that are associated with the business of pharmacy. Fully established in 1930, the FDA has made significant strides in the safety and efficacy of drug products that crowd the U.S. market and their mission statement clearly evokes their purpose.

The FDA is responsible for protecting the public health by assuring the safety, efficacy and security of human and veterinary drugs, biological products, medical devices, our nation's food supply, cosmetics and products that emit irradiation.

In 1938 the U.S. Congress enacted the Federal Food, Drug and Cosmetic Act. This one piece of legislation catapulted the United States into a champion of public health and safety as well as becoming the cornerstone for the FDA. The FDA, which is under the administrative power of the Department of Health and Human Services, has helped to bring about great change in the field of pharmacy. For example, the Durham-Humphrey Amendment of 1951 created two separate categories of drugs: prescription and non-prescription. An even greater achievement may be the Kefauver-Harris Amendment of 1962, which placed tighter restrictions on the development and marketing of new drugs and also gave the FDA sole power in regulating prescription drugs as well as the marketing behind those drugs.

While changes continue with the U.S. market, the security afforded to its citizens goes without question. Throughout the years, it has been the FDA who has sought to work openly with legislators and pharmaceutical companies alike to bring to the citizens of the United States the safest drug regimens while maintaining effectiveness and cost as well.

DEA Administrative Laws

Title II of the Comprehensive Drug Abuse Prevention and Control Act of 1970 (Controlled Substance Act)

Enacted in 1970 under the Nixon administration, the Comprehensive Drug Abuse Prevention and Control Act set about to create legislation that would monitor the manufacture, importation, possession, use, and distribution of controlled substances. This piece of legislation was a confirmable response to the United States' staunch allegiance to fight the continually mounting war on illicit drugs. This legislation not only called for tighter restraints on controlled substances, but also created five separate classifications of controlled substance based upon each drug's degree of potential addiction.

The Controlled Substance Act also forced more accountability. Manufactures, pharmacies, pharmacists, and prescribers are all regulated in one way or another by the statues under the Controlled Substance Act. DEA registration numbers and the DEA 222 form are just two ways in which the DEA helps to preserve the integrity of this law.

Controlled Substance Classifications

Controlled substances are drugs that have been recognized by the DEA to be dangerous and/or possess a greater potential for abuse. There are five classifications or schedules of controlled substance, each classification being a step down based upon medical use and abuse potential.

1. Schedule I (C1)
   a. Drugs that hold the potential to be highly abusive
   b. Not accepted for safe medical use in the Unites States
   c. Includes drugs such as heroine, marijuana, and GHB (gamma-hydroxybutyric acid. Better known as the "date rape drug")
2. Schedule II (CII)
   a. Drugs that hold a high potential for abuse
   b. Accepted in the United States as a form of medical treatment (typically for the treatment of acute pain)
   c. A new prescription must be written each time it is filled.
   d. Includes drugs such as hydrocodone, morphine, oxycodone, hydromorphone, and anabolic steroids
3. Schedule III (CIII)
   a. Drugs that hold a potential for abuse, but potential is less than CII
   b. Accepted in the United States as a form of medical treatment (typically for the treatment of severe pain)

   c. Prescriptions for CIII drugs are not refillable after 6 months from the original date of the prescription

   d. Includes drugs such as codeine and are most often combined with an analgesic (acetaminophen)

4. Schedule IV (CIV)

   a. Drugs that still hold a potential for abuse, but potential is less than CIII

   b. Accepted in the United States as a form of medical treatment

   c. Prescriptions for CIV drugs may be refilled up to five times in 6 months

   d. Includes drugs such as diazepam, lorazepam, and alprazolam

5. Schedule V (CV)

   a. Drugs that have a low abuse potential relative to CIV

   b. Accepted in the United States as a form of medical treatment

   c. Includes drugs such as cough remedies that may have small amounts of codeine as a key ingredient

While the formation of drug classifications was a key element of the Controlled Substance Act, the use of DEA registrant numbers also came into play. Under DEA regulations, a person or entity that wishes to manufacture, dispense, or distribute controlled substances must register with the DEA and obtain an authorized DEA registrant number. This law applies to manufactures, pharmacies, wholesalers, and practitioners.

DEA practitioner registration numbers are perhaps the most commonly exampled form of DEA registration in pharmacy and will likely be the one most technicians will have the greatest interaction with. The DEA states their definition of a practitioner, under the Controlled Substance Act, as "a physician, dentist, veterinarian, hospital, or other person licensed, registered or otherwise permitted by the United States or the State in which he or she practices to dispense controlled substances in the course of professional practice." In reference to "other person," it may include practitioners such as a physician's assistant or a nurse practitioner. The ability of these professionals to prescribe controlled substances is relegated to their State Board of Pharmacy, but if they are permitted to do so, they must still obtain a DEA registrant number.

The method for assigning DEA registrant numbers begins with a nine-character number that contains two-alphabet letter and seven digits. Any physician, dentist, or veterinarian will have a DEA number that begins with the letters A, B, or C. Professionals that the DEA classifies as mid-level practitioners, physician's assistants, and nurse practitioners will have a DEA number that begins with the letter M. The second letter in the DEA registrant number will typically be the first initial of practitioner's last name. Again, this is typically the case, but there may be some exceptions. The next digits are numbers that are randomly generated by a computer and exclusive to the registrant. The final or ninth position is a number, when calculated, will verify registration.

Verification of a registrant DEA number involves a fairly simple calculation and while it certainly works to validate a number it can be subject to forgers who also know how the process works. If at any time the validity of a DEA number is in question, it is always best to verify the information with the prescriber and/or the DEA. Here is the calculation used to verify a DEA prescriber registration number.

- Add together the first, third, and fifth digits
- Next, add together the second, fourth, and sixth digits
- Multiply the second sum by 2
- Add together the first sum and the second sum
- If calculated correctly, the right-most digit should be the same as the last digit in the registrant's DEA number

> **DEA Prescriber Registration Verification Example**
> **AA5836727, Joshua Andrews, MD**
>
> Registration begins with an A, B, or C for physicians
>
> Add **(5 + 3 + 7) 15**, and then add together
>
> **(8 + 6 + 2) 16** and multiply by **16 × 2 = (32)**
>
> Then add together the first sum and the second sum
>
> **15 + 32 = 47**. The digit to the most right should
>
> be the same as the last digit in the registrant number; in this case **(7)**
>
> This DEA process of validation verifies this registrant number.

DEA 222 Form

The DEA 222 form is another tool the DEA uses to track controlled substances. Any time a Schedule I or II controlled substance is purchased or returned between a wholesaler and a pharmacy or a pharmacy-to-pharmacy, a DEA 222 form must be done. This process, which can now be completed online through the DEA Web site, www.deaecom.gov, involves a triplicate form that must be completed by both the seller and the purchaser. The DEA has very specific criteria that must be met when completing a 222 form.

- Form must be completed in triplicate with the pharmacy keeping the third copy of the form.
- The first and second copies of the form go to the supplier.
- The supplier will then keep copy 1 for their records and send copy 2 to the DEA as record of transaction.
- DEA form must be signed by the pharmacy's assigned Power of Attorney. Typically, this may be the lead pharmacist or the pharmacy director, but it is usually a person in an administrative position.
- The supplier may refuse any DEA 222 form, which has mistakes, cross-outs, or alterations of any kind. If a supplier refuses a DEA 222 form, they must remit copies 1 and 2 back to the pharmacy with an explanation for the refusal.
- A pharmacy may cancel a CII order or any part of a CII order but must notify the suppler in writing. The supplier will then strike a line through the item(s) to be eliminated from the order and write void across the line.

DEA 106 Form

As you may recall, the central purpose of the DEA is to provide tighter restraints and regulatory control over drugs that have the potential for abuse. Drug diversion or illegal purchase of illicit drugs for illegal means is a criminal act, which the DEA does not take lightly. Unfortunately, pharmacies and wholesales can also be a means for drug diversion. In order to combat this issue any time, if a pharmacy or wholesaler experiences a loss or theft of controlled substances, they must contact the DEA office and the local police as well as complete a DEA 106 form.

The form may be completed in written form or electronically through the DEA's Drug Diversion Control Program's Web site at http://www.deadiversion.usdoj.gov. Failure to complete any of these procedural steps can result in fines and/or criminal charges for the pharmacy and/or the wholesaler depending upon where the loss or theft occurred.

Combat Methamphetamine Epidemic Act

In September 2006, the U.S. Congress passed the Combat Methamphetamine Epidemic Act. The legislation was a direct reaction to the emergent issue of illegal methamphetamine distribution and use. Pseudoephedrine, which is an over-the-counter (OTC) antihistamine, became one of the core ingredients in the production of the illicit street drug known as "meth." Since pseudoephedrine was a common OTC product, the curators of this illicit drug had no problem procuring the ingredients they needed. In turn, the illegal sale and use of methamphetamine skyrocketed. In 2005 it was estimated that methamphetamine cost the U.S. tax payer 23 billion dollars. Since the inception of the Combat Methamphetamine Epidemic Act in 2006, there has been an epic decrease in illegal methamphetamine activity in the United States.

Under the Combat Methamphetamine Epidemic Act, pharmacies and other retail outlets such as grocery stores need to relegate OTC drugs that are ephedrine, pseudoephedrine, or phenylpropanolamine based on behind-the-pharmacy counter or they must be locked in a cabinet out of the site of customers. There are also restrictions placed on the number of grams a customer can purchase and the number of grams a pharmacy can sell on a daily basis. These rules also apply to mail-order pharmacies.

Along with the limit on purchases and sales of these drugs, there must be a listing of the purchases recorded either electronically or written on a logbook. Purchasers need to present a Federal or State issued photo ID, such as a driver's license, and sellers must verify that the information on the ID matches the information on the logbook. Logbook information must include the name of the drug, amount purchased, name and address of person who made the purchase, as well as the date and time of the purchase. Any one who purchases these drugs and provides false information on the logbook is subject to a fine of 250,000 dollars or a prison term of up to 5 years. The pharmacy must also provide a written warning concerning the consequences of providing false information. The pharmacy must keep record of the logbook for at least 2 years from the last signed date in the logbook.

In order for pharmacies to sell the drugs affected by the Combat Methamphetamine Epidemic Act, they must provide proof of self-certification and training concerning the new legislation. If the seller has more than one outlets that sell these drugs, then they must provide proof of certification and training at all outlets. The training information, which is provided by the Attorney General's office, can be found on an Internet site delivered by the Department of Justice. In addition to the training and certification, which must be completed by all employees involved in the selling of these drugs, the seller must also provide a written statement to the Attorney General's office, acknowledging their understanding of the legislation's requirements. Failure to comply with any of these requirements can result in the pharmacy's inability to sell these drugs through their retail outlets. Pharmacies must also relinquish logbooks and certifications at will to federal, state, and local authorities, if they are requested.

A complete listing on the limits for consumer purchase and retail sales can be viewed on the DEA Web site at http://www.deadiversion.usdoj.gov/meth/cma2005.htm.

Final Notes

The establishment of the DEA brought about change within the pharmacy profession, which has provided more control and patient safety concerning controlled substances. Primary to these changes was the passing of the Comprehensive Drug Abuse Prevention and Control Act of 1970. This legislation provided a systematic categorization of controlled substances based upon their medical use and their potential for abuse. It also established a registrant system as a means to verify the authenticity of those prescribing, distributing, and manufacturing drugs.

While the Controlled Substance Act is perhaps the most influential piece of legislation enacted through the DEA, the Combat Methamphetamine Epidemic Act, enacted in September 2006, has had far-reaching results as well. According to a July 2010 report distributed through the White House, nearly 1400 or 30% of known meth labs across the United States have been shut down since the inception of the Combat Methamphetamine Epidemic Act—more proof of the DEA's importance in the profession of pharmacy.

A full explanation of the Controlled Substance Act as well as more details concerning the Combat Methamphetamine Act can be viewed at http://www.deadiversion. usdoj.gov. Viewing these very important pieces of legislation is central to the education of a pharmacy technician. Taking the time to familiarize one's self with these laws only increases the professionalism of a pharmacy technician.

FDA Administrative Laws

The Federal Food, Drug and Cosmetic Act of 1938

The creation of the FDA has been as important to the development of the pharmacy profession as the DEA. Officially established in 1930, the FDA, which is a branch of the Department of Health and Human Services, has been a defender of changes for the safety and efficacy of drugs both for humans and for animals. The Federal Food, Drug and Cosmetic Act of 1938 was a re-write of the Food and Drug Act of 1906 and created the most radical changes to the profession of pharmacy. Along the way, several amendments to this act have enhanced its far-reaching ability for change.

Prior to the passing of the 1938 Federal Food, Drug and Cosmetic Act, the U.S. Congress had only made an uninspired attempt at regulating the safety and usefulness of drugs produced and imported to the United States. One of the first attempts at regulation came in 1848 with the passing of the Drug Importation Act. The Drug Importation Act gave the U.S. Customs Services the right to inspect drugs, which were imported from overseas. If the Customs Services felt the drugs were "tainted" or of "low quality," then they had the right to refuse admittance of the drug into the United States. This law was somewhat effective for drugs coming into the United States, but did not regulate those drugs, which were being produced in this country.

In 1906, under President Theodore Roosevelt's administration, the Food and Drug Act was enacted. This law, which made it illegal for states to sell or buy drugs, food, or drinks, which were knowingly mislabeled or contaminated, became the undertone for which the Federal Food, Drug, and Cosmetic Act would later be build. The Food and Drug Act of 1906, while it had good intentions, fell markedly short of protecting the citizens of the United States. Part of the reason for its failure came because of poor regulation at the state and federal levels. In 1933, 3 years after the inauguration of the FDA, a re-write of the 1906 Food and Drug Act was recommended, but it wasn't until 1938 that this actually happened.

The passing of the Federal Food, Drug and Cosmetic Act was primarily Congress's reaction to the 107 deaths of people who had taken elixir sulfanilamide that mistakenly contained diethylene glycol, a relative to antifreeze. The passage of the Federal Food, Drug and Cosmetic Act of 1938 became the first authentic attempt to regulate the safety and efficacy of food, drug, and cosmetic products available in the United States. This act not only required products to be deemed safe for human and animal use, but also mandated factories to be open to FDA inspection.

In 1941, 300 people died from the use of an antibiotic, sulfathiazole, being compromised with the sedative phenobarbital. The FDA jumped into action, creating landmark controls on the manufacturing and quality of consumer products. The result of these changes came to be known as Good Manufacturing Practices (GMP), a footnote of the Food, Drug and Cosmetic Act.

GMP entails manufacturers to provide a level of quality assurance to the consumer as well as confidence in the security of the product. Regulations, record keeping, cleanliness, a qualified work staff, unhampered machinery, as well as a system for procuring quality assurance standards are just some of the elements associated with GMP. While the FDA sought to keep these practices open-ended, they are still under the regulatory mandate of the FDA.

The next considerable piece of legislation to the Food, Drug and Cosmetic Act came in 1951. The Durham-Humphrey Amendment of 1951 took direct aim at the profession of pharmacy. This amendment brought about the institution of two separate classifications of drugs: prescription and non-prescription. The Durham-Humphrey Amendment defined the safety of drugs by categorizing prescription drugs as medications that needed oversight by a licensed physician and therefore needed a written prescription; all other drug would be labeled as non-prescription or OTC.

In addition, prescription drugs would need to contain a label from the manufacture, which was clearly visible and specified, "Federal law prohibits dispensing without a prescription." Furthermore, a label containing directions dictated by a prescriber and transcribed by a pharmacist would be placed on the drug's container. This piece of legislation also allowed for the refill of certain medications.

In 1962, there were seven physicians who worked as investigative drug officers for the FDA. One was a woman by the name of Frances O. Kelsey, MD, PhD. It was Dr. Kelsey's sound judgment and medical expertise that helped to avoid a situation, which had horrific potential. During the early 1960s, Thalidomide was a sedative, being used for morning sickness, distributed by Chemie Grunenthal, a German company. Thalidomide, it was later found, was responsible for thousands of deformed babies in Western Europe. It was the actions of Dr. Kelsey that kept this tragedy from happening in the United States. Even though the manufacturers of Thalidomide had applied for approval in the United States, Dr. Kelsey remained skeptical of its safety and refused to approve it for use in the United States.

Dr. Kelsey was central in not allowing Thalidomide to be approved for use in the United States; the second action came from the U.S. Congress. In 1962, the Kefauver-Harris Amendment was passed. The Kefauver-Harris Amendment required all drugs marketed in the United States to not only be safe for use, but also prove their usefulness.

Under this new amendment to the Food, Drug and Cosmetic Act, drug companies were required to perform extensive testing in order to prove the drug's safety and use before the FDA could give approval. Along with these new application requirements, drug companies were required to provide informed consent to those who were part of clinical studies as well as report any adverse effect. Kefauver-Harris went even further by giving the FDA complete regulator control over new drug applications as well as overseeing prescription drug advertising; non-prescription drug advertising is controlled by the Federal Trade Commission.

The Kefauver-Harris Drug Amendment also brought about the formation of the Advisory Committee on Investigational Drugs. The Advisory Committee on Investigational Drugs assists the FDA on policies and procedures regarding products seeking FDA approval in the United States. Today, the standards set forth by the FDA for drug approval are considered the rule by which all other countries seek to mimic.

The Fair Packaging and Labeling Act of 1966

As is the case in all of history, progression is inevitable. This is no less the case in the profession of pharmacy. In 1966 the Fair Packaging and Labeling Act asked products shipped throughout the United States to have labeling, which was forthright and instructional to the consumer. According to rules agreed upon by the FDA and FTC (Federal Trade Commission), all interstate consumer products must include the following:

- Must clearly identify the product by name
- Provide the name and address of the manufacture, distributor, or packer
- Provide net weight of product based upon the standards set forth by the Office of Weights and Measures
- FDA would be responsible for product which fall under the categories of food, drug, cosmetics, or medical device; all other products would fall under the responsibility of the FTC

There are few exceptions to these rules, most of which are associated with industrial products. It should also be noted that insecticides and other forms of poisonous pest controls fall to the authority of the Environmental Protection Agency.

Poison Prevention Packaging Act of 1970

Further measures of drug safety came in 1970 with the passing of the Poison Prevention Packaging Act of 1970 (PPPA). The PPPA, which actually falls under the supervision of the Consumer Product Safety Commission, was targeting the deaths of children under the age of 5 years due to accidental poisoning. The PPPA required all prescription drugs, non-prescription drugs, as well as products considered to be household hazards to have child-resistant closures.

This act as it pertains to the pharmacy profession involves the use of child-resistant containers for prescription medications. While the majority of prescriptions are filled using child-resistant containers, there are a few exceptions:

- A prescriber may request non-child-resistant closures for a patient but must do so for each prescription, each time it is prescribed.

- A patient may request non-child-resistant closures for a prescription or for all of their prescriptions. It is a recommended best-procedure practice to have the patient sign a waiver stating they have requested non-child-resistant containers for their prescriptions.

- Child-resistant containers are not required for prescriptions used in a hospital or institutional setting as long the medication is being administered by a licensed health-care professional.

- Child-resistant containers are, however, required for prescription that are to be administered at a nursing home or long-term care facility.

The language of the PPPA involves several exemptions to the statues in the act. A detailed explanation of the PPPA can be viewed on the Consumer Product Safety Commissions Web site at http://www.cpsc.gov/businfo/pppa.pd.

While the PPPA was a step in the right direction for patient safety, the next significant piece of legislation would not come until 1982, and unfortunately, it came on the heel of a national disaster.

In 1982, the greater Chicago area became hostage to what has become known as the "Tylenol Murders." In 1982, seven people, ages 12–35, died after taking Extra-Strength Tylenol. All of the incidences happened in the Chicago area and police soon found the connection. The common factor in all of the deaths was Tylenol. Upon further investigation the people found each of the victims had taken Tylenol laced with potassium cyanide. In fact, investigators would later find out that the amount of potassium cyanide inserted into the Tylenol capsules, 65 mg, was 10,000 times the 5–7 mcg needed to cause death. To this day, the Tylenol murders remain unsolved, but from tragedy arose legislation, which sought to keep an event such as this from ever happening again.

Anti-Tampering Act of 1983 provided the following consumer safety standards:

- Most OTC products and cosmetics need to have tamper-resistant packaging.

- Tamper-resistant indicates there must be some form of barricade so that when broken it signals to the consumer there is a chance the product has been tampered with.

- Product must state that it has tamper-evident packaging.

- In addition to packaging requirements, stiff penalties and mandatory jail sentencing were put in place. Severity of the crime determines the severity of the punishment.

Orphan Drug Act 1983

On the heels of the Anti-Tampering Act came the Orphan Drug Act of 1983. The Orphan Drug Act established incentives for drug manufactures willing to develop new drugs for diseases defined as rare. A rare disease as described by the U.S. Congress is defined as "a disease affecting fewer than 200,000 people." The Orphan Drug Act gave drug companies enticements that would help build a stronger market for drugs that treated diseases which otherwise might not be developed. Part of the incentives spelled out in the act include the following:

- A 7-year period where the drug developer had marketing exclusiveness of the orphan drug.
- A 50% tax credit toward costs aligned with the cost of clinical testing and research.
- Grants for clinical testing and research for new drug therapies.

1997 Congress built upon the Orphan Drug Act incentives, which included adding the following:

- Drug companies who developed orphan drugs would be exempt from the normal FDA imposed drug application fees. In 2001 the typical application fee could cost up to $500,000.
- If the orphan drug being developed is for an illness, which is considered to be "life threatening," then approval could be expedited.

The Orphan Drug Act of 1983 has proven to be a successful tool in combating diseases, which might otherwise go without notice. Since the law's beginning in 1983, 350 drugs have been effectively developed and marketed in the U.S. consumer market. This is a long way from the less than 10 drugs, which had been developed in the decade prior to 1983.

Drug-Price Competition and Patient Term Restoration Act of 1984

Prior to the 1984 Drug-Price Competition and Patient Term Restoration Act, drug companies who wanted to produce and market generic forms of prescription drugs needed to go through an approval process, which was just as rigorous as one for the approval of a new drug. In order to try and decrease the cost of medications and make the market more competitive, Congress introduced legislation, which would make the approval process for generic drug less of a labor-intensive process.

Spearheaded by California Representative Henry Waxman and Utah Senator Orrin Hatch, the law essentially called for a more competitive market for prescription drugs by allowing manufacturers of generic drug to prove only a drug's "bioequivalence," eliminating the need to proceed through the mounts of paperwork and testing associated with developing a new drug.

The second half of this law allowed brand name drug manufacturers to acquire an extended 5-year period on new drug patents as well as offering monetary inducements for new drugs being developed. According to the language of the law, these were to be a measure of reimbursement for the lengthy time process necessary for new drug approval. Since the enactment of this law, some have argued that it gives the manufacturers of brand name drugs a greater ability to keep their drugs from the generic market, extending drug patents for drugs, which would then be imposed to generic markets. However, the law has made the process for producing generic drug less of a demanding process, allowing more generic drugs to be produced and sending savings onto the consumer.

Food Drug and Modernization Act of 1997

The Food Drug and Modernization Act of 1997 was the FDA's answering toward a move to the twenty-first century. Under this act, the FDA sought to clarify information to the consumer and encourage new drug development. Some of the results of the act include the following:

- Fast-tracking new drug applications, in particular those that dealt with life-threatening illnesses.
- Detailed explanation of the pharmacy's role in extemporaneous compounding as well as allowing states to negotiate the standard for process.

- "Caution Federal law prohibits dispensing without a prescription" was shortened and replaced by "Rx only."
- The warning label, "Maybe habit forming," was removed from some drugs.
- Drug manufactures were rewarded with 6 months of extended exclusivity in exchange for more intense pediatric studies of drugs.

These are just a few of the accomplishments of the Food, Drug and Modernization Act of 1997. A full text of the law can be viewed at:www.fda.gov/Regulatory Information/Legislation/FederalFoodDrugandCosmeticAct

Adverse Events Reporting System 1998

The FDA put the Adverse Events Reporting System, which is not actually legislation, but rather a process, into action in 1998. This system bears mentioning due to the innovative way it evolved as an advocate of patient medication safety.

The Adverse Events Reporting System (AERS) is a computer system database for storing and tracking medication errors or adverse drug events. The information in this system is an accumulation of data dating back to 1969. As of December 2010, the AERS contained over 4 million events. AERS helps to track drugs, which may be a risk to the public due to either the composition of the drug or how it is being administered. The AERS breaks down the yearly statistics by:

- Domestic and foreign drug events
- Drug events reported by consumers and health-care workers
- Patient outcomes

Where AERS is the database used to store collected information, MedWatch is the system used to engage the reporting process. Any consumer or health-care professional may make a report to MedWatch. There are three avenues for report an adverse drug event:

- Call the MedWatch reporting line at 1-800-FDA-1088.
- File a report online at www.accessdata.fda.gov/scripts/medwatch/medwatch-online.htm
- File a MedWatch 3500 form and mail or fax (1-800-FDA-0178).

Anyone who makes a report to MedWatch is protected under the restraints of HIPAA, so questions concerning autonomy should be answered. Since its introduction, MedWatch and its database, AERS, have been at the forefront of patient safety by instituting recalls and partnering with drug companies to ensure products reach the U.S. consumers that are up to FDA standard and cause no intentional harm.

Ethics: The Solid Base for All Professions

The practice of pharmacy is one of the most heavily regulated industries of our time. How, then, does the professional pharmacy technicians reconcile their actions with their own moral, ethical, and legal standards. What does it mean to be moral, or ethical, and what are legal standards? Very often these terms have very personal meaning. For example, what might be moral or ethical to one person may not be moral or ethical to another person. Legal standard, on the other hand, is just a stand set by the law.

As we stated earlier, morals and ethics can be very personal, and in reality, have similar, but different meanings. Morals are defined by the Merriam Webster dictionary as "concerning or relating to what is right or wrong in human behavior." For example, most people would consider being trustworthy and dependable as moral traits. People who have been able to establish themselves as having these types of traits are generally thought to know the difference between what is right and what is wrong. They would, in most cases, be considered a moral person.

Ethics are not far removed from morals. In fact, many people believe one cannot exist without the other. As with the term *morals*, the Merriam Webster dictionary establishes a clear definition of the term *ethics*. Ethic as defined by Merriam Webster dictionary is "rules of behavior based on ideas about what is morally good and bad." Ethics are built upon our idea of what is right and wrong, or moral. Ethics may also be thought of as a standard of conduct for a given profession. The practice of pharmacy is built upon ethical standards that not only require practice within the legal standard, but also what is morally responsible, and ultimately best for the patients the profession serves.

John, for example, is a certified pharmacy technician with a local community pharmacy. John has noticed that business has decreased significantly since a large retail chain moved in down the street. One day John overhears another technician spreading gossip about the large retail chain while they are conversing with a loyal customer. The technician continues to spread disparaging remarks about the retail chain to two more customers. This pattern of bad behavior continues throughout the week till John finally decides he must stop the gossip.

John doesn't want his coworker to get in trouble but knows it is unethical to spread rumors about another business just to increase your own business. John feels he only has one choice, so he decides to approach his manager with the situation. Eventually, John's morals, or his sense of right and wrong, had bothered him so greatly that his ethical standards felt compromised. In order to correct the solution, John had to do what he felt was right.

Pharmacy technicians must realize that not every situation they may encounter will have a rule or regulation that dictates their proper response or behavior. For example, pharmacy law does not usually mandate that a pharmacy choose the best-priced medication for a patient, but pharmacy ethics do. One must also remember that a profession's ethical standards may not necessarily be aligned with one's own personal moral or religious beliefs.

Each technician has many decisions to make every day. These decisions profoundly affect the people we serve, and the people we work with, including the pharmacists we assist. Our decisions and actions must be well thought out, carefully considered, and not just knee-jerk, emotional, or blindly legal behaviors.

Code of Ethics

The American Association of Pharmacy Technicians (AAPT) has adopted the following pharmacy technician code of ethics in order to help guide the pharmacy technician in decision-making and professional behavior.

Preamble

Pharmacy technicians are health-care professionals who assist pharmacists in providing the best possible care for patients. The principle of this code, which applies to the pharmacy technicians working in any and all setting, is based on the application and support of moral obligations that guide the pharmacy profession in relationships with patients, health-care professionals, and society.

Principles

I. A pharmacy technician's first consideration is to ensure the health and safety of the patient and to use knowledge and skills to the best of his or her ability in serving others.

II. A pharmacy technician supports and promotes honesty and integrity in the profession, which include a duty to observe the law, maintain the highest moral and ethical conduct at all times, and uphold the ethical principles of the profession.

III. A pharmacy technician assists and supports the pharmacist in the safe, efficacious, and cost-effective distribution of health services and health-care resources.

IV. A pharmacy technician respects and values the abilities of pharmacists, colleagues, and other health-care professionals.

V.   A pharmacy technician maintains competency in his or her practice and continually enhances his or her professional knowledge and expertise.

VI.   A pharmacy technician respects and supports the patient's individuality, dignity, and confidentiality.

VII. A pharmacy technician respects the confidentiality of a patient's records and discloses pertinent information only with proper authorization.

VIII. A pharmacy technician never assists in the dispensing, promoting, or distributing of a medication or medical devices that are not of good quality or do not meet the standard required by law.

IX.   A pharmacy technician does not engage in any activity that will discredit the profession will and expose without fear or favor, illegal, or unethical conduct in the profession.

X.   A pharmacy technician associates with and engages in the support of organizations that promote the profession of pharmacy through the use and enhancement of pharmacy technicians.

Final Thoughts

The practice of laws and ethics is essential to the pharmacy profession state of well being. Laws and regulations can be complex and, at times, incomprehensible, but understanding their purpose and the reasons why they were created will help to educate the pharmacy technician, creating a safer experience for the patient. The practice of pharmacy is regulated by both federal and state agencies, but it is impossible to list the specifics of pharmacy law in each individual state. It is highly recommended that pharmacy technicians visit their State Board of Pharmacy Web sites in order to gain a comprehensive understanding of their state's pharmacy laws and regulations.

The State Board of Pharmacy is also an excellent source of information when contemplating a career as a pharmacy technician. A visit to the State Board of Pharmacy Web site will provide a list of requirements to practice as pharmacy technician in that state as well as the rules governing pharmacists and pharmacy technician duties.

National pharmacy technician certification exams focus solely on federal pharmacy regulation simply because of the wide range of diversity with individual state pharmacy law. This chapter provides a thorough review of federal pharmacy laws in order to assist the certification candidate with the best possible study guide.

CHAPTER REVIEW QUESTIONS

1. The two federal authorities responsible for the development of laws pertaining to drugs in the United States are the _____ and the _____.
   a. DEA/FDA
   b. CIA/FDA
   c. FDA/CIA
   d. FBI/DEA

2. The _____ created _____ categories for controlled substance.
   a. Pure Food Act/Six
   b. Humphreys Act/Six
   c. Durham Act/Five
   d. Controlled Substance Act/Five

3. A registrant DEA number contains _____ digits, _____ alpha letters, and _____ numbers.
   a. 7, 2, 9
   b. 9, 2, 7
   c. 5, 7, 2
   d. 10, 8, 2

4. The DEA _____ form must be used any time CI or CII controlled substance are transferred from a wholesaler to a buyer or when they are _____.
   a. 242/sold
   b. 222/sold
   c. 222/returned
   d. 242/returned

5. The DEA _____ form is used any time there is _____ or _____ of controlled substances.
   a. 105, loss, and theft
   b. 105, gain, and loss
   c. 106, loss, and gain
   d. 106, loss, and theft

6. _____ of 2006 requires that any OTC drug product containing ephedrine, pseudoephedrine, or phenylpropanolamine be kept behind the pharmacy counter and out of the reach of the general public.
   a. Illegal Drug Act
   b. The Combat Methamphetamines Epidemic Act
   c. Cocaine Addition Act
   d. Federal Prescription Act

7. All prescription medication must contain the words, "Federal law prohibits dispensing without a prescription" or _____.
   a. Prescription only
   b. Generic allowed
   c. Brand only
   d. D.A.W.

8. The Poison Prevention and Packaging Act of 1970 requires the use of _____ caps for all prescription medications dispensed from a pharmacy unless otherwise indicated by the patient or the patient's physician.
   a. Child-resistant safety caps
   b. Amber containers
   c. Recyclable
   d. Un-used

9. _____ created incentives for research done to develop drugs for diseases that affected less than 200,000 people each year.
   a. The Affordable Care Act
   b. The Orphan Drug Act
   c. Pure Food Act
   d. Movement Against Meth Act

10. The FDA is a branch of the _____ _____.
    a. Centers for Medicare and Medicaid
    b. U.S. Justice Department
    c. U.S. Department of Health and Human Services
    d. District Justice

chapter 4

Sterile and Non-Sterile Compounding

Learning objectives for this chapter will include:

- Describing infection control measures.
- Explaining the requirements for safe handling and disposal medications.
- Describing documentation procedures.
- Explaining product sterility.
- Describing the equipment used during sterile and non-sterile compounding practices.
- Describing sterile compounding procedures.
- Describing non-sterile compounding procedures.

Keeping Sterility Intact

Infection control is of primary concern to many professions these days, and the practice of pharmacy is no different. In recent years, the sterility of compounded medications has taken the national spotlight. Unfortunately, in most cases, the attention comes only after tragedy has struck, the most recent and visible incident being the deaths and injury that came from the New England Compounding Center (NECC) in Framingham, Massachusetts. Contaminated epidural steroid injections resulted in 48 deaths, and an additional 720 patients needed to be treated for fungal meningitis. Not only did this catastrophic event enforce the importance of compounded drug sterility and the role of infection control, but also pushed forward federal legislation to prevent such an incident like NECC from happening again.

Sterile intravenous or IV compounding has long been a vital part of the practice of pharmacy. Pharmacists and pharmacy technicians alike compound thousands of sterile IV products for patients each and every day. Hospitals, outpatient clinics, home health agencies, and long-term care facilities are just a few of the patient-care areas that may be serviced by compounded sterile products (CSPs). Oftentimes patients who require IV or parenteral administration are extremely ill or have body systems that have been compromised. Hence, it is essential that aseptic technique should be followed.

When talking about aseptic technique, we would be negligent not to include the standards of USP<797>. The United States Pharmacopeia (USP) is "a scientific, nonprofit organization that sets standards for the identity, strength, quality and purity of medicines, food ingredients and dietary supplements manufactured, distributed and consumed worldwide" (US Pharmacopeial Convention). Chapter 797 of the United States Pharmacopeia (USP) specifically deals with the standards that should be used during the sterile IV compounding process. It is, for all intents and purposes, the Bible of sterile IV compounding. It is important to note that while USP is not a branch of the federal government, the federal Food and

Drug Administration does have the authority to enforce the standards associated with USP<797>. So for this reason it is imperative that all pharmacy staff, and in particular, pharmacy-compounding staff, have a full and educated understanding of USP<797>.

In order to understand the standards associated with USP<797>, we must first understand the concept of aseptic technique. USP<797> becomes useless without the use of aseptic technique, and without aseptic technique CSPs cannot be reliably and verifiably produced.

So what is aseptic technique and how does it fit into the standards set by USP<797>? Aseptic technique, as defined by the language of USP<797>, is as follows: "a mode of processing pharmaceutical and medical products that involves the separate sterilization of the product and of the package (containers-closures or packing material for medical devices) and the transfer of the product and its closure under at least ISO Class 5 condition" (USP<797>).

While we have not yet delineated the conditions associated with ISO Class 5, aseptic technique, simply stated, is a process designed to prevent microbial contamination of compounded drugs and the packages they are transferred to or stored in so that a safe, reliable product can be delivered to the patient.

Aseptic Technique

Understanding how to accomplish proper aseptic technique when compounding sterile IV products is essential in order to provide the patient with a safe and reliable product. There are several aspects to accomplishing proper aseptic technique and one of the first steps is having a well-established comprehension of the tools used in the completion of sterile IV compounding.

Syringes, needles, alcohol swaps, 70% isopropyl alcohol, filter needles, filter straws, empty sterile IV bags, empty sterile vials, premix solution bags, tubing and filtration sets, the list could go on and on, but these are just a few items found within a sterile IV and chemotherapy compounding area. Pharmacy technicians working within a sterile IV and chemotherapy compounding environment soon come to understand that proper use of these instruments is as important as understanding the drugs they are compounding.

For the intent of this text, aseptic technique will be associated with the procedures used to compound parenteral medication. The term *parenteral* effectively means any drug that does not go through the body's digestive tract, unlike a drug that may be taken by mouth such as a tablet or capsule. Parenteral drugs can be administered or delivered to the body in various ways. One of the most common, and perhaps most recognized ways is intravenously or IV. When a parenteral drug is given to a patient via IV administration, the drug is introduced to the body through the veins. IV drugs are oftentimes given when immediate release of the drug is required or when the patient is unable to tolerate or ingest the drug orally. Parenteral drugs may also be administered as intramuscular, intrathecal, intradermal, intrapleural, intra-arterial, intraocular, intraperitoneal, subcutaneous, or as an epidural.

ROUTE OF ADMINISTRATION	APPROVED ABBREVIATION	EXAMPLE
Intravenous—*into a vein*	**IV**	Antibiotics, such as Ancef
Intramuscular—*into a muscle*	**IM**	Vaccines, such as a flu vaccines
Subcutaneous—*underneath the skin*	**Sub-Q or sub-q**	Opioids, such as morphine
Intra-arterial—*into an artery*	**IA**	Vasodilators, such as epinephrine
Intrathecal—*into the body through the space under the arachnoid membrane of the brain and spinal cord*	**IT**	Some chemotherapy drugs, such as methotrexate and cytarabine

(continued)

ROUTE OF ADMINISTRATION	APPROVED ABBREVIATION	EXAMPLE
Intraocular—*into the eye*	**IOL**	Diuretics, such as mannitol
Intraperitonel—*into the body through the peritoneum*	**IP**	Some chemotherapy drugs, such as Taxol
Epidural—*into the body through the dura mater that surrounds the brain and the spinal cord*	**No abbreviation**	Opioids, such as Dilaudid
Intradermal—*into the body through the skin*	**ID**	Allergy and tuberculosis testing
Intrapleural—*into the body by the pleura or pleural cavity or the membrane area within the lungs and thorax*	**No abbreviation**	***(Need to add here)***

Intravenous solutions are the most commonly compounded parenteral solutions. Most of us have seen an IV bag hanging from a patient's IV pole or have had IV solutions ourselves, so they are easily recognized. However, there are various forms of IV solutions. An IV solution that has been prescribed for a patient will, of course, enter the body through a vein. Intravenous solutions are administered into the body by either a peripheral or central vein.

Peripheral veins, or the veins from your hands, arms, feet, and legs, are typically used to administer IV solutions. Central lines or central venous lines are more complicated than peripheral because they are placed into the body through either the jugular, a large vein within the neck, or the subclavian vein, a large vein just beneath the clavicle, the superior vena cava, which collects blood from the head, arms, and chest and discharges it into the right atrium of the heart, or the femoral vein, which is located in the upper thigh and pelvic area.

Another difference between peripheral and central lines is in not only where they are placed, but also how they are placed. A physician, registered nurse, or paramedic usually places peripheral lines. Central lines need to be placed in the radiology department by a radiologist, a nurse specially trained for central line placement, or a radiology technologist trained in central line placement. Pain medication and a mild sedative are given to keep the patient calm during the procedure. The radiologist then administers a local anesthetic in the area where the central line is to be placed. The radiologist then inserts a needle underneath the skin to create an opening or tunnel for the central line to be placed. The central line is then placed in the opening, with only the tip of the line resting in the intended vein. In neonates, central lines are placed within the umbilical vein.

Central lines are generally placed when the patient must be on an extended drug therapy, such as chemotherapy, IV antibiotic therapy, total parenteral nutrition (TPN), dialysis, or another drug, which may be too caustic to smaller veins within the body. Central lines, while sparing the patient multiple needle sticks, do pose the potential for several other serious issues, the most prevalent being the potential for infection. However, patients with central lines may also be at an increased risk for blood clots and air embolisms, as well as the potential for a hole or tear to the central line and dislodging of the central line. If any of these situations takes place, then it is important that the patient receive medical attention as soon as possible to avoid any further complications.

One final parenteral line, which needs to be discussed, is a peripherally inserted central catheter (PICC) line. PICC lines are central lines that are placed peripherally, meaning, the catheter is placed into veins of the upper arm. Placement of PICC lines is often less invasive for the patient and can be placed by a registered nurse that has been specifically trained in the procedure or by a physician. An ultrasound is used to locate the appropriate vein for insertion. The patient is given a numbing agent, such as lidocaine, and the catheter is placed into the selected vein where it is directed into a large vein in the chest. Once the catheter has been placed, a chest X-ray will be taken to verify placement of the PICC line.

PICC lines, just as with other central lines, are placed for various reasons, extended IV antibiotic drug therapies, TPN, chemotherapy, or even for patients who may require routine blood sampling. Patients who have had a PICC line placed may also be at an increased risk for infection as well as blood clots, blockage of the catheter, dislodging, or moving of position. If any of these situations arises, as with other central lines, the patient should seek medical attention as soon as possible.

IV INFUSION SITE	PLACEMENT OF IV LINE	POTENTIAL PROBLEMS
Peripheral	Placed in the veins located in the arms, feet, legs, and hand	Infection, dislodgement, air embolism, blood clots
Central	**Adults**—jugular vein, subclavian vein, superior vena cava, or the femoral vein **Neonates**—umbilical vein	Infection, dislodgement, air embolism, blood clots, tear or hole in catheter of central line, movement of line placement
PICC	Placed in the veins of the upper arm	Infection, dislodgement, air embolism, blood clots, tear or hole in catheter of central line, movement of line

How an IV solution is administered is as important as what and where the solution is infused. IV solutions may be administered as either an IV push, as a continuous infusion, or as an intermittent infusion. IV push or IVP is an infusion that is given over a specified amount a time, typically over several minutes, and generally does not have a volume greater than 10 ml. For example, Claforan (cefotaxime), a third-generation cephalosporin antibiotic, may be administered as an IVP over a period no greater than 3–5 minutes. IVPs are compounded in syringes for ease of use. They are compounded with a minimal amount of diluent and then drawn into a syringe with the appropriate dosage. Once all air bubbles have been eliminated, a safety cap is placed on the product, labeled with the correct patient and dosage information, checked by the pharmacist, and sent out for administration to the patient. Once the IVP has reached the patient for administration, the nurse uncaps the syringe and attaches it to a port on the patient's IV infusion line, then gradually pushes the medication over the appropriate time.

Intravenous piggybacks or IVPBs are intermittent infusions also commonly referred to as small volume parenteral (SVP). IVPBs or SVPs are often used for medication that are to be administered over a timed interval. IV antibiotics are generally given as an IVPB. For example, Ancef (cefazolin) is a first-generation cephalosporin antibiotic. The recommended dose of cefazolin in a non-compromised adult is 1 g every 8 hours. Since the 1 g dose is to be given every 8 hours, it would be considered an intermittent dose and therefore a small volume parenteral.

Where intravenous drugs that are given by IV push or as an IV piggyback deal in small volumes, typically no greater than 250 ml, but can be as much as 500 ml, LVPs or large volume parenterals are considered to be continuous infusions, because the volume is normally greater than 500 ml. LVPs are administered by a rate, rather than by a specific time interval. An IVP or an IVPB may be administered with an explicit number of doses given over scheduled intervals, every 8 hours or every 12 hours, etc., where an LVP will be ordered as a rate per hour. A good example would be 1000 ml of normal saline with 20 mEq of potassium administered to the patient at a rate of 120 ml per hour. In other words, the patient will be receiving 120 ml of the LVP every hour and at the current rate the patient would need another LVP in approximately 8 hours.

INTRAVENOUS INFUSION TYPE	VOLUME	EXAMPLE
Intravenous Push or IVP	*Generally less than 10 ml of solution administered over several minutes*	*Some antibiotic and chemotherapy agents. Administration push rate depends on drug.*
Intravenous Piggyback (IVPB) also known as small volume parenteral	*Generally less than 500 ml of solution given over a specific, timed interval*	*Most IV antibiotic. Typically with a volume of 500 ml or less on a scheduled time, such as every 8 hours*
Large Volume Parenteral (LVP) also known as continuous infusion	*Generally 500 ml or more of solution, administered as a specific rate per hour*	*Electrolytes and Total Parenteral Nutrition (TPN) are two good examples. Typical order rate may be 120 ml per hour per bag volume.*

Syringes, Needles, and Compounding Hoods

As it is with any profession, there are certain instruments or tools that are common to the practice of sterile IV compounding. Syringes, needles, IV tubing, and compounding hoods are all tools of the trade, and the process of sterile IV compounding cannot be carried forward without them. Syringes and needles may be some of the most familiar tools of the trade. Syringes and needles come in various sizes. It is important to understand the difference in syringe and needle sizes as it can directly affect the accuracy of the sterile product being made.

Syringes may be made of glass or plastic, but most commonly, plastic. Use of glass syringes within a sterile IV and chemotherapy compounding environment is rare, and are often only used in instances when a patient has a known allergic reaction to plastic or if drug stability is in question by using a plastic syringe. There are seven common sizes for syringes: 1 cc, 3 cc, 5 cc, 10 cc, 20 cc, 30 cc, 60 cc.

There are two common types of syringes:

- Tuberculin syringes, which measure a maximum of 1 cc and are most often used to administer insulin. Tuberculin syringes may also be referred to as insulin syringes or slip-tip syringes, because the needle slips into the barrel of the syringe upon administration.
- Leur-Lok syringes are the most identifiable type of syringes within a sterile IV compounding environment. Leur-Lok syringes are threaded at the tip of the syringe barrel in order to hold the needle securely to the tip of the barrel during compounding or administration.

Syringes used in sterile IV and chemotherapy compounding should have measurement marks pre-printed on the outside barrel of the syringe. As the volume size of a syringe increases, for example, 10–30 cc, the accuracy of the syringe's measurements decreases. A good demonstration of this difference would be the measurement accuracy from a 5 cc syringe to a 30 cc syringe. On a 5 cc syringe, each line represents a measurement increment of 1 cc, whereas on a 30 cc syringe each line represents a measurement increment of 2 cc, making it more difficult to estimate finite measurements. As a general rule when choosing a syringe for withdrawing IV medications for compounding purposes, always choose the syringe that is closest to the volume to be drawn in order to provide the most accurate measurement. The one exception to this rule concerns hazardous drugs or chemotherapy agents. When reconstituting or withdrawing hazardous drugs or chemotherapy agents, it is recommended that an oversized syringe, not more than 10 cc, be used as a safety precaution and to prevent the risk of spillage when expelling access air from the syringe. A good rule of thumb states that the volume of the hazardous drug or chemotherapy agent should take up no greater than three-fourth of the chosen syringe's total volume capabilities. Choosing a syringe in this way also reduces the risk of spillage and contamination should the plunger of the syringe disconnect from the barrel of the syringe.

Tuberculin syringes or slip-tip syringes measure a maximum volume of 1 cc and generally have a permanent needle attached to the tip of the syringe. The needle of a tuberculin or slip-tip syringe is held onto the syringe by pressure and friction. These types of syringes have a great risk of needle and syringe separation and should never be used to compound hazardous drugs or chemotherapy agents due to the increased risk of spillage and contamination.

There are seven basic parts to a syringe:

- The Leur-Lok tip is where the needle will attach and lock. The Leur-Lok tip should never be touched in order to prevent the risk of contamination and maintain product sterility and integrity.

- The barrel houses the medication prior to injection or administration. This section of the syringe is where calibration marks will be found. Smaller syringes, 1–5 cc, will have calibration marks of 1 cc increments, and larger syringes, 10–60 cc, will have calibration marks of 2 cc increments.

- The top collar is located at the base of the barrel and is used to assist, along with the flat-end lip, to ensure the plunger remains untouched during the withdrawal and injection process.

- The plunger is used to push air from the syringe and should never be touched during withdrawal or injection of a product due to the increased risk of contamination to the final product.

- The plunger piston is a black rubber cap at the top of the plunger that is used to line up with calibration marks in order to obtain the correct volume of product required. The plunger piston should also remain untouched in order to maintain sterility and integrity of the product.

- The flat-end lip is located at the base of the plunger and used to assist, along with the top collar, to ensure the plunger remains untouched during the withdrawal and injection process.

The second most recognized element of a sterile IV and chemotherapy compounding environment is the needle. Needles come in various sizes and are measured by the size of the needle opening or bore. A needle's bore or opening decreases as its gauge size increases. For example, while a 25 gauge (G) needle may sound as if it has a larger bore or opening than an 18 gauge (G) needle, the converse is true. A 25 G needle will have a much smaller opening (bore) than an 18 G needle, allowing fluid to be injected or withdrawn more freely than the 25 G needle. The 18 G needle is most commonly used in the sterile IV and chemotherapy compounding environment. However, products that have a high viscosity or resistance of flow may require the use of a high gauge needle.

Needles are made from aluminum or stainless steel and may range in gauge sizes 13, the largest bore or opening, to 27, the smallest bore or opening. Needle gauge sizes 16 through 18 are the most common sizes used in sterile IV and chemotherapy

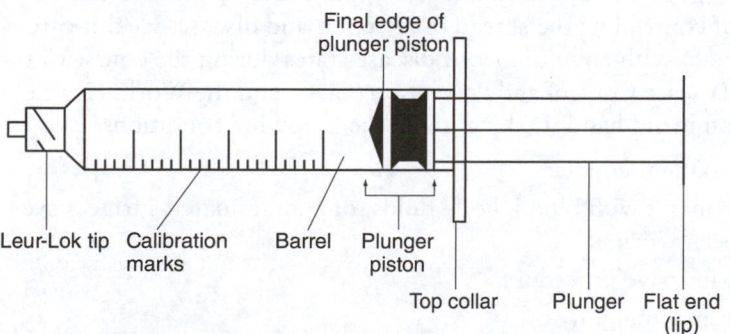

Figure 4.1 Diagram of a syringe

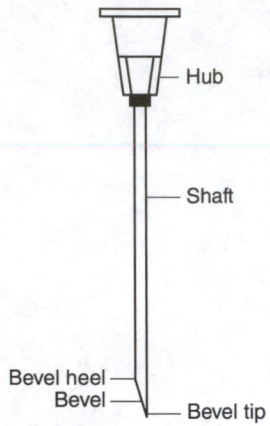

Figure 4.2 Image and diagram of a needle

compounding. The smallest gauze sizes are generally categorized for use with tuberculin or slip-tip syringes, which are used to administer insulin or allergy injections.

There are four basic parts to a needle:

- The hub, which attaches to the Leur-Lok tip, must never be touched in order to maintain product sterility and integrity.
- The shaft, which is made of aluminum or stainless steel, is the largest part of the needle. As with the hub, the needle shaft should never be touched in order to maintain product sterility and integrity.
- The bevel heel houses the bore or opening. This part of the needle is where the needle's slant begins to form the tip of the needle. Once again, this area should never be touched in order to maintain product sterility and integrity, and also to prevent accidental exposure to needle sticks.
- The bevel tip is at the end of the bevel heel and is the sharpest area of the needle. Caution should always be taken concerning the bevel tip, not only for matters of product sterility and integrity, but also as a matter of safety to prevent accidental exposure to needle sticks.

Filter needles and filter straws are used anytime there is risk of particulate contamination to a compounded product. Particulate contamination may happen when a vial becomes cored or when using a glass ampule as part of the compounding process. Coring occurs when a needle enters a vial and a piece of rubber stopper is displaced into the vial's liquid. In most cases, this happens for one of two reasons: the needle gauge may be too large for the vial and product size or the vial may have been entered into with the bevel down rather than up.

Glass ampules offer an entire different reason for employing the use of a filter needle. Glass ampules, while not used as commonly as glass vials, store medication prior to administration. Medication within a glass ampule does not require the use of dilution and often contains smaller quantities of the medication, typically 5 cc or less. Manufacturers that house products in glass ampules will usually place a painted ring around the break off point or neck of the ample to indicate where the ample should be broken for entry.

Transfer Needles and Devices

Transfer needles and devices are often used when multiple doses of a drug need to be pulled from a vial. The use of transfer needles and devices reduces the risk of product contamination that may be associated with multiple needle sticks to the same vial. Transfer needle and devices can be used with multi-dose vials and large- or small-volume IV solutions.

Infection Control Measures

Infection control measures play a large role in the practice of pharmacy as well as the language of USP<797>. In fact, aseptic technique and infection control rely heavily upon each other. If a pharmacy technician is unable to maintain sterile aseptic techniques, then infection control will most certainly become a concern. One of the simplest ways of adhering to aseptic technique and fostering proficient infection control measures is by performing proper hand-washing procedure.

This act may seem like a simple thing, but hand washing is one of the most efficient ways of controlling the spread of infection and disease. Health-care workers may come in contact with any number of disease states during the course of their day. The Centers for Disease Control and Prevention (CDC) and the World Health Organization (WHO) recommend hand washing under the following conditions:

- Before patient contact
- After contact with blood, body fluids, or contaminated surfaces even if gloves have been worn
- Before invasive procedures
- After removing gloves

- Before eating and before returning to workstation
- After using a rest room

Of course these are some generalized conditions and the pharmacy technicians may not encounter some of these situations; still it is a basic guideline that should be put into practice by all health-care workers.

USP<797> addresses hand-washing procedures under Personal Protection Equipment (PPE). Hand washing and the use of PPE are two of the most essential elements of aseptic technique and infection control. Like many procedures in the field of pharmacy, the donning of PPE and hand washing have specific processes that must be followed in order to prevent cross-contamination.

The sterile compounding room should only be for personnel that have been trained specifically for that area of the pharmacy. Staff members that have not been trained to work within the sterile compounding area should not be permitted into the clean room area. Keeping this area sterile is essential for compounding procedures and additional personnel only heightens the risk of contamination.

When donning personal protective equipment, always start at the bottom and work your way to the top. When removing personnel protective equipment, work in reverse, from the top to the bottom. Be certain to always place discarded PPE in the appropriate bin, which should be located in the anteroom. Listed further is the recommended order for donning PPE as per USP<797>:

- Members are not permitted to work within the sterile compounding area if they have open sore or infected wounds.
- Members are not permitted to work within the sterile compounding area if they have an upper respiratory infection.
- Members must remove all outer clothing, such as coats and hats, as well as all visible jewelry rings, necklaces, and earrings. If staff members cannot remove a ring it must be cleaned thoroughly and covered by a sterile glove.
- Gowning and garbing prior to proceeding to the clean room should be from the dirtiest area of the body to the cleanest area of the body:
  - shoe covers (then)
  - hair covers (then)
  - facial hair cover if appropriate (then)
  - facial mask
- Hand washing should follow in this manner:
  - Hand washing should be done in a no-touch sink.
  - Antibacterial soap or detergent should be used.
  - Hand washing should start at the hands and nails and progress to the elbows, being careful to scrub finger and underneath nail beds.
  - Hand-washing process should take no less than 30 seconds.
  - Non-shedding paper towel should be provided to dry hands and forearms.
- After proper hand washing, staff should slip on a non-shedding gown that fits securely around the wrist.
- The final step of gowning and garbing should be placing sterile gloves on so that they form one continuous surface with the gown sleeves:
  - Gloves should be re-sanitized with sterile 70% isopropyl alcohol (IPA).
    - This process should be repeated each time the gloves come in contact with a non-sterile surface.
- When leaving the clean room area, hand washing as well as the replacement of protective equipment, shoe covers, hair cover, facial cover, facemask, and gown should be done. Non-shedding gown may be left in the ante-area and used for a period of no more than 24 hours or during 1 shift.

Compounding Non-Sterile Medication

Compounding has always been a basic part of the practice of pharmacy, even though it has changed a great deal through the years. In the early twentieth century, most prescriptions were compounded in the pharmacy. However, safety and consistency issues arose. For example, without set standards, a prescription for a 500 mg/5 ml suspension may have been compounded at one pharmacy as 500 mg/5 ml and at another as 600 mg/5 ml. The number of compounded prescriptions steadily decreased over the decades with the increased availability and mass production of medications.

Today, manufacturers are required by the FDA to follow Good Manufacturing Practices (GMP). GMPs ensure that a 500 mg/5 ml suspension actually contains 500 mg/5 ml. Currently, most pharmacies compound a prescription only if the medication is not available from a manufacturer. When a prescription is compounded for a specific prescription or patient, it is called extemporaneous compounding. When a pharmacy compounds medications in anticipation of receiving a prescription, it is called batch compounding or batching. Batch compounding adds to the pharmacy's inventory and is not intended for a specific prescription or patient.

The number of custom compound pharmacies is currently on the rise. Physicians, medical institutions, and patients are realizing, more than ever, the importance of tailoring an individual's medications to meet his or her specific needs. A majority of pharmacists who are going back to compounding are doing it for the love of science and interest in their patients' well-being. Pharmacists and technicians must ensure that correct drug, dose, and directions are provided, but compounding can provide the best outcome for the patient.

The following eight factors should be considered when compounding pharmaceuticals:

1. **Organization and Personnel.** The entire pharmacy, including all personnel involved in the manufacturing process, is responsible for producing not only a safe product, but also one that does what it is intended to do. The pharmacists involved have the authority to approve or reject any product manufactured in their facility. The pharmacy also has the responsibility to train technicians or verify that they have the knowledge and skills to perform the duties required.

2. **Facilities.** Compounding and repacking work areas should be well lit and clean. These areas should be located away from high-traffic areas, public spaces, or any chemical that might interfere with compounding activities. Ventilation and temperature control also need to be considered.

3. **Equipment.** Equipment must be kept clean and in proper working condition at all times. Pharmacy technicians are usually assigned the task of filling, cleaning, and servicing any automated dispensing or compounding systems in a pharmacy practice.

4. **Control of Components and Drug Product Containers and Closures.** An appropriate supply of finished product containers (vials, lids, suppository molds) and actual drug or drug component containers (sterile water bottles, simple syrup containers) must be available, and stored in a clean, dust-free environment.

5. **Production and Process Controls.** It is important for good quality control that the medication is made to specific standards and in the same specific way and proportion each and every time it is manufactured. Recipes may be stored in computers, in notebooks, on cards, and so on. The recipe source should include all ingredients (active and inactive) as well as information on the manner in which the ingredients are combined to ensure strength and purity.

6. **Packaging and Labeling Controls.** It is a good manufacturing practice to monitor packaging labels constantly to ensure that they contain all the required information and that the information is in the right form. Finished packaging should also

be inspected for any defects, such as leaks, cracks, or defective seals. This control process should be addressed in detail in your pharmacy's policies and procedures manual.

7. **Holding and Distribution.** The pharmacy is most likely compounding and manufacturing more than one medication order at a time. Therefore, the finished products must be stored or quarantined in such a manner that the medication will not be used until after final verification by the pharmacist. Temperature, humidity, and light must be considered in medication storage.

8. **Records and Reports.** All compounding processes must be documented and retained, according to state pharmacy law, because there may be a time when a product or even a product container has been recalled and needs to be tracked. Information that needs to be recorded and stored may include:
   - Production dates
   - All components used, including manufacturer's, lot numbers, and expiration dates
   - Facility lot number
   - Facility expiration date
   - Identification of equipment used
   - Weights and measures of components used
   - All in process quality controls
   - Statement of actual yield
   - Complete labeling control records, including samples of labels
   - Description of drug product containers and closures
   - Identification of person(s) performing each step of the process, including final verification

Non-Sterile Compounding Equipment

It is a primary duty of a pharmacy technician to maintain all pharmacy equipment. This is especially important in compounding pharmacies. All equipment must remain clean, adjusted, and ready for use at all times. The pharmacist cannot wait while a piece of equipment is located, calibrated, or sanitized. Compounding technicians often use this equipment themselves and must understand its uses and maintenance requirements.

Balances

A Class A (or Class III) prescription balance has two pans and is used for weighing small amounts of drug substances, 120 g or less. The smallest readable amount that can be weighed is 10 mg. This is called the balance's readability. The capacity range (CR) for a Class A balance is 60 or 120 g, depending on the balance. The balance's variance or sensitivity requirement (SR) is 6 mg. This is the amount of substance it takes to move the pointer one-division mark.

A digital balance is a one-pan balance; the drug is measured inside the wind cover. This type of balance is quickly replacing the prescription balance because it is more accurate and easier to use.

Weights

A Class A prescription balance is used with a set of weights. Weights should be stored in their original boxes with clearly marked compartments. Forceps, preferably plastic tipped, should always be used when handling the weights, because oil from a person's hands can affect the accuracy of the weights. When the scale is in use, the area on which it is placed should be clean, dry, level, and away from air ducts and fans to minimize air movement. When the weights are not in use, they should be properly covered and stored.

Weigh Papers and Boats

Weigh papers are small, flexible papers that are used to measure and transport powders and semisolid substances. One side is coated with wax to prevent absorption and help to facilitate complete removal of the substance from the paper.

Weigh boats are rigid plastic containers that are used to measure and transport powders and semisolid substances. Most weigh boats have raised edges that make it difficult to completely remove some substances, especially semisolid substances. Therefore, when measuring semisolid substances, such as ointments, creams, and pastes, it is best to use weigh paper rather than a weigh boat. Both weigh papers and weigh boats are available in a variety of sizes.

Graduated Cylinders

A graduated cylinder is designed to have a narrow diameter that is the same from the top to the base. This type of "graduate" can be made of glass or plastic and is most commonly used as a liquid measuring device in a pharmacy. Selecting the proper graduate depends on the quantity of substance to be measured. The technician should select a cylinder that is only slightly larger than the quantity to be measured. The substance to be measured should never constitute less than 5% of the graduate's capacity.

Compounding Slabs and Ointment Paper

Compounding or ointment slabs are made of ground glass that is approximately 0.5 to 1 inch thick. They have nonabsorbent surfaces and are used to mix solid and semisolid substances. Most slabs are approximately 12×12 inches.

Parchment or ointment paper can be used instead of a compounding slab. The advantage to using parchment paper is that there is no need for a clean up. The paper is discarded after use. The disadvantage is that the paper can absorb water when creams are being mixed.

Spatulas

Spatulas are available in stainless steel as well as hard rubber and are used to count tablets and pills, transfer ingredients to weigh boats and papers, as well as mix liquids and semisolids. The hard rubber spatulas can be porous and can absorb some of the substance. The stainless steel spatulas are less porous but may become corroded by substances such as iodine.

Mortars and Pestles

The most common and recognizable type of pharmacy compounding equipment is the mortar and pestle. Mortars and pestles are used to grind, crush, pulverize, and mix pharmaceutical ingredients. The mortar is a cup-shaped vessel. The drug or drug products to be ground, crushed, pulverized, or mixed are placed in the mortar. The pestle is then used as the tool for grinding, crushing, pulverizing, or mixing the drug or drug products.

Glass is preferred for mixing liquids and semisoft dosage forms and are nonporous and do not stain. Wedgewood has a coarse surface and is best used for particle reduction. However, it is extremely porous and stains easily. Wedgewood pestles have wooden handle. Porcelain or ceramic mortars and pestles have glazed surfaces and are considered to be the standard for pharmacy compounding and particle reduction. The mortar and pestle should always be made of the same material, no matter which type is used.

CHAPTER REVIEW QUESTIONS

1. Chapter _____ of the United States Pharmacopeia is the chapter that deals with the use of aseptic technique and procedures during _____.
   a. USP 800, non-sterile compounding
   b. USP 800, sterile IV compounding
   c. USP 757, non-sterile compounding
   d. USP 797, sterile IV compounding

2. _____ drugs are injected into the body's system through a _____ and _____ drugs are injected in a _____.
   a. Intravenous/muscle, sublingual/vein
   b. Intravenous/vein, intramuscular/muscle
   c. Sublingual/vein, intramuscular/muscle
   d. Intravenous/muscle, sublingual/muscle

3. Syringes may be made of _____ or _____, but are most commonly made of _____.
   a. Glass, plastic, plastic
   b. Plastic, glass, glass
   c. Plastic, glass, rubber
   d. Glass plastic, rubber

4. There are _____ basic parts to a syringe.
   a. Four
   b. Six
   c. Seven
   d. Three

5. According to the CDC and WHO, one of the simplest things you can do to prevent spread of infection is _____.
   a. A flu vaccine
   b. Proper hand washing
   c. PPE
   d. Antibiotics

6. When donning PPE you should start with the _____.
   a. Gown
   b. Head cover
   c. Gloves
   d. Shoe covers

7. Hand-washing procedures should be done for no less than _____.
   a. 30 seconds
   b. 1 minute
   c. 45 seconds
   d. 1.5 minutes

8. A Class A is the same as a _____ prescription balance.
   a. Class II
   b. Class IV
   c. Class III
   d. Class I

9. Compounding or ointment slabs are made of _____ and approximately _____ to _____ inch thick.
   a. Ground glass, 0.5–1 inch
   b. Porcelain, 1–1.5 inch
   c. Ground glass, 0.75–2 inch
   d. Porcelain, 0.5–1 inch

10. _____ are rigid plastic containers that are used to measure and transport powders and semisolid substances.
    a. Weight rings
    b. Weight boats
    c. Weight bowls
    d. Weight containers

5 Medication Safety

Learning objectives for this chapter will include:

- Describing error prevention strategies during data entry.
- Explaining package inserts and medication guide requirements.
- Describing issues that require a pharmacist's intervention.
- Identifying look-alike/sound-alike medications.
- Identifying and defining high-alert medications.
- Identifying common strategies for medication safety.

Medication safety is essential to health and well-being of the patients that the practice of pharmacy serves. While it is true that there are specific tasks that only a pharmacist can perform, medication safety and awareness is a universal task. Pharmacists and pharmacy technicians alike should be educated equally on safe medication practices, not only for the patient's safety, but also for their own.

In order to understand safe medication practices we should first understand the definition of medication error. The FDA defines medication error as "Any preventable event that may cause or lead to inappropriate medication use or patient harm while the medication is in control of the health-care professional, patient or consumer." The FDA further details medication error by stating that "Such events may be related to professional practice, health care products, procedures, and systems, including prescribing: order communications; product labeling, packaging, and nomenclature; compounding; dispensing; distribution; administration; education; monitoring; and use."

As we can see, the FDA definition of a medication error allows for a wide array of scenarios, but the key line within the definition is *preventable event that may cause or lead to inappropriate medication use or harm.* Unfortunately, every pharmacist and pharmacy technician will make or be a party to a medication error at some point in their career. One of the reasons this becomes true is due to the daily stresses of our work environments.

External stresses, such as staffing issues, prescription or drug orders that are written indecipherably or missing information, or an unusually busy day, are all factors that can make our attention wane. Internal stresses may also break our attention, thus creating a greater risk for medication error. The constant ringing of the telephone, any equipment that fails, or even drug shortages and recalls can be internal stresses. Pharmacies can become overwhelming businesses within a very short expanse of time. It is no wonder external and internal stresses are often blamed, at least in part, as the reason why a medication error occurred.

While external and internal stresses most certainly play a key role in many medication errors, they are not the sole reason why errors occur. Medication errors can happen at any or even several times before an order or prescription reaches the patient. Of course, the goal is not only to prevent the error from reaching the patient, but also to prevent it from occurring in the first place.

The Institute for Safe Medication Practices (ISMP) is an organization that champions the development of medication safety. ISMP estimates that two of every three patients that visit a physician for illness leave the physician with a prescription. Given the population of the United States alone, this translates into more than 3.4 billion prescriptions every year. This number does not even begin to account for the countless number of refill and emergency medications filled each year, so as you can see, the risk of a medication error can be quite daunting.

This chapter will provide some strategies for preventing medication errors as well as understanding what constitutes a high-risk medication, and recognizing medication issues that need to be brought to the attention of the pharmacist. Safety of the patient should always be the first priority. Pharmacy technicians that know how to enact safe medication practices will help in assisting and enforcing the overall safety of the patient.

Preventing Errors from the Beginning: Data Order Entry

As already stated, two out of every three patients that visit a physician will walk away with a written prescription. In a hospital or institutional setting, the physician will assess the patient and then transcribe the patient's orders to the health system's computers. Either way, whether it's a prescription or a patient order, any medications ordered for the patient will first need to be entered into the pharmacy's computer.

Data order entry is one of the first processes in filling a patient prescription. It is also one of the most common ways medication errors can occur. Physician orders that are not written correctly, a prescription that has missing dose information, patients that have a JR or SR as part of their legal name, sound-alike/look-alike medications, missing or incorrect patient information, these are all situations where a data order entry error might occur.

So how do we keep data entry errors from happening in the first place? One of the first and most important ways is by remembering the *five rights of safe medication practices*. The *five rights of safe medication practices* is taught to nursing students as a precursor to administration of patient medications; however, it is a medication safety practice that has been adopted by all health profession disciplines. The *five rights of safe medication practices* are as follows:

- **Right patient**
- **Right drug**
- **Right dose**
- **Right route**
- **Right time**

Remembering these five patient rights when receiving patient medication orders in a hospital or institutional setting will allow the pharmacy technician to be proactive in preventing data entry errors. In addition to the five patient rights just listed, pharmacy technicians receiving medication orders within a hospital or institutional setting should make certain that the prescriber has signed the medication order, or in some cases as when a nurse takes a verbal order, signs as the prescriber's authorizing agent. Patient medication orders that do not have a prescriber's signature will need to be addressed by the pharmacist. Remembering these simple medication practice ideals will help to provide the patient with a safe and effective treatment as well as allow the pharmacy technician to alert the pharmacist of any potential issues related to the patient's medication therapy.

Another valuable tool for eliminating data entry order errors in a hospital or retail setting is Computerized Physician Order Entry (CPOE). Most hospitals and institutional facilities use the CPOE to prevent data order errors. When health systems use the CPOE, the prescriber will enter the patient orders directly into the computer. The order will then be forwarded to the pharmacy where the pharmacy technician, or in a large number of cases, the pharmacist, will review the order before a patient label is printed for dispensing.

CPOE provides several patient medication safety measures including the following:

- Standardized order entry throughout the health system.
- Order entry sets can be specialized for specific prescribers.
- All health system departments can view current and pending patient orders, which allows for the elimination of medication conflicts such as scheduling issues, patient testing, and so on.
- Prescribers and other health system professionals are able to see the patient's medication history, as well as view clinician guidelines that may help in preventing dosing errors.
- CPOE systems check for patient allergies, contraindications, and dosing issues, and alert the prescriber or the pharmacist during the order entry process.
- Prescribers use *electronic signature,* which provides a much more secure ordering process.
- Depending on the facility's capabilities, prescriber's may be able to order patient medications with a tablet or even a smart phone.
- ICD-9 and ICD-10 codes, which provide more accurate billing processes, are typically linked to CPOE.
- CPOE also enables the health system to collect data concerning patient order entry, alerting them of any current or potential problems within system.

As effective as CPOE has become over the last decade, it does not come without its own set of issues and precautions. One of the greatest issues is the sense of false security that CPOE can provide. While computerized systems largely benefit the patient during medication order entry, they are not error free.

Any number of issues can present themselves. Pharmacists and pharmacy technicians alike must be aware that the potential for medication order entry error may still exist. CPOE is linked to the health system's formulary. If an error was instituted during entry of a formulary item, spelling error, NDC number error, incorrect dose, and so on, the error will get carried across the facility, which in turn may cause multiple medication order entry errors.

Another example of a potential error may be that a very busy prescriber may unintentionally choose the wrong medication for the patient, or possibly override an alert that could prove dangerous or even fatal to the patient. Poorly trained staff will also inhibit the effectiveness of CPOE. All staff involved with the process of CPOE should be thoroughly trained. Pharmacy staff will be largely involved in the process of CPOE and should also be aware that the potential for medication order entry error may still exist. Pharmacy technicians that keep this in mind will help to prevent medication errors as well as provide the patient with the best care possible.

Pharmacy technicians that work within a retail or community setting should also be alerted of the *five rights of safe medication practices.* Unlike a hospital or institutional setting, the retail or community pharmacy technician will most likely be the patient's first point of contact. When the pharmacy technician receives the prescription from a patient, they must check to ensure that the prescription contains the following information:

- Date the prescription was written
- Patient's information: name, address, and date of birth

- Prescriber's information: name, address, and DEA registration number
- Drug name, strength, and form
- Medication instructions, that is, *1 tablet B.I.D* or *take 1 tablet every 6 hours*
- Quantity of drug to be dispensed
- Number of authorized refills if applicable
- Hand written signature of the prescriber

If the pharmacy technician receives a new patient prescription that has any of the aforementioned information missing, they will need to ensure that the missing information is obtained. If any of the patient's information is missing, the pharmacy technician may simply write it down by checking with the patient. If any other information, which cannot be checked with the patient, is missing, the pharmacy technician will need to alert the pharmacist.

It is essential that all patient, prescriber, and drug information is completed when receiving new prescription orders. Not only does it eliminate any potential data entry and filling order error, but it may also eliminate the chance of an error being repeated. State boards of pharmacy will also address incomplete patient, prescriber, and drug information during any random or scheduled inspection. A few extra minutes thoroughly examining a new prescription order may save the patient, the prescriber, and the pharmacy staff from unwanted and potentially dangerous medication safety issues.

As previously mentioned, the ISMP has been a driving force for the call of safe medication practices. ISMP regularly alerts the medical community of potential medication safety hazards, but also provides ways of solving potential issues of harm. Some good examples include the following:

- Look-alike/sound-alike medications
  - Drugs that are commonly confused with one another and should be stored separately from one another.
  - www.ismp.org/tools/confuseddrugnames.pdf
- High-alert medications
  - Medications that have a high risk of harm if used incorrectly
  - www.ismp.org/tools/institutionalhighAlert.asp
  - www.ismp.org/communityRx/tools/ambulatoryhighalert.asp
- Tall man lettering
  - Mixing upper and lower case lettering in the medication's name
  - www.ismp/tools/tallmanletters.pdf
- Separation of inventory
  - Placing medications that are high-alert medications, such as chemotherapy drugs or narcotics, in areas that are away from other formulary items will prevent harmful or fatal errors from happening.
  - Narcotics must be maintained under a locked storage system.
- Leading and trailing zeros
  - Use of extra zeros within a dose only provides for a greater potential of error. For example 1-g dose should be written as 1 g and not 1.0 g. If the period between the 1 and the 0 is illegible, the prescription may be mistaken for 10 g and not 1 g.
- Limited use of error prone abbreviations
  - Certain medical abbreviations are prone to error and should not be used. For example, the medication directions q1d (once daily) might be misinterpreted as qid (four times daily) and should be written simply as "Use daily".
  - www.ismp.org/tools/errorproneabbreviationlist

- Do not crush list
  - Some medications when crushed may inhibit the drug's releasing mechanism, causing too much or not enough of the drug to be released into the patient's system.
  - www.ismp.org/tools/DoNotCrush.pdf
- Pediatric concentration list
  - Pediatric dosing can be troublesome as well, and while pharmacy technicians are not permitted to dose or give recommendations on dosing, they should be aware of potential pediatric dosing hazards.
  - www.ismp.org/Tools/PediatricConcentrations.pdf

Joint Commission, an independent accrediting body for hospitals and other health institutions, also has been proactive in the elimination of medication errors and increasing patient safety. Joint Commission's National Patient Safety Goals are a set of patient goals evaluated and released each year by Joint Commission, which hospitals and health systems accredited by Joint Commission must seek to provide. Some of the goals related to the practice of pharmacy include.

- Identifying patients correctly
  - Use of two patient identifiers—patient name, date of birth, and medical record number
- Improve staff communications.
  - Make sure the patient information is received by the right staff member in a timely manner—for example, patient allergies or patient medication histories.
- Use medications safely.
  - Label all medication, including those to be used as part of a procedure.
  - Take additional safety precautions with patients using blood thinners such as Coumadin or heparin.
  - Document and pass along correct patient medication information.
    - Employ the use of medication reconciliation.

A full list of Joint Commission's National Patient Safety Goals can be viewed at www.jointcommission.org/assets/1/6/HAP_NPSG_Chapter_2014.pdf. Please keep in mind that National Patient Safety Goals are evaluated on a yearly basis and may change from year to year.

Patient package inserts, medication guides, and auxiliary labels are yet a few more tools the practice of pharmacy uses to guard against medication errors and provide patient safety. We have already seen how organizations such as ISMP and Joint Commission foster an attitude of urgency concerning patient medication safety. The practice of pharmacy continues this practice with the use of additional patient packaging guidelines.

Under federal mandate all prescription drugs sold to the public must contain eight essential criteria known as Consumer Medication Information (CMI). Overseeing of this mandate known as the *Prescription Drug Product Labeling: Medication Guide Requirements* is undertaken by the Federal Food and Drug Administration (FDA). A prescription medication must contain the following information:

- Drug name, directions for use, and how to monitor for improvement
- Contradictions and what to do if they apply
- Specific directions about how to use and store medications, and overdose information
- Specific precautions and warning about medications

- Symptoms of serious and frequent possible adverse reactions and what to do
- Certain general information, including encouraging patients to communicate with health-care professionals, and disclaimer statements
- Information that is scientifically accurate, unbiased, in tone and content, and up-to-date
- Information in an understandable and legible format that is readily comprehensible to consumers

Prescription medications are not the only drug products with federally mandated labeling requirements. In May 2005, the FDA enacted mandatory labeling guidelines for all OTC or nonprescription drug products sold to the public. Monographs, which define specific drug information and safety requirements for OTC drugs, must be clearly visible on the drug product's label. Drug monographs must include the following information:

- A drug's active ingredients including strength and form
- A drug's indications as well as warnings and directions for use
- A drug's inactive ingredients
- Drug storage information
- Drug manufacturer's contact information

Drug labeling requirements such as those listed above help to protect the public from possible misuse due to lack of information, and ultimately provide a safer, more effective use of OTC drug products. Pharmacy technicians should be aware of OTC labeling requirements in order to assist the pharmacist in providing the best possible care for the patient.

From time to time the FDA released warnings concerning OTC or prescription medications in order to protect and inform the public about specific adverse effects that accompany therapy of a particular drug. Black box warnings are the highest warning the FDA gives to prescription medications. OTC medications do not have black box warning, and would simply be recalled if the potential for extreme harm to the public were found.

Black box warnings or boxed warnings get their name from the black boxed warning the FDA mandates of prescription drugs that have been found to have severe or potentially fatal effects. In accordance with FDA standards, if a prescription drug exhibits any of the following criteria, a black box warning will be issued for the drug:

- Serious reaction to include:
  - Death
  - Life-threatening reaction
  - Hospitalization or prolonged existing hospitalization
  - Persistent or significant incapacity resulting in substantial disruption of the ability to conduct normal life function
  - Congenital normality or birth defect
- Otherwise clinical significant adverse reaction
  - Specific drug and drug reaction need to be taken into consideration.
- Anticipated adverse reaction
  - Drugs that are considered to be high-alert medications, such as heparin, will carry a black box warning.
- Adverse reaction with unapproved use
  - Drugs are approved for specific uses and indications; when a drug is used for something other than its indication, an unforeseen reaction might occur.

The following image is an example of the FDA's black box warning. This particular black box warning is concerning the antidepressant Prozac or its generic fluoxetine.

PROZAC®
FLUOXETINE CAPSULES, USP
FLUOXETINE ORAL SOLUTION, USP
FLUOXETINE DELAYED-RELEASE CAPSULES, USP

WARNING

Suicidality and Antidepressant Drugs—Antidepressants increased the risk compared to placebo of suicidal thinking and behavior (suicidality) in children, adolescents, and young adults in short-term studies of major depressive disorder (MDD) and other psychiatric disorders. Anyone considering the use of Prozac or any other antidepressant in a child, adolescent, or young adult must balance this risk with the clinical need. Short-term studies did not show an increase in the risk of suicidality with antidepressants compared to placebo in adults beyond age 24; there was a reduction in risk with antidepressants compared to placebo in adults aged 65 and older. Depression and certain other psychiatric disorders are themselves associated with increases in the risk of suicide. Patients of all ages who are started on antidepressant therapy should be monitored appropriately and observed closely for clinical worsening, suicidality, or unusual changes in behavior. Families and caregivers should be advised of the need for close observation and communication with the prescriber. Prozac is approved for use in pediatric patients with MDD and obsessive compulsive disorder (OCD). (*See* WARNINGS, Clinical Worsening and Suicide Risk, PRECAUTIONS, Information for Patients, *and* PRECAUTIONS, Pediatric Use.)

Medication Safety Caps and Auxiliary Warning Labels

There can be no doubt, safety of the patient is the first concern of all health-care professionals. Pharmacy in particular has taken on this task in a number of ways, many of which we have already been discussed. However, the federally imposed mandate for medication safety measures, such as childproof caps for prescription medications as well as childproof caps and sealed containers for OTC medications, has done more for patient medication safety than any other piece of federal legislation.

The Poison Prevention Packaging Act (PPPA) of 1970 was enacted to protect children from accidental poisoning by household products. Under the control of the Consumer Product Safety Commission (CPSC) the act requires that all household products, such as cleaning materials as well as prescription medications and specific OTC medications, have childproof caps before being marketed to the public. The OTC products that are mandated to have a childproof cap include:

- Aspirin
- Methyl salicylate, for example, wart removers such as Compound W
- Iron
- Acetaminophen
- Diphenhydramine
- Ibuprofen
- Loperamide
- Mouthwash
- Lidocaine – product with more than 5 mg of lidocaine in a single packet
- Dibucaine – products with more than 0.5 mg of dibucaine in a single packet
- Naproxen – 250 mg or more in a single dose
- Ketoprofen – 50 mg or more in a single dose

- Fluoride – products that contain 50 mg of elemental fluoride or 0.5% fluoride in a single package
- Minoxidil – products that contain more than 14 mg in a single package
- Nonprescription drugs – any oral drug that contains an active ingredient once only available by prescription such as the antihistamine Claritin

A great number of drug manufacturers have enacted childproof safety standards for all of their products and as the call for stricter safety practices increases so will the packages themselves.

Childproof caps on prescription medication are mandated unless otherwise indicated by the prescriber or requested by the patient. Patients that may have difficulty in opening prescription caps, such as those with arthritic hands, may choose to have their prescriptions filled with non-childproof lids or containers. Patients requesting non-childproof lids or containers must sign a consent acknowledging their request. The signed request will be kept on the patient's profile until changed by the patient or otherwise considered invalid.

Medication safety is of utmost importance to the practice of pharmacy and many times goes well beyond just the patient. Grandchildren, pets, and other individuals within a household may easily ingest medication that might be harmful to them. Safety caps are a preventive measure and the lack of safety caps only increases the risk potential.

Drug Utilization Review: Helping to Notify the Pharmacist

Drug Utilization Review (DUR) or Medication Utilization Review (MUR), as it is sometimes called, may not seem as if it is a medication measure, but in truth, it is a very effective medication safety tool. The pharmacist ultimately conducts DURs, but the pharmacy technician's ability to recognize patients that are in need of this invaluable service is critical.

DURs are a comprehensive review of a patient's medication therapy. This is an extremely useful tool in the practice of pharmacy and medicine, because it not only summarizes the patient's medication therapies, but also gives the pharmacist a diagnostic view of what the provider is prescribing as well as how the pharmacist has dispensed the patient's medications.

The evaluative classifications of DURs are as follows: prospective, concurrent, and retrospective. Each one of these classifications has a very specific purpose, which allows the pharmacist to evaluate the patient's drug therapy during explicit periods of time during their drug therapy.

- **Prospective**—This allows the pharmacist an overall view of the patient's drug therapy prior to dispensing any new medications the provider may have prescribed.
- **Concurrent**—From this vantage point, the pharmacist is monitoring the patient's current drug therapy. Continuous monitoring will allow the pharmacist to alert the provider of potential therapy issues or therapies the patient may not be tolerating well.
- **Retrospective**—This is an effort of continued monitoring by the pharmacist after the patient has taken the prescribed medication therapy. Again, monitoring the patient's medication therapy allows the pharmacist to alert the prescriber of issues that may be harmful to the patient or suggest therapies that may provide a better outcome for the patient.

As we have reiterated several times throughout this text, the pharmacy technician is an indispensable member of the pharmacy team; however, pharmacy technicians are *never* permitted to offer advice or information concerning medications to patients or other health-care professionals. Pharmacy technicians that are able to alert the pharmacist of patients in need of drug utilization review help to foster an attitude of preventive care for the patient, and ultimately assist the pharmacist in creating the best possible care for the patient.

Another area where the pharmacy technician becomes invaluable to the safety of patients is Adverse Drug Events (ADE). ADEs are situations where a medication error has caused injury or harm to a patient. An ADE may arise after the patient has taken a single dose or multiple doses. ADEs are important to the protection of the patient, because they are used as an informative and cumulative tool by the FDA to track medications that have the potential for causing harm to patients.

Although the FDA requires drug manufacturers to thoroughly test and research new medication before they are marketed to the public, some adverse reactions are not reported until after the medication has been dispensed to the general public. MedWatch, which is sub-group of the FDA, gathers ADE reports to one central site as an informative tool for prescribers, pharmacists, and other health-care providers.

Pharmacy technicians should be acutely aware of ADE reporting as its importance is key to continued medication safety for the patient. Pharmacy technicians should be attentive toward patients that may have experienced an ADE by reporting the patient's issues and/or symptoms to the pharmacist. Making the pharmacist aware of a potentially harmful medication event will allow the pharmacist to consult with the patient and proceed with further investigation if necessary.

Finally, pharmacist–patient consultation is perhaps one of the most effective methods of proactive medication safety. There are several situations that could arise where a consultation with the pharmacist is in order. For example, Janie is a certified pharmacy technician that works at a local community pharmacy in her hometown. It is a small town, which means seeing a familiar face is not unusual. In fact, Janie knows most of her customers by name. One day Mrs. Corrie comes to the pharmacy counter and tells Janie she has had a cold for quite some time. Mrs. Corrie goes on to explain her symptoms to Janie, and then asks Janie if she could recommend an OTC medication to relieve her symptoms.

Janie, who is quite familiar with Mrs. Corrie's medication profile, knows Mrs. Corrie takes several heart and blood pressure medications. Janie also knows that many OTC cold preparations are contraindicated with the medications Mrs. Corrie takes. Knowing this information about Mrs. Corrie, Janie politely tells Mrs. Corrie it would be best for her to consult with the pharmacist. Janie shows Mrs. Corrie to the consultation area, asks Mrs. Corrie to have a seat, and then relays the information to the pharmacist. The pharmacist thanks Janie for her efforts and goes to speak with Mrs. Corrie.

This is a situation that could have turned out very differently had Janie simply directed Mrs. Corrie to the cold remedy aisle. Because Janie was familiar with Mrs. Corrie's medication therapy, and because she was aware of the possible contraindications of mixing heart and blood pressure medication with OTC cold and flu remedies, she did the best possible thing for Mrs. Corrie by advising her to consult with the pharmacist.

Safe and effective drug therapies are the building blocks for progressive and effective patient care experiences. Pharmacy plays one of the largest roles in safe medication practices. Pharmacy technicians should be aware of the tools available for carrying out safe medication practices. CPOE, medication safety caps and guidelines, auxiliary labels, prescription and patient order requirements, documentation of patient information, as well as DURs and ADEs are always used by pharmacies to help protect the patient.

CHAPTER REVIEW QUESTIONS

1. The five rights of safe medication practice are _____, _____, _____, _____, and _____.

   a. Right physician, right drug, right dose, right route, and right time
   b. Right patient, right day, right dose, right route, and right time
   c. Right patient, right drug, right dose, right route, and right term
   d. Right patient, right drug, right dose, right route, and right time

2. CPOE stands for _____ _____ _____ _____.

   a. Computerized Patient Order Entry
   b. Computerized Physician Order Entry
   c. Computerized Patient Oddity Entry
   d. Computerized Person Order Entry

3. Under federal law, all prescription drugs sold to the public must have _____ essential criteria known as _____.

   a. Seven, Consumer information management
   b. Six, Consumer medication information
   c. Eight, Consumer medication information
   d. Eight, Consumer information management

4. In May 2005, the FDA enacted mandatory labeling guidelines for _____.

   a. Over-the-counter medications
   b. Prescription drugs
   c. Generic drugs
   d. Legend drugs

5. Childproof caps on prescription medication are mandated unless otherwise indicated by the _____ or requested by the patient.

   a. Pharmacist
   b. FDA
   c. DEA
   d. Prescriber

6. The evaluative classifications of DURs are _____, _____, and _____.

   a. Prospective, consult, and retrospective
   b. Prescription, concurrent, and retrospective
   c. Prospective, concurrent, and retrospective
   d. Prospective, concurrent, and refills

7. Two out of every three patients that visit a physician will walk away with a _____.

   a. Clear diagnosis
   b. Written prescription
   c. Health-care bill
   d. Outpatient order

8. The FDA defines a medication error as any _____ event that may cause or lead to _____ medication use or patient harm while the medication is in control of the health-care professional, patient, or consumer.

   a. Preventable, inappropriate
   b. Reportable, inappropriate
   c. Preventable, appropriate
   d. Reportable, appropriate

9. _____ such as staffing issues may be a factor associated with an increased risk for medication errors.

   a. Internal stresses
   b. Extracurricular activities
   c. Administrative duties
   d. External stresses

10. _____ medications are medications that have an increased risk for harm if used incorrectly.

   a. Expired
   b. High-alert
   c. Over prescribed
   d. Low-alert

6 Pharmacy Quality Assurance

Learning objectives for this chapter will include:

• Quality assurance practices for pharmacy inventory and medication management systems, such as National Drug Code (NDC) numbers, bar coding, and data order entry procedures.

• Risk management guidelines and regulations.

• Communication channels in the practice of pharmacy, patients, coworkers, administration, and other health-care providers.

• Productivity, efficiency, and customer assurance measures.

What Is Quality Assurance?

As it is with many things, when trying to understand how to achieve good quality assurance measures, one must first understand the definition of the term *quality assurance*. Quality assurance in the health-care profession is a promise to patients that they will receive care of the highest standard that will not only keep them from harm, but also help them achieve and maintain a state of continued well-being.

In the practice of pharmacy, quality assurance is not only a measure that should be strived for on a continued basis, but also one that should be constantly evolving to meet the changing needs of patients and the profession of health care. As patient safety measures improve and regulation expands, so should the practice of pharmacy. The pharmacy technician will be in the grips of improvement and change. As we have already seen, the role of the pharmacy technician in the practice of pharmacy is not only mandated, but is also in a chronic stage of transformation.

Gone are the days when the pharmacy technician was simply an "extra" hand to the pharmacist. Today pharmacy technicians are taking on tasks that were once performed only by the pharmacist, and even positions of authority. The good news is that the role of the pharmacy technician is now growing. With the advent of new health-care regulations, such as the Affordable Care Act, pharmacists will be required to perform more clinical processes. This, of course, opens the pharmacy technician up to a wide array of tasks, many never performed by technicians before.

Knowing all of this, it is easy to understand why quality assurance is so imperative in the practice of pharmacy. One of the important pieces to providing patients with care that exhibits quality assurance is the use of effective communication. Effective communication goes well beyond speaking with the customers or patients; effective communication is knowing how to approach a problem, getting the problem solved, a chain of command, and of course, communicating with other health-care professionals. An inability to perform any one of these tasks within the communication chain will cause a break, which will eventually lead to the disintegration of quality assurance.

Communication in Quality Assurance Measures

Whether a pharmacy technician works in a retail or institutional pharmacy, he or she needs to be skilled in the administration and management of pharmacy practices. A major skill needed in both practice settings is good communication skills. Technicians must be able to understand and be understood to avoid medication and procedural errors. Although technicians in retail settings communicate primarily with patients and technicians in institutional settings communicate primarily with other health-care professionals, the skills needed for good communication are the same.

Communication skills are vital to the delivery of pharmaceutical care in all pharmacy settings. A skilled pharmacy technician must be able to communicate effectively with other trained health care professionals and patients who have little or no knowledge about their prescriptions.

Although listening is sometimes considered a passive activity, to understand properly what is being said, a person must be actively involved in listening. This is important because not all communication is verbal. Nonverbal forms of communication, such as body language, which includes facial expressions, posture, hand motions, eye contact, and physical proximity, are valuable communication indicators to the listener. Voice tone and pitch are also important components. For example, you may ask a patient how he is doing and he may answer "Just fine," but you can tell by his body language and expression that he is not "just fine."

A good communicator is also aware of communication barriers that may inhibit the message from being fully understood. Communication barriers can include physical or emotional impairments as well as cultural and language differences. A skilled technician must be able to recognize these barriers and accommodate them.

An excellent technique for technicians to ensure that patients comprehend them is to ask open-ended questions. For example, after you have given a patient detailed instructions, ask her to tell you how she is going to take a medication. A simple smile or a nod does not indicate understanding, but repeating instructions back correctly does indicate comprehension.

Cultural and language differences can also be barriers to effective communication. One culture may find things such as eye contact or standing within 18 inches of another person uncomfortable. Patients from some cultures may be offended if you address them by their first name. Although English is the most used language in the United States, many patients may have some other language as their native language. As an English-speaking technician, you must be aware of language differences that may cause miscommunication and medication errors. For example, *once* in English means "one time," whereas in Spanish it is the number 11. Think of how often we use *once* in our directions to patients. What would be the difference if they hear it as "eleven"?

The truth of the matter is that we live in a multicultural world, and being able to adapt to the needs of the patients pharmacies serve is not only critical to the health and well-being of the patient, but also essential to good quality assurance measures in the practice of pharmacy.

The Business of Pharmacy

Any business that wishes to succeed must operate in such a manner that the revenue (the money coming into the business) exceeds the expenses (the money that it costs to do business). Every employee is an important part of this process. Pharmacists and technicians must provide pharmaceutical care for their patients while managing the business in a profitable manner.

While profitability is an important part of any business model, including the practice of pharmacy, it is only one factor of business. Going back to matters of quality assurance, a pharmacy, retail or institutional, cannot succeed without a solid business model, and of course, a good business model includes measures of quality assurance. In the practice of pharmacy this includes measures dealing with risk management, regulations, and protection of the patient, as well as solid plan for profitability. While profitability is not the only measure of a successful pharmacy, it is an essential marker. If a pharmacy is unable to remain profitable, it will be forced to close its doors, which does a disservice not only to the patient, but to the employees as well.

So, how do you keep a pharmacy profitable and maintain quality assurance matters? The answer is not as difficult as it may seem. It cannot be repeated enough; communication is a key element in the success of a pharmacy as well as the career of the pharmacy technician. Understanding this simple concept will not only allow the pharmacy to prosper, but will also allow the career of the pharmacy technician to thrive. Keeping this in mind, we need to understand some very basic business concepts and practices.

Basic Business Concepts and Practices

A pharmacy that cannot succeed is useless not only to its customers and patients, but also to its employees. Success in the practice of pharmacy involves more than just profitability, but profitability also allows the pharmacy to continue to operate, which needs to happen in order to continue to serve customers and patients, and to keep pharmacists and pharmacy technicians employed. It may seem like a very basic, common sense concept, but the reality is that poor execution of business practices can bring a pharmacy to its knees very quickly.

Documentation in the practice of pharmacy is indisputably one of the most essential pieces of quality assurance. In many cases, documentation in the practice of pharmacy is a mandated task. Patient records, prescription monitoring, pharmacy technician and pharmacist licensing and registration, wholesaler purchasing and receiving, as well as requirements from the state board of pharmacy, DEA, and FDA are all part of a very important, mandated documentation process. So, it should come as no surprise that the business end of pharmacy, as it applies to matters of quality assurance, demands clear and accurate documentation.

Keeping a Record of Business

Accounting records must be kept for tax purposes as well as for general business use. While a separate department most often conducts financial matters in an instructional or health system pharmacy, the pharmacy's staff is still responsible for documentation of what comes into and out of the pharmacy. If an institutional or health system pharmacy has poor documentation practices, the results will become apparent within the space of the fiscal year.

A fiscal year will not typically run the same period as a calendar year, which is January 1st through December 31st. Fiscal year is generally based upon quarterly periods. For example, General Hospital's fiscal year runs from July 1st to June 30th of the following year, and the new fiscal year will begin again on July 1st of that same year. It is a business practice that is used for taxes and accounting purposes. In the practice of pharmacy this is also a time when the pharmacy's inventory is scrutinized and challenges of profitability are addressed.

Pharmacies use a variety of systems to record financial items. As we stated earlier, institution and health system pharmacies generally have a separate department within the health system that controls accounting practices for the pharmacy, but in a retail setting, particularly small or local retail pharmacies, the accounting practice is handled by an outside firm that is hired by the pharmacy. Some pharmacies contract with accounting agencies; others have in-house employees that keep the books. No matter which method is used, it is important to maintain current, accurate financial records using a process that is flexible, easily understood, inexpensive, not time-intensive, and convenient to use.

Product pricing is important to the success of business of pharmacy; this can be said for both institutional and retail pharmacy. Most nonprescription items are priced based on a percentage markup. Different markup values are often used for different product categories. For example, a 1-ounce tube of antibiotic ointment may be marked up 40%. If the tube costs the pharmacy $1.40, then 40% of the cost will be added to obtain the selling price. The formula for calculating markup is

$$\text{Selling price} = \text{cost} + (\text{cost} \times \text{markup})$$
$$\text{Selling price} = \$1.40 + (\$1.40 \times 0.402)$$
$$= \$1.40 + \$0.562$$
$$= \$1.96$$

The markup on costume jewelry may be 100%. For example, a necklace may cost the pharmacy $10.00. We would add 100% of the cost back to the cost to obtain the selling price:

$$\text{Selling price} = \$10.00 + (\$10.00 \times 1.02)$$
$$\text{Selling price} = \$10.00 + \$10.00$$
$$= \$20.00$$

However, $19.95 sounds less expensive than $20.00, so let's sell the necklace for $19.95. Most retail prices traditionally end in either five or nine.

Again, while the practice of pharmacy is about caring for and protecting the patient it serves, if a pharmacy is not able to meet the basic quality assurance matters, it will not be profitable. If a pharmacy is unable to remain profitable, it will be forced to close its doors, leaving behind a customer and patient base in need of care, and pharmacists and pharmacy technicians unable to provide that care. Understanding the basics of business may not seem to be an essential piece of quality assurance in the practice of pharmacy, but in reality it has a great deal to do with successful implementation of quality assurance measures.

Policies and Procedures

The practice of pharmacy has changed vastly over the past decades as a result of new drugs, delivery systems, automation, government regulations, and the growth of professional organizations. The American Society of Health-System Pharmacists (ASHP) was one of the first organizations to develop standards of practice for hospital pharmacy. Today, the ASHP states the minimum standards as follows: "An operations manual governing pharmacy functions (e.g., administrative, operational, and clinical) shall exist."

All pharmacies are required to have written policies and procedures (P&Ps) for all pharmacy-related operations. These written documents are gathered together in one book or manual called a policy and procedures manual. This manual should contain all applicable P&Ps as well as long-term goals for the pharmacy.

P&Ps are not just for the pharmacy. Every department in the institution or organization will have P&Ps specific to their operations and departmental needs. There will also be an institutional or organizational policy and procedures manual. Departmental policies and procedures should not conflict with the organization's P&Ps.

Policies and procedures are also sometimes referred to as standards of practice or standard operating procedures (SOPs), and these two terms may be used interchangeably. Pharmacy technicians must be familiar with the P&Ps or SOPs of their respective pharmacies: Their job depends on it.

A *policy* can be defined as "a definite course or method of action selected from among alternatives and in light of given conditions to guide and determine present and future decisions." Policies are written statements that provide a framework for action and are considered broad guidelines for the pharmacy. The following statement is an example of a policy.

The Pharmacy Department, due to the nature of its responsibilities and functions, shall have strict standards of employee conduct and behavior.

Pharmacists and pharmacy technicians are expected to conduct themselves as professionals. This departmental policy very clearly relays this sentiment. Policies will very often also have a consequence attached to them that spells out the ramifications of not following a defined policy. For example, the consequence for not following the referenced policy go something like this, *employees that are unable to conduct themselves as expected or are unable to conduct the responsibilities and functions associated with their position, will be put on verbal warning.*

A *procedure* can be defined as "a particular way of accomplishing something or of acting; a statement of a series of systems to implement the policies of the department or organization." A procedure is a written instruction that describes the sequential steps necessary to complete a specific task. A good example of a procedure follows:

PROCEDURE

1. Conduct

a. All pharmacy department employees are to conduct themselves in a courteous and professional manner at all times.

b. When dealing with the public or with other hospital employees, each employee is a representative of the entire pharmacy department and the institution. A helpful and polite manner shall be maintained at all times. Conditions and situations that could lead to potential conflicts or disagreements should be referred to a supervisor.

Besides being required, a well-written policy and procedures manual has many benefits, including that it

1. Improves both inter- and intradepartmental communication
2. Creates standards of care
3. Provides a mechanism for documenting standards of care
4. Enhances staff orientation and training
5. Improves and maintains staff morale
6. Enables management to systematically, objectively, and efficiently measure staff and departmental performance
7. Provides a source of information
8. Encourages cost-effective use of resources
9. Provides an administrative tool for planning, developing, and improving pharmacy service

The manual should contain information telling employees how to perform day-to-day tasks as well as the procedure to follow in case of emergencies. It should provide guidelines covering the responsibilities of each employee position as well as specifying the chain of command of employees. The policies and procedures manual should be created when the business is formed and should be updated on a regular basis.

Institutional pharmacies have a *pharmacy and therapeutics (P&T) committee,* which consists of pharmacy personnel and other institutional staff. The main responsibility of the P&T committee is to create and maintain the drug formulary, but it can also play an important role in developing P&Ps. Because the practice of pharmacy is constantly evolving, the formulary and P&Ps must be updated frequently.

An additional responsibility of the P&T committee is to implement these changes by notifying the staff to ensure that everyone stays current with respect to developments in pharmaceuticals. This may be accomplished by seminars, bulletins, and newsletters. The committee also provides a means for drug-use evaluation, medication-error reporting, and adverse-reaction reporting.

Business practices and policies and procedures are only a small part of what constitutes quality assurance. As we stated at the beginning of this chapter, communication is a large piece of quality assurance. Poor communication can be problematic, increasing the risk for error or harm to the patient. Pharmacy technicians should be able to understand not only how to communicate with patient, customers, and other health-care workers, but also what is entailed in the communication process known as chain of command.

Chain of command is the order of authority and authorization within an institution. Every business practice or institution, including the practice of pharmacy, has a chain of command. In the practice of pharmacy, chain of command within the pharmacy generally begins with the pharmacy manager or the pharmacist in charge. After the pharmacy manager the authority generally falls on the pharmacist and then the pharmacy technician. In some cases, depending upon the size of the pharmacy, an assistant pharmacy manager or coordinator may be in place, in which case they would fall in line behind the pharmacy manager, but before the pharmacist.

If a pharmacy, such as large institutional pharmacy, offers various pharmacy services, there may be a pharmacist assigned as the managing person for those services. For example, if an institutional pharmacy offers anticoagulant services as part of their outpatient care, there may be one pharmacist that manages these particular services; however, that pharmacist will generally report to the assistant pharmacy manager or directly to the pharmacy manager.

Many facilities are placing pharmacy technicians in positions of management and authority. A pharmacy technician manager or coordinator oversees the tasks and duties of even the other pharmacy technicians employed within the pharmacy. The duties of a pharmacy technician manager or coordinator might involve tasks such as weekly work schedules, payroll, hiring of new pharmacy technician, implementation of new process, training procedures, and departmental meetings. The assistant pharmacy manager or the pharmacist in charge oversees the pharmacy technician manager's authority, but generally, all issues related to pharmacy technicians would go through the pharmacy technician's chain of command.

It is important for pharmacy technicians to understand and comply with their pharmacy's chain of command procedures. Pharmacy technicians are expected to hold themselves to a high ethical and moral standard, and conduct themselves just as any other health-care professional might do. Following a pharmacy's chain of command policy helps to enforce professionalism, but also establishes and re-enforces the need for quality assurance measures within the pharmacy.

So far, we have been able to determine that quality assurance involves several elements: solid business practices, effective communication, adherence to policies and procedures, and implementation and respect for chain of command. One more measure of quality assurance deals with the execution of safety measures used to protect customers, patients, and staff.

Measures of Safety Affecting Quality Assurance

Earlier in the text, we talked about medication safety measures. The practice of pharmacy is constantly changing, and part of the reason for this continued change is the protection of customers, patients, and staff. Patients and other health-care professionals rely on the knowledge and experience of the pharmacist and the pharmacy technician. It is assumed that those that work within the pharmacy will provide the patient with the safest, most effective treatment available. Other health-care professionals rely on the pharmacy to help maintain the safety and well-being of patients. A good example would be automated dispensing cabinets.

Automated dispensing cabinets, such as Omnicell or Pyxis, allow other health-care professionals to retrieve medications for their patients in a timely and safe manner. The safer and more efficient a delivery system is, the better the treatment experience is for the patient, which, of course, falls directly to matters of quality assurance. However, safety mechanisms, such as automated dispensing cabinets, can only be as effective as the persons responsible for their operation.

Bar code scanning is a safety measure that is universal among health-care systems and retail pharmacies. During the bar coding scanning process, the drug's National Drug Code (NDC) number is scanned into the pharmacy's computer system. The NDC number allows the computer to recognize a specific drug by manufacturer, strength, and form. If this information is incorrectly entered into the computer system, the error may continue across the entire health-care system or retail setting. Undeniably, this will eventually end in a medication error. It is for this reason that careful attention and consideration must be paid when entering a drug's NDC number into an institutional or retail pharmacy's computer system.

The Drug Listing Act of 1972 required manufactures to provide the FDA with a list of all drugs produced by them, which resulted in the formation of the NDC. The NDC number is a number unique to a particular drug product or device. An NDC number must accompany any drug or device a manufacturer produces for consumption by the public.

The NDC number is composed of 10 digits, broken into three segments, and each segment contains very specific information about the drug or device. The first set of numbers, which is four to five digits long, refers to the drug manufacturer. The next set of numbers, which is three to four digits long, identifies the product, and the final one or two digits signifies the quantity of the product. For example,

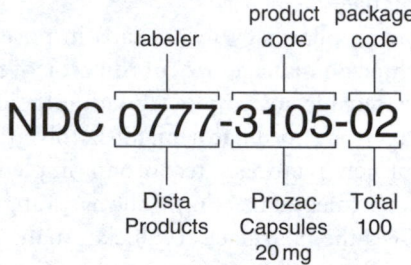

This NDC number is for the drug Prozac. From the NDC number we can tell the manufacturer of the drug is Dista Products. The drug product is Prozac 20 mg capsules, and the number of capsules in the bottle or package is 100.

Not only is the NDC number useful in identifying drugs or devices during bar coding procedures, but it also assists in drug recovery during product recall situations. During a drug recall situation, the manufacturer or FDA sends out a bulletin stating a mandated recall of a drug. Drug recalls are categorized as Class I, II, or III recall; Class I being the most severe and III being the least.

A Class I drug recall is the most serious recall due to the drug's potential for severe or irreversible harm, with even potential of death to those that consume it. A Class II is not as severe as a Class I, but still has the potential for a serious side effect. Class II recalls involve drugs whose side effects are serious, but temporary. Class III recalls are not as severe as Class II and I, but still have the potential for harm. Class III recalls may involve issues such as manufacturing or packing defects, and while the potential for harm is present, it is unlikely.

Use of the federally mandated NDC number has protected the lives of thousands of patients, and is a demonstration of another effective measure in quality assurance. Pharmacy technicians should be inherently aware of the processes associated with bar coding, NDC numbers, and drug recalls. Measures such as these protect patients and solidify the effectiveness of a pharmacy team that has made a point of enacting solid quality assurance standards.

Final Matters of Quality Assurance

Quality assurance in the practice of pharmacy involves the protection, care, and security of the patients we have chosen to serve. Not only are measures of business, communication, chain of command, and safety essential to quality assurance, but also are matters of consistency. Whether a drug is produced by a larger manufacture or compounded with a pharmacy, it should be consistently the same in all aspects.

Drugs compounded in a pharmacy should be following strict policies and procedures. Caution must always be taken to reduce the risk of infection to patients and staff. Personal Protective Equipment (PPE) is an effective utilization tool for this along with being aware of recommendations for handling hazardous drugs, particularly when dealing with sterile compounded drugs. USP<797> recommendations for compounding sterile drug products should *always* be maintained. Pharmacy technicians that are not familiar with these recommendations should contact their supervisor before attempting sterile compounding procedures.

Products dispensed from a pharmacy are also required to maintain proper labeling. A prescription dispensed to a patient from a retail setting must contain the following information:

- The name, address, and phone number of the pharmacy
- The name of the patient
- The prescription serial number
- The date the prescription is filled
- Drug names, strength, and quantity
- The patient directions for use of the medication, including any required auxiliary labels
- The prescriber
- The initials of the pharmacist that checked the prescription
- The number of allowable refills, if applicable

Prescriptions missing any of the required information are considered invalid and should not be dispensed to the patient. Again, protection of the patient is always the first concern in the practice of pharmacy, and quality assurance cannot be obtained without first seeking protection of the patient.

SUMMARY

Pharmaceutical care for the patient is the ultimate goal of all pharmacy services, no matter the location, the business plan, or the profit margin. All pharmacy personnel should remind themselves daily that pharmaceutical care is the responsible provision of drug therapy for the purpose of achieving definite outcomes that improve a patient's quality of life.

CHAPTER REVIEW QUESTIONS

1. Good communication skills in the practice of pharmacy are essential not only for a pleasant working environment but also for the safety of the patient. Communication barriers can be a constant threat to the process of communication: They include
   a. Physical, cultural, language, music
   b. Cultural, money, physical, emotional
   c. Emotional, cultural, physical, language
   d. Music, emotional, physical, cultural

2. Fiscal years are based upon _____ and typically run from _____ to _____.
   a. Days, June 29th, July 1st,
   b. Weeks, June 1st, July 30th
   c. Days, April 15th, December 30th
   d. Quarters, July 1st, June 30th

3. The term *procedure* is defined as,
   a. A particular way of accomplishing something or of acting
   b. The way we feel about accomplishing an act
   c. Standards of acting or performing
   d. Feeling obligated to accomplish a deed

4. The main duty of a health organization's P and T committee is to
   a. Discipline pharmacists and pharmacy technicians for poor performance
   b. Establish communication standards between pharmacy staff
   c. Create and maintain a drug formulary for the organizations
   d. Allow prescribers to relay patient's needs to pharmacy staff

5. The NDC number consists of _____ digits and is broken down into _____ separate segments.
   a. 11, 4
   b. 10, 3
   c. 4, 11
   d. 10, 2

6. Chain of command refers to
   a. The order in which a prescription should be filled
   b. The number of employees a store or facility might have
   c. The number of managers a store or facility might have
   d. The order of authority or authorization in an organization

7. During the use of bar code scanning, the drug's _____ is scanned to ensure the correct drug is being used.
   a. Invoice
   b. NDC number
   c. Prescription label
   d. Authorization code

8. A Class I drug recall has the potential to cause _____ or possibly _____ if consumed by a patient.
   a. Severe harm, death
   b. Severe harm, paralysis
   c. Paralysis, death
   d. Death, blindness

9. Class III drug recalls involve _____.
   a. Broken tablets or manufacture defects
   b. Manufacture defects or drug seals
   c. Broken tablets or drug seals
   d. Manufacturing defects or packaging defects

10. The second set of digits of an NDC code can contain up to _____ numbers and identifies the _____.
    a. Four, manufacturer
    b. Four, drug product
    c. Three, manufacturer
    d. Three, drug product

Medication Order Entry and Fill Process

7 chapter

LEARNING OBJECTIVES

Learning objectives for this chapter will include:

- Understanding the requirements of error-free order entry.
- Interpreting data for order entry, prescription, and prescriber's orders.
- Listing the requirements for labeling a prescription or prescriber's order as well as the labeling requirements for compounded products.
- Obtaining the right packing for a drug product.

Anatomy of a Prescription: Understanding Necessary Information and Processes

There can be no doubt that the prescriptions and the medication orders are two primary elements to the practice of the pharmacy. It is for this reason that accuracy of these two pieces of information must be accurate to ensure that the patient has a safe and effective treatment experience. Pharmacy technicians must be able to identify the information necessary on a prescription or medication order.

A prescription is a written, verbal, or electronic order from a prescriber to a pharmacist for a drug or a drug device to be dispensed to a patient. A prescription may be handwritten and given to the patient or the health-care professional for presentation at the pharmacy of the patient's choice or communicated directly to the pharmacist through telephone or verbal order given by the patient's prescriber or the prescriber's authorized agent, such as a nurse. Only a licensed, registered pharmacist is permitted to take a verbal prescription or medication order. Prescription or drug orders may also be sent by fax or electronically to the pharmacy for processing.

Essential Information

There is specific information a prescription must contain before being filled and verified for dispensing the medication to the patient. There are 10 essential elements that make up a prescription order.

- **Prescriber Information**—This includes the prescriber's name, address, phone number, state license number, as well as DEA number. It should be noted that the prescriber's DEA number is not required for prescriptions that do not involve controlled substances. For example, a prescription for the hypertension medication lisinopril would not require the prescriber to have his or her DEA number on the prescription.
- **Patient Demographics**—This includes the patient's name, address, and date of birth. This information is not only required for verification of patient profile information and insurance processing, but it also prevents errors that might occur due to similar names, such as a situation involving Senior or Junior.

- **Drug Name and Strength**—It is important to remember that many drugs are available in various strengths and forms. Confusion on which drug strength to fill only leads to delay in care for the patient as well as creating the potential for medication error.
- **Drug Quantity**—A specified quantity of the prescribed drug must be indicated on the prescription in order to provide the patient with enough medication to complete the necessary therapy. It is important to remember that CII drugs may only be filled for a 30-day supply.
- **Route of Administration**—Just as many drugs have various strengths, many have multiple routes of administration. Route of administration is important to ensure that the patient receives a route of administration appropriate to the patient. For example, an infant prescribed an antibiotic would be unable to swallow a capsule, so a liquid would be ordered.
- **Sig/Directions**—Instruction on how the patient should take the prescribed medication helps to eliminate errors and gives the patient clear directions on the use of the medication.
- **Number of Refills**—If applicable, the prescription must have the number of refills permitted. Prescription refills are only permitted for a period of 1 year from the date the prescription was originally filled. CII prescriptions are not permitted to have refills.
- **Indication for Brand/Generic**—The prescriber must indicate on the prescription if the patient is permitted to receive brand name drug or a generic equivalent. If the patient must receive the brand name drug, the prescriber must write *Brand Necessary* or *Dispense as Written*. Filling a prescription with a generic equivalent but indicating instead that the brand was filled is considered insurance fraud and punishable by federal law under HIPAA. In many states the pharmacist may provide the patient with a generic equivalent unless otherwise indicated.
- **Prescriber's Signature**—A prescription must contain the signature of the prescriber ordering the medication. If a signature has not been written on the prescription, the pharmacist may call for verbal verification and sign as the prescriber's authorized agent, the one exception being CII prescription medications.

From the Prescriber, to the Pharmacy, to the Patient

The typical oath of a prescription from the time it is written by the prescriber to the time it is dispensed to the patient is as follows:

- The prescriber writes the prescription and gives it to the patient or the patient's agent. The prescriber or the prescriber's authorized agent may also give the pharmacist a telephone or verbal order for the patient.
- The patient or the patient's agent takes the prescription to the pharmacy.
- The pharmacy technician checks the prescription for completeness—10 essential elements for a prescription.
- The pharmacy technician enters the prescription into the pharmacy's computer system where the billing process begins and the prescription label is generated.
- The pharmacy technician then goes to the pharmacy shelf and selects the correct drug as indicated in the patient's prescription order. At this time the pharmacy technician will verify the prescription label against the prescription order or hard copy.
- The pharmacy technician fills the prescription order for the indicated quantity either by counting or pouring or compounding the prescribed drug.
- Once the correct amount of drug is filled and placed in the appropriate drug vessel, the pharmacy technician once again verifies the drug label and then places it on the prescription container.

- The pharmacy technician will place the required drugs on one side, where it will await pharmacist's verification before being given to the patient.
- The pharmacist will verify the prescription against the prescriber's order and check for any discrepancies on the drug label as well as attach any auxiliary labels that may be required. Once the prescription has been verified and signed off by the pharmacist, it is ready to be dispensed to the patient.

Once this process is complete, the pharmacy technician will complete the billing process, bag the prescription, and place it in a bin for the patient to take. When the patients come to pick up their prescription the pharmacy technician will ask the patients if they need consultation with the pharmacist. If the patients indicate that they need consultation with the pharmacist or if the pharmacy technician determines there are factors that may require pharmacist consultation, the pharmacy technician will inform the pharmacist of the consultation.

In a hospital or institutional setting the medication processing will be slightly different than in a retail setting. In a hospital or institutional setting the prescriber will assess the patient and diagnose the illness. Once the patient's diagnosis has been established, the prescriber will order the patient's treatment therapy. This usually entails the prescriber using a process known as Computer Physician Order Entry (CPOE).

Health systems that use CPOE help to decrease the risk of medication error by having the prescriber input the patient's medication treatments directly into the computerized health system. The order will then be transmitted to the pharmacy, where it will be verified by a pharmacist. Once the pharmacist has verified the order, a label will be printed.

The pharmacy technician will retrieve the patient prescription label and fill it with the indicated medication. After the pharmacy technician fills the medication the pharmacist will verify the order for accuracy before the medication is delivered to the nursing unit. The nurse will scan the medication at the patient's bedside and verify it against the patient's Medication Administration Record (MAR) before administering the drug to the patient.

The safety processes implemented in a pharmacy are critical for protecting the patient from potential harm. When one of these steps is interrupted or omitted, the risk to the patient is increased exponentially. Pharmacy technicians should take care to make correct filling and dispensing processes are kept intact in order to save the patient from any harm.

An important part of maintaining the processes for filling and dispensing patient medications involves patient profiles and medication records.

Patient Profiles and Changes

Pharmacy technicians are responsible for setting up and maintaining patient profiles. These profiles, besides being confidential legal records, give the pharmacist a complete view of the patient's diagnosis and treatment history. Information on a patient profile should include:

- **Patient Demographics**—Complete name (Sr., Jr., II, etc.), patient identification or medical record number, address, date of birth, sex, name of parent or legal guardian if applicable.
- **Insurance and Billing Information**—Insurance company, phone number, group number, patient identification number, and any other information that specifically identifies that patient.
- **Medical History**—Any past or present information related to the patient's condition and treatment, as well as any known allergies. If the patient had any reactions or severe allergic reactions, this information would be indicated on the patient's profile. The type of reaction should also be indicated on the patient profile, such as *difficulty breathing when taking drug products that contain codeine* or *hives with the use of any antibiotic containing penicillin*. Information such as this is essential for protection of the patient and the admittance of this information could have fatal consequences for the patient.

- **Prescription History**—This is a list of medications the patient has taken in the past or is taking at present. This information may also be listed within the patient history. Prescription histories allow the pharmacist to develop complete and accurate Drug Utilization Reviews (DUR), which are mandated for all Medicare patients. Prescription histories should also include any OTC or herbal medications the patient may be taking as some OTC and herbal medications are contraindicated with certain prescription medication.
- **Prescription Preferences**—Whether the patient prefers brand or generic medications, or whether they want nonchild resistant containers with easy-off lids.
- **Refusal of Information**—Whether the patient has ever refused to sign pharmacy documents, including but not limited to, HIPAA and insurance forms.

Patient profiles in hospital pharmacies may also include the patient's account number, room number, diagnosis, as well as names of practitioners, allergies, and dietary restrictions. The profile may indicate barriers that may impede treatment processes for the patient such as language difficulties or disabilities. This information then becomes part of the patient permanent hospital or medical record information.

One of the most important items in a patient's profile is the patient's name. Several challenges arise when a patient goes by a nickname or has changed a name as a consequence of marriage, adoption, or divorce. To avoid dispensing a prescription to the wrong patient or adding multiple incomplete profiles for the same patient to the computer, pharmacy technicians should verify they have the correct patient by comparing the name against the date of birth, or by verifying the patient's address or phone number in the patient's profile. By performing this simple double-check, technicians can ensure that the correct prescription is being processed for the correct patient.

Technicians need to ensure that the patient's profile is always kept up to date with the correct information. When reviewing the prescription, technicians should always ask patients if there have been any changes to their profile information, such as a change of address or phone number or even a name change. Pharmacy technicians should also verify insurance information at this time, as insurance carriers may change due to an employment or benefits change.

Drug Interactions

A drug interaction occurs when a substance or condition affects the pharmacologic activity of a drug. In most cases, the interaction causes an increase or decrease in the drug's effect, or sometimes a completely different, unintended effect. Most pharmacy computer systems have automatic warning systems that will alert the technician of possible adverse reactions. A qualified and competent pharmacy technician will have a working knowledge of these potential problems. It is imperative that any time the computer alerts the technician to a potential problem, reaction, or allergy, the technician immediately informs the pharmacist. It is out of the scope of practice for a technician to override most of these alerts. Some of the most common warnings/alerts include:

- **Therapeutic Duplication**—A therapeutic duplication warning is an indication that the patient has more than one active prescription for the same medication or has two different medications that produce the same or similar effect. This is common among patients who have more than one doctor writing prescriptions for them.
- **Drug–Drug Interaction**—A drug–drug interaction alert is an indication that the patient has a medication in his or her profile that will cause an unfavorable reaction if it is taken along with the new prescription. A common drug–drug interaction occurs with warfarin and aspirin.
- **Drug–Food Interactions**—A drug–food interaction indicates that the medication being prescribed interacts with certain foods.
- **Drug–Disease Interactions**—A drug–disease interaction occurs when a past, current, or present patient medical condition precludes use of the drug.

- **Drug–Lab Interactions**—In a hospital setting, certain medical tests may interfere with the patient's medications, therefore requiring temporary suspension of the patient's drug therapy.
- **IV Incompatibility**—An IV incompatibility alert indicates that there is a potential interaction if two or more IV drugs are mixed together in the same container. For instance, total parenteral nutrition (TPN) with both calcium and phosphate would trigger an alert, because mixing these substances together can cause a precipitate to form.

REMEMBER

All warnings and alerts should be forwarded to the pharmacist for further investigation and possible consultation.

Processing Prescriptions

After a technician receives a prescription, the challenge is to get the right medication to the right patient in the right form and strength at the right time, and at the same time, charge the responsible party. Although each pharmacy may differ in one aspect or the other, there is a basic procedure for processing and filling a prescription.

1. Review the prescription or medication order to ensure that it is complete. Reviewing the prescription includes making sure that the patient is in the database and collecting any changes that need to be made to the patient's profile (demographic, history, insurance/billing).

2. Review the patient's profile in relation to the new order you are processing. Is the patient already on similar medications? Can this new medication react unfavorably with any other medication he may be taking? Has the patient reported any allergies that may be triggered by this medication? Although the pharmacy's software automatically checks for interactions, the main responsibility lies on the technician and ultimately the pharmacist to protect the patient and follow the prescriber's directions.

3. Select the prescribed medication in the right dosage form, strength, and quantity from the formulary database in your pharmacy's computer. The best way to choose the correct medication is to choose by the National Drug Code (NDC). The NDC number is a 10-digit, three-segment, permanent and unique number assigned to the drug by the U.S. Food and Drug Administration (FDA) when it first becomes available in the United States.

   - The first segment is called the *labeler code* and identifies the manufacturer or distributor of the drug.
   - The second segment is called the *product code* and identifies the dosage form, strength, and formulation.
   - The third segment is called the *package code* and identifies the type and size of the drug package.

   By matching the number on the label with the number on the stock bottle, the technician ensures that the correct drug has been selected.

4. Next, generate the prescription label. The directions typed on the label must be exactly the same as the prescriber intended, as well as clear enough for the patient to understand and follow. These directions should answer the following questions:

   - What should the patient do with the drug? (e.g., take, apply, instill)
   - What should the patient take, apply, or instill? (e.g., take *one tablet,* apply *ointment,* instill *2 drops*)

- How should the patient take, apply, or instill the drug? (e.g., take one tablet *by mouth*, apply ointment *to rash*, instill 2 drops *in each eye*)
- How often should the patient take, apply, or instill the drug? (e.g., take one tablet by mouth *two times daily*, apply ointment to rashes *every 8 hours*, instill 2 drops in each eye *4 times daily*)

Most computer systems designed for prescription dispensing use a series of sig codes. These sig codes or abbreviations are designed to save time and to standardize label language. For example, if you type, "1t po tid prnp," the label will read, "Take 1 tablet by mouth three times daily as needed for pain."

The following table lists some of the most common abbreviations/sig codes used in prescription processing and transcription of sig codes to complete patient directions.

ABBREVIATION/SIG CODE	DEFINITION
A	before
ac	before meals
ad	right ear
a.m.	morning
amp	Ampule
a.s.	left ear
a.u.	both ears or each ear
BID	two times daily
cap	capsule
cc	cubic centimeter
CHF	congestive heart failure
DW	distilled water
ECT	enteric coated tablet
fl or fld	fluid
fl. oz	fluid ounce
GI	gastrointestinal
gr	grain
gtt	drop
gtts	drops
HA	headache
HBP	high blood pressure
h or hr.	hour
HT or HTN	hypertension
IA	intra-arterial
ID	intradermal
IM	intramuscular
IV	intravenous
IVP	intravenous push

ABBREVIATION/SIG CODE	DEFINITION
IVPB	intravenous piggyback
lb.	pound
mcg or µg	microgram
mEq	milliequivalent
mg	milligram
mg/kg	milligrams per kilogram
ml or mL	milliliter
ml/hr	milliliters per hour
n&v or n/v	nausea and vomiting
NS	normal saline
NTG	nitroglycerin
od	right eye
os	left eye
ou	both eyes or each eye
P	after
pc	after meals
p.m.	evening
po	by mouth
pr	rectally
prn	as needed
Q	every
q4h	every 4 hours
q6h	every 6 hours
q12h	every 12 hours
q24h	every 24 hours
qd	every day
qh	every hour
QID	four times daily
qs	a sufficient quantity
sl	sublingual
SOB	shortness of breath
ss	one-half
sq or subq	subcutaneous
stat	immediately or now
supp	suppository
susp	suspension
tab	tablet
tbsp	tablespoon

(*continued*)

ABBREVIATION/SIG CODE	DEFINITION
TID	three times daily
ud	as directed
ung	ointment
UTI	urinary tract infection
wk	week

SIG CODES ENTERED INTO COMPUTER BY THE PHARMACY TECHNICIAN	PATIENT DIRECTIONS
T 1c po bid × 3w	Take one capsule by mouth twice daily for 3 weeks.
G 1 tsp po q12h prn cong	Give one teaspoon by mouth every 12 hours as needed for congestion.
AAA ud for itching	Apply to affected area(s) as directed for itching.
I 1–2 gtts os qid	Instill 1–2 drops into left eye four times daily.
I 1P po q12h	Inhale one puff by mouth every 12 hours.

5. After you double-check the information entered into the computer system and know that the information is complete, you can print the label. The label, like the prescription itself, by law must contain certain information, including:
   • The name and address of the pharmacy (some states also require the pharmacy phone number)
   • The serial or prescription number (as assigned by the computer program)
   • The date the prescription was filled (the expiration date is based on the date the prescription was written)
   • The name of the prescriber
   • The name of the patient
   • The name of the drug (some states require both brand and generic names)
   • The quantity of drug being dispensed
   • Refill information
   • Directions for use, including dose and frequency (directions must *not* contain abbreviations)
   • Precautions or warnings

6. In many cases, the pharmacy computer will not print a label until the prescription has been charged to the correct party. If the patient has insurance, then the insurance provider has to be billed for this prescription. If the following information has been double-checked, this process will be completed quickly.
   • Patient name and patient or person code
   • Group number and patient ID number
   • Correct number of days' supply
   • NDC number for the medication being dispensed

7. Select, count, and pour the correct medication. Again, the correct medication is verified based on the NDC. A good rule of thumb to ensure that you have the correct drug (other than by NDC) is to read the label thrice: once when the drug is selected off the shelf, once when the drug is counted and poured, and once more when the drug is returned to stock. In addition, it is common practice to count twice for accuracy, especially when counting controlled substances.

8. Set up the original prescription or medication order, the stock bottle(s) used, and the finished product for the pharmacist's final approval and verification. For a compounded prescription, the pharmacist will also have to see the recipe sheet you used. Upon successful verification, the pharmacist will approve the medication for dispensing.

9. Store the finished product properly, including patient information sheets, receipts, and notes the pharmacist may need when counseling.

Refilling Prescriptions

A refill is an authorization from the prescriber to fill a prescription exactly as written in addition to the first time it is presented at the pharmacy. A refill allows the patient to receive the medication additional times without the prescriber having to write a new prescription. The expiration date for refills is the same as for the original prescription, and the prescription cannot be dispensed after that date even if the patient has refills remaining.

If the patient has prescription insurance, most plans will pay for a refill only if the patient has used at least 75% of the prescription. The 75% rule is based on the number of days' supply that the technician entered into the computer. Therefore, it is imperative that the days' supply is calculated and entered correctly, or the patient's insurance may not pay for a refill. For example, if the patient receives a 30-day supply of medication on the first day of the month, she must wait at least until the 23rd day of the month before requesting a refill. If she requests a refill earlier, the insurance company will probably reject the claim.

Transferring Prescriptions

The laws governing the transfer of prescriptions between pharmacies differ in various states and depend on the class of drug involved. In most states, it is the pharmacist's responsibility to transfer prescriptions. However, technicians must understand and be familiar with the laws in the state where they practice. Your supervising pharmacist is a great resource to help guide you in transferring prescriptions to or from the pharmacy.

Where it is permitted, a prescription may be transferred for one fill or for the entire prescription. It is important to document the transfer. Both the transferring and the receiving pharmacies must keep specific documentation. Check with your state board of pharmacy for specific requirements regarding the transfer of prescriptions in your state.

Once the pharmacy's records show that the prescription was transferred and has already been filled or refilled, it must be returned to stock. Likewise, any insurance billing claim must be reversed, because two pharmacies cannot charge an insurance company for the same prescription. In such a case, the claim would be rejected.

Working Together with the Pharmacist

Assisting the pharmacist is at the core of being a pharmacy technician. With the exception of patient counseling, receiving new prescriptions, and performing the final verification of a prescription, a pharmacy technician can do almost any task in most pharmacy practice settings. Of course, the pharmacy technician always works under the direct supervision and authority of a pharmacist. Today's fast expanding health-care industry has a great requirement for skilled and knowledgeable technicians who possess in-depth understanding of the prescription process as well as a working knowledge of drugs, interactions, and computer systems, among other things.

Pharmacy technicians perform a wide array of tasks essential to the care and well-being of the patient. In the past, pharmacists performed the majority of the duties associated with the practice of pharmacy.

Duties that were once allocated to the pharmacist are now being taken over by the pharmacy technician. The push for greater pharmacy-based involvement in direct care of the patient is the initiative for many health systems as well as the Affordable Care Act (ACA). The following is just a sample of the tasks commonly performed by technicians in two of the main practice settings (retail and hospital):

- Answer basic questions that do not require professional judgment, such as item location or referral to the pharmacist.
- Answer the phone.
- Check, order, receive, and restock pharmacy inventory.
- Clean and maintain pharmacy equipment.
- Compound nonsterile pharmaceuticals.
- Deliver medications to patients and other medical personnel.
- Fill medication orders.
- Inventory and restock "crash cart" medications.
- Inventory, restock, and maintain pharmacy robotics and technology.
- Operate cash registers.
- Perform pharmaceutical calculations.
- Prepare and process insurance claims.
- Prepare medications.
- Prepare prescription labels.
- Prepare sterile intravenous admixtures, including IVPB, LVP, IVP, chemotherapy, and TPN.
- Provide excellent customer service.
- Receive and process refill requests.
- Receive new prescriptions and review for completeness.

Pharmacy technicians should understand that as pharmacy practices change, particularly with the increased requirement for patient medication counseling and pharmacist-based drug therapy intervention and planning, the pharmacy technician will take on a much larger role in the practice of pharmacy.

It was once thought that skills of the pharmacy technician required critical analysis or professional judgment. While the pharmacist always has the last word on drug verification and that pharmacy technician is never permitted to dispense drug information, professional judgment does become a necessary skill for the pharmacy technician.

Professional judgment in regard to the pharmacy technician may be as simple as a technician recognizing a patient who needs consultation, to more complex, such as identifying a patient drug dosage that may need to be questioned or verified. Whatever the case may be, professional judgment is an essential piece of the pharmacy technician's career, and continued development of professional judgment allows the practice of pharmacy to provide the pharmacy technician's career growth.

Policies, Procedures, and Technicians

Throughout this chapter we have learned how the skills of the pharmacy technician assist with assuring a safe medication experience for the patient. Measures such as maintaining patient profile, verifying patient information, addressing prescriptions and drug orders for completeness, as well as sustaining an accurate and safe data entry process help to eliminate medication errors, protecting the patient and affording them the best possible outcome.

Another piece of the puzzle that allows pharmacists and pharmacy technicians to provide the patient with a positive experience as well as establish pharmacy services are policies and procedures (P&Ps). Policies and procedures are valuable guides for any employee, especially pharmacy technicians. All employers will have their own P&Ps, in a written or electronic manual that must be readily and easily accessible to employees. Common policies and procedures include the following:

- Hiring requirements
- Employee benefits
- Expected employee behavior and standards
- Monitoring of patient allergies
- Management of toxic or dangerous drugs
- Proper procedures for protecting patients from errors
- Proper handling and distribution of drugs
- Proper handling of cytotoxic drugs
- Correct aseptic technique for compounding and admixtures
- Emergency procedures for disasters: fire, earthquake, tornado, and so on

P&Ps are not intended to put restrictions on the pharmacy technician, but instead to give clear and precise directions that will guide the technician in proper pharmacy protocol, the safe handling of drugs, and safety protection, all of which can protect pharmacy technicians from career-ending errors. However, if a policy or procedure is ambiguous or unclear, the pharmacy technician should always consult the pharmacist for clarification.

SUMMARY

Finally, none of the procedures investigated in this chapter become useful in patient care without the employment of three indispensable qualities: quality assurance, quality control, and quality improvement. Without these three qualities in place, procedures become invalid and useless to the care of the patient.

Quality assurance (QA) can be defined as the ongoing set of activities used to assure that the processes used in the preparation of drug products meet predetermined standards of quality. QA programs determine that facilities, systems, and written policies and procedures are adequate and are followed to assure that all final products meet the institution's requirements. You can think of QA as the *overall plan* for maintaining quality.

Quality-assurance mechanisms are divided into two important categories that should not be confused: quality control and quality improvement. Both are critical to the operation of a pharmacy, but each has its separate place in the ongoing quest to improve patient health care and safety.

Quality Control (QC) is a process of checks and balances (or procedures) that are followed to ensure that end products meet or exceed specified standards (i.e., zero errors and zero problems). Quality control is the *day-to-day management* of quality in the pharmacy, which is necessary to prevent defective products from reaching the patient.

Quality Improvement is an ongoing process that monitors, evaluates, and identifies problems by study, reports, charting, and collecting all of the pertinent information. Technicians often play a valuable role in this process by helping to collect, organize, and chart quality-improvement data.

Pharmacy technicians that keep these three quality measures intact when creating patient profiles, verifying patient information, validating a prescription or medication order for completeness, or employing patient data entry alleviate the potential for patient drug errors and other issues related to inaccurate patient information.

CHAPTER REVIEW QUESTIONS

1. The 10 essential elements of a prescription order include patient demographics, prescriber information, drug name and strength, drug route of administration, number of refills, indication of brand or generic, number of refills, directions for taking the drug, _____, and _____.
   a. Quantity of drug, pharmacist's name
   b. Technician's name, pharmacist's name
   c. Quantity of drug, prescriber's number
   d. Quantity of drug, prescriber's name

2. Today's health-care systems often use CPOE, which stands for
   a. Cooperative physician operating equipment.
   b. Computer prescriber oriented efficacy.
   c. Computer prescriber order equipment.
   d. Computer physician order entry.

3. When completing patient demographic for a patient's profile always remember to include the patient's _____.
   a. Full name, including any indication to Jr. or Sr. status
   b. Patient's preferred name, including any nickname the patient goes by
   c. Spouse's name as it may be needed for verification purposes
   d. Occupation for worker compensation claims and conversation purposes

4. Drug interactions occur when
   a. Two like prescription drugs are intermixed.
   b. A substance or condition affects the pharmacologic activity of a drug.
   c. A drug is combined with another drug and a chemical reaction occurs.
   d. Patients take more than one prescription drug at a time that counteracts other prescription drugs.

5. The first segment of an NDC number per FDA requirements must
   a. Be no less than five digits long.
   b. Be written in numeric and alphabetic code.
   c. Identify the country of origin.
   d. Identify the drug manufacturer.

6. Patient profiles should include all prescription and _____ drugs the patient may be taking to avoid any potential drug interactions.
   a. Diet
   b. Over the counter
   c. Liquid
   d. Mail order

7. If a patient is to receive a brand name drug _____ or _____ must be written on the prescription by the prescriber.
   a. No other drug is permitted, brand only
   b. Brand only, medically necessary
   c. Medically necessary, dispense as written
   d. Dispense as written, brand name only

8. When a patient is taking two or more prescriptions that work in similar ways for the same disease state it is known as
   a. Fraud.
   b. Duplication of therapy.
   c. Inaction of therapy.
   d. Completed therapy.

9. When a pharmacy technician receives a new order or prescription into the pharmacy, they should first
   a. Check the prescription for medical errors.
   b. Call the patient and let them know when it will be ready.
   c. Call the drug company and ask for verification.
   d. Check the prescription for completeness.

10. When a past, current, or present patient medical condition precludes use of a certain drug, we call this
    a. A prescribing error.
    b. Poor judgment.
    c. Drug–disease interaction.
    d. Drug–drug interaction.

Pharmacy Inventory Management

8 chapter

Learning objectives for this chapter will include:

- Defining the term *inventory* and understanding the differences between inventory management and inventory control.

- Discussing the role of a formulary in maintaining drug inventories.

- Describing and comparing the various inventory management systems used in a pharmacy setting.

- Listing the steps for returning expired drugs or drugs ordered by mistake.

- Describing the drug recall process.

- Comparing the processes used in ordering controlled substances as well as the inventory limits associated with controlled substances.

- Describing and explaining the Controlled Substance Act (CSA), including the five drug classes.

- Describing the two primary types of inventory management systems: manual and point-of-sale (POS).

- Explaining how to assist with special ordering and receiving procedures.

- Explaining medication storage and distribution.

- Discussing the safe handling of cytotoxic drugs and hazardous materials.

- Discussing special concerns concerning investigational drugs.

- Explaining bulk compounding and repackaging of pharmaceuticals.

Inventory Control

In the practice of pharmacy, inventory control is one of the most important responsibilities of pharmacy technicians, and the quality and quantity of products can mean the difference between life and death for patients. One can easily understand why monitoring purchase, storage, and stock levels of drugs and supplies becomes so essential to the well-being of the patients pharmacies serve. In fact, one might say it is as essential as dispensing the right drug to the right patient.

In order to meet patient's needs, medications need to be on hand and uncompromised. However, some medications can be quite expensive and costly to store, especially if it is a medication meant only for a specific disease state. All medications are required to have expiration date, and should never be used beyond the expiration date stamped on the manufacturer's label. It is for this reason that inventory control can be a balancing act, requiring detail to attention and time management.

In order to purchase medications, a pharmacy must have a license from the Drug Enforcement Agency (DEA). Once the pharmacy has applied for licensure, the DEA will assign the pharmacy a number specific to that pharmacy. Next, the pharmacy will need to choose a drug wholesaler or supplier. Pharmacies may purchase medications directly from the manufacturer, but this becomes a very paper-laden and time-consuming process. Imagine completing a purchase request form for each and every medication stocked in your pharmacy; the process would be endless.

The use of wholesalers for pharmacy inventory purchasing allows the inventory process to flow much more efficiently, and, in the long run, provides a cost-saving measure to the pharmacy as well. If more time is spent on labor order medications, paperwork, manufacturer's Web sites, or speaking with the manufacturer's representatives, then less time is spent on the actual control of the inventory and more time is spent on labor.

When a pharmacy agrees to purchase 80–90% of all its pharmaceuticals from a single wholesaler, then that wholesaler is termed a prime vendor. The wholesaler acts as an intermediary in procuring pharmaceuticals and other supplies for the pharmacy at special prices. This agreement still allows the pharmacy to make special purchases from other vendors when necessary. The wholesaler gets shipments directly from numerous manufacturers and can provide their products to the pharmacy all charged on one convenient invoice.

Although the pharmacist in charge is ultimately responsible for overseeing inventory management and control, the day-to-day management tasks, such as ordering, receiving, and control processes, are generally handled by the pharmacy technician.

There are thousands of medications on the market today that one would be counterproductive to stock all of them in any one pharmacy setting. So how does a pharmacy know what to stock? The answer is a formulary. A formulary is a list of all medications and devices approved for dispensing in a pharmacy.

In hospitals, the formulary is crafted from the pharmacy and therapeutics (P&T) committee. The committee, generally consisting of physicians, pharmacists, nursing staff, and administrative staff, meets several times a year to discuss the medications their hospital uses to treat disease states. It is the committee's responsibility to keep up with the ever-changing information dealing with disease states and the medications that treat them. The committee will agree upon an approved list of medications to be used as the hospital's formulary.

In most retail settings, a buyer or head pharmacist usually makes the decision on formulary for the pharmacy as part of his or her position authority. However, in an independent retail setting it is the owner's responsibility to make formulary decisions.

There are six key components that influence the decision-making process for formulary.

- Drug availability
- Dosage form
- Strength or concentration
- Accepted therapeutic use
- Correct dosages
- Federal, state, or local policy affecting the use of a medication, that is, a restricted antibiotic

Medication costs are also a concern when creating a formulary. While cost certainly isn't the only factor considered when formulary comes into play, it does have a great deal to do with its creation, particularly in smaller hospital systems and individually owned retail pharmacies. Budgets need to be allotted and a pharmacy's formulary takes up a large part of that budget. Not keeping budgetary guidelines in place when dealing with the creation of a pharmacy's formulary could cause financial concerns in the future.

Inventory Management Systems

With the exception of the creation of the formulary, pharmacy technicians maintain all aspects of a pharmacy's inventory. Using the formulary as a guide, the technician must ensure that adequate stock of all medications and medical devices is available between deliveries. The technician must monitor stock levels, expiration dates of stock, drug product recalls, drug storage conditions, as well as drug shortages and back orders.

Maintaining a formulary that will provide a health system or retail setting patients with a safe and effective medication therapy is always the goal. Pharmacy technicians that monitor a pharmacy's inventory complete the task through a process known as inventory control or inventory management. Two specific types of inventory management systems are used by pharmacies: manual and point-of-sale (POS).

Smaller pharmacies are more likely to use a manual inventory management system, and large retail and health-system pharmacies will most likely use the POS management system. POS formulary management is a computerized system that allows the pharmacy to manage formulary as an automated process.

A computerized or POS inventory system works much like a balance sheet, as each drug or device on the pharmacy's shelves are tracked from the time it is ordered to the time it is dispensed. As drugs or devices are dispensed, the computer subtracts them from the pharmacy's inventory. POS systems automatically create drug orders based on the pharmacy's use.

A pharmacy technician that uses a POS system does not need to do a physical inventory before each order, but must review the computer-generated order for accuracy before it is transmitted. If demand for a medication increases, the technician can adjust the order accordingly. The *minimum order point* is the amount of a product left on the shelf that will automatically trigger a reorder. The *maximum order level* indicates the maximum quantity of a drug that should be on the shelf at any given time.

Order levels are determined based on a drug's usage, and these levels reflect the smallest and largest quantities of a drug or device to be kept on the pharmacy's shelves. Once the minimum quantity is reached, the computer automatically adds the item to the order.

A pharmacy's inventory can be quite costly to maintain. In order to keep cost and waste to a minimum, inventory must be kept at a level that will ensure the pharmacy has a sufficient supply of inventory available to complete patient drug orders and prescriptions, but not so much that inventory loss becomes an issue. Very often when excessive inventory is ordered, particularly if it is a drug or a device that is rarely dispensed by the pharmacy, there is a greater risk of drug expiration, and this only adds to waste for the pharmacy.

Take this case scenario into consideration: Mary knows that her pharmacy dispenses about 100 units of warfarin each week. She sets them minimum order point for 25 units. When the computer recognizes that the stock of warfarin has fallen below 25 units, it will automatically order the drug product. Mary notices through her daily order reports that the pharmacy has begun to use more warfarin; she can increase the minimum order point. Conversely, if Mary's report shows a decrease in sales, she can decrease the minimum order point. Mary's careful watch over the inventory's controls will not only help to ensure that patients receive their orders from the pharmacy in a timely and efficient manner, but also help the pharmacy negate pharmaceutical waste, which is always of value.

A manual system requires all inventory activities to be done by hand. A daily inventory must be done for ordering purposes. Usually this entails the inventory person, typically a pharmacy technician, to physically "scan" the pharmacy's shelves for items that are low in stock and need to be reordered for the next day. Most pharmacies will have a "want book" available for pharmacists and technicians to write down items that need to be ordered for the following day. Pharmacies that implement a manual process may also have minimum and maximum numbers listed on the drug's shelf. Having minimum and maximum numbers available to staff decreases the risk that too much or not enough stock will be ordered.

An all-inclusive physical inventory is taken at regular intervals, typically prior to the end of a pharmacy's fiscal year, and decisions are made concerning the adjustment of the pharmacy's minimum and maximum order levels. Pharmacy technicians that are responsible for maintaining pharmacy inventory through a manual process often know their pharmacy's inventory so well that very little order adjustment is required.

Purchasing

Whether the order was compiled electronically or manually, the technician must arrange for the purchase. Several options are available to all pharmacies. A pharmacy may purchase drugs directly from the manufacturer, from a wholesaler, or from other vendors. Pharmacy management, and not the pharmacy technician, will make the decision on vendor choice. Although this decision may ultimately fall on the pharmacy manager or the pharmacist in charge, the inventory technician may be consulted as part of the decision-making process.

The first step in placing a drug order is creating a purchase order (PO). A PO contains information specific to a particular drug, and the inventory order process cannot proceed without them. A PO must contain the following minimum information:

- Name of the drug or device to be ordered
- Dosage form
- Package size
- Concentration or strength
- Quantity of each package
- Drug identification or National Drug Code (NDC) number

The purchase order number will also contain the pharmacy's name, address, phone number, and customer identification number. Electronic ordering will automatically transmit the pharmacy's information along with the actual order. In many cases, manual ordering is done on preprinted forms with several copies for each order.

If the pharmacy is ordering from a manufacturer, the pharmacy must fill out the PO and send it directly to the manufacturer. Once the PO is received the manufacturer will fill the order and send it to the pharmacy. A PO sent directly to the manufacturer is known as a *direct purchase order*.

In purchasing there is strength in numbers, and sometimes pharmacies band together and make a commitment to a manufacturer to purchase large quantities of drugs or devices over a period of a year or more. The manufacturer in turn reduces the cost of the drugs or devices to the pharmacies within the group. Pharmacies within a committed buying group are known as a *purchasing group*.

Most retail pharmacies purchase inventory through wholesale purchasing. The wholesaler purchases drugs and devices from many different manufacturers and warehouses them at one location. Most pharmacies are able to purchase 85–95% of their inventory from this single source. They usually cannot purchase 100% of their inventory from any one supplier, because of special order item or items that may be needed, but not supplied by their wholesaler.

Receiving an Order

Once the order has been placed the pharmacy awaits its arrival. Most wholesalers supply on a daily basis, and some may deliver more frequently, depending upon the demands of the retailer and the wholesaler's delivery schedule. Some wholesalers even provide weekend delivery for pharmacies, particularly those that are open 24/7. On the other hand, ordering direct from the manufacturer takes longer, depending upon the ordering relationship between the pharmacy and the manufacturer.

Drug orders are delivered in unmarked, sealed medication totes or boxes. Included with the drug order will be corresponding packing slips and invoices. Packing slips are used by the wholesaler to pull and pack drug orders. Invoices are used to bill the pharmacy for the drug order.

Controlled drugs are listed on a separate invoice and packed in a separate container from other drugs on the order. After the order has been delivered, the pharmacist must verify the controlled substance order before it is placed into stock. If there are any discrepancies, the wholesaler will be called immediately.

Chemotherapy and hazardous drugs are separated from other drugs in the order. Chemotherapy and hazardous drugs need to be handled safely in order to prevent patients, staff, or delivery personnel from any harm. As with all other drug order totes, totes that contain chemotherapy drugs should be sealed. Additionally, totes containing chemotherapy or hazardous drugs should be examined carefully for damage before being placed on pharmacy shelves. Products that are damaged should not be moved to pharmacy shelves, but rather carefully placed in a yellow biohazard bag and returned to the wholesaler.

Items that must be kept frozen or need refrigeration will also be delivered from the wholesaler in separate totes. Frozen and refrigerated items should be examined for damage, verified against the order receipt, and placed in the appropriate freezer or refrigerator as soon as possible in order to prevent contamination to the drug product. Refrigerated or frozen drug products that "feel" as if they are warm to touch or have thawed during the delivery process should be placed in appropriate storage units, but separated from other products already in the storage unit. At this point, the inventory technician should consult the pharmacist in charge.

Along with the invoices, stickers are often included with the order. These stickers facilitate easier reordering, especially under a manual system, because important information is printed on each specific item's sticker. As items are checked line by line against the invoices, price stickers are affixed to the product itself. When affixing stickers, it is important not to cover any information such as the drug name, strength, lot number, or expiration date. Most inventory stickers include the following information:

- Wholesaler's item number
- Date of receipt
- Net cost
- Average wholesale price
- Invoice number

Careful checking of each item is imperative to ensure that only those items received are added to the pharmacy's inventory. Receiving an item into inventory that was not actually shipped is one of the most common errors under a POS system. The result is a shortage of medication that may or may not be realized until that particular mediation is needed for a patient.

Receiving and stocking inventory are two of the most important responsibilities of the entire pharmacy inventory operation. Mistakes made during this process can easily jeopardize the health of patients and produce costly consequences. It is important that all stock be completely checked against the invoice when it is delivered. The following is a step-by-step approach that should be followed when receiving inventory:

1. Make sure that the name and address on the boxes are correct. Drug deliveries often end up at wrong locations, especially with a chain store delivery.
2. Make sure that the shipping manifest of the carrier matches the actual number of boxes delivered. All boxes should be accounted for. If the invoice indicates that five totes are to be delivered, the inventory technician should verify that five totes are being delivered.
3. Retrieve the manufacturer or warehouse invoice and /or packing slip. If any box or container is marked to be refrigerated or kept frozen, immediately place the contents in the refrigerator or freezer to avoid damage to the drug product. Special orders, chemotherapy, and investigational drugs should also be handled according to facility protocol.
4. The following information should be checked against the purchase order invoice:
   - Name of the drug
   - NDC

- Strength or concentration of the drug
- Dosage form
- Quantity
- Expiration dating (Checking the expiration date is extremely important. Drugs with short dating should be returned to the supplier for items with longer expiration dating.)

5. Once the order has been confirmed as correct, the new stock is almost ready to be placed on the pharmacy shelves. Before placing stock on shelves, attach inventory labels to the drug product. In most cases the inventory label will be attached to the bottom side of the drug bottle, but this will vary according to the policies and procedures of the pharmacy.

6. Finally, after the new stock has been verified, and the appropriate inventory label has been placed on the bottle, it can be placed on the pharmacy shelf. Pharmacy technicians placing new stock on pharmacy shelves should remember to always rotate the stock, so that the product expiring first is always at the front. Rotating stock is essential in cutting pharmacy waste. Any stock found to be expired or damaged should be removed from the pharmacy shelves immediately.

These routine audits may be done on a monthly or quarterly basis, depending on facility protocol. Written documentation showing the results of these audits should be kept available for review if needed.

Removing Stock from Inventory

One of the main priorities of inventory control is to make sure that the inventory is in usable condition and safe for patient use. Recalled, expired, and improperly stored drugs must be immediately removed from the pharmacy inventory.

Routine expiration date and/or storage audits must be conducted of the medication inventory stock in both retail and hospital pharmacies, because the pharmacy is responsible for medication control of the entire facility. During these audits the technician checks for drugs that have expired or will soon expire, as well as for any drugs that may be stored improperly.

In hospitals, inventory audits are commonly called *unit inspections*. The central pharmacy, satellite pharmacies, nursing units, patient-care areas, and any other locations where drugs are stored in the facility must be included in these audits. Routine inventory audits may be done on a monthly or quarterly basis, depending on facility protocol. Written documentation showing the results of these audits should be kept available for review if needed.

Recalls

In compliance with Article 20 of the FDA's Pharmaceutical Good Manufacturing Practices, an alert system must be in place to notify proper authorities in the event of a pharmaceutical recall. The goal of the alert system is to protect the public's health from potential risks caused by using defective or unsafe pharmaceutical products.

A drug recall is an event in which a manufacturer or supplier agrees to remove and correct marketed products that are in violation of applicable laws, may be defective, or may pose a potential risk to the health of the public. There may be many different reasons for recall of a pharmaceutical product. Common reasons for recalls include quality defects, contamination, and counterfeiting.

Recalls are classified according to the relative degree of health hazard of the product being recalled. Recalls are divided into three groups: Class I, Class II, and Class III.

- In Class I recalls, the use of or exposure to a particular product is likely to cause serious adverse health consequences or even death. It is the most severe of the three classes.

- In Class II recalls, the use of or exposure to a particular product may cause temporary harm or medically reversible adverse health consequences, or the likelihood of serious adverse health consequences is very remote.
- In Class III recalls, the use of or exposure to a particular product is not likely to cause serious adverse health consequences.

In the event of a recall, the FDA forwards a recall notice containing pertinent information the pharmacy needs to take appropriate action. Recall notices include the following information:

- Recall classification
- Recall number
- Product name
- Dosage form and strength of the medication
- Packaging information (size)
- Batch or lot control numbers affected by the recall
- Expiration dates
- Brief description or reason for the recall
- Product manufacturer's name and address

Upon receiving such information, the inventory control manager should check the information given in the recall against the inventory in stock. Any recalled products in stock should be promptly removed from the inventory. Appropriate instructions will be included with the recall information as to what actions to take in returning the recalled product(s) to the manufacturer or drug wholesaler.

Returns

Every wholesaler or drug manufacturer has his own policies for accepting returned merchandise and drug products for either replacement or credit. First, authorization must be obtained from the supplier for the return, and then that supplier's specific return procedure must be followed.

Controlled substances, those drugs in Classes II–V, will have very specific requirements for returns in accordance with DEA regulations. Any controlled substances that are to be returned to the wholesaler or manufacturer should be returned strictly to the specifications enforced by the DEA.

Expired Drugs

Despite product rotation and careful ordering controls, a drug will sometimes expire before it can be dispensed. In some cases, these drugs may be returned to the supplier for credit. In other cases, they must simply be destroyed. Authorizations forms need to be completed before the products can be packaged and shipped. Pharmacies sometimes hire a "returns company," which, for a fee, goes through all the pharmacy shelves and collects expired and unusable drugs, fills out the appropriate paperwork, and packages the drugs for shipment back to the supplier.

Controlled Substances

Under the federal Controlled Substances Act (CSA), any drug considered to be a controlled substance, falls under one of five classifications. Controlled substances are classified as Schedule I, II, III, IV, or V drugs. The factors that determine where a drug is ranked for scheduling purposes include medicinal value, harmfulness, and potential for abuse. A pharmacy technician should be aware of the schedules of drugs and their potential for danger or abuse.

Drugs in Schedule I have no medicinal value. Drugs in this class are illicit or "street" drugs such as heroin, cocaine, and LSD.

Schedule II includes a number of drugs that pharmacies dispense on a daily basis. These drugs have been found to have medicinal value, but are highly addictive. Included in this class are stimulants such as methylphenidate (Concerta, Ritalin) and severe-pain medications such as hydrocodone (Norco, Vicodin), oxycodone (Percocet, Tylox), morphine sulfate (Avinza, Roxanol), meperidine (Demerol), and fentanyl (Sublimaze). The Schedule II medications are kept under lock and key. A daily verified count of Scheduled II medications should be done at least once a week. Verifying the number of Scheduled II medications against the inventory record helps to address issues related to counting or diversion. Obtaining Schedule II drugs for patient use is more complex than obtaining other drugs.

Medications in Schedule III (e.g., Tylenol with codeine, testosterone), Schedule IV (e.g., Valium, Xanax, Lunesta), and Schedule V (e.g., cough syrups with codeine) require a different level of control because of their lower risk of danger and abuse potential. Schedules III–V also have been proven to have medicinal value, and still have the potential for addiction, but are not considered to be as addictive as Schedule I or II drugs.

Schedule III-C drugs, which include pain medications as well as antianxiety and antidepressant agents, still require high security levels. Although obtaining them may not be as complex as obtaining Schedule II drugs, they are still controlled substances and are regulated more than noncontrolled drugs. That being said, it is still wise to do regular audits of Scheduled III drugs in order to address counting issues or to ward against potential diversion.

Distribution throughout the facility should be monitored properly so that all controlled substances can be accounted for at all times. Excellent and up-to-date record keeping is a must in order to maintain an accurate count of all drugs with controlled status.

Pharmacies that employ manual accounting systems use paper documentation of controlled-drug distribution. All documentation must be kept on file in the pharmacy. If a pharmacy uses an automated dispensing system, such as Pyxis or Omnicell, computerized records are available for documentation purposes. Regardless of the documentation method used, it is imperative that scheduled drugs are tracked and accounted for in through an efficient manner.

Most health-system pharmacies as well as some retail settings have converted to computer-generated documentation, which can be more efficient than manual documentation, but pharmacy technicians should still be aware that errors can occur during the data entry process, or even when a scheduled drug is removed incorrectly from the system. Errors such as these can be difficult to track and correct, but for the purpose of DEA-mandated documentation, the pharmacy needs to make every effort possible to make sure all controlled substances, Schedules II–V, are accounted for.

When controlled substances are distributed from the pharmacy to a nursing unit or other patient-care area, they are logged from inventory onto a "sign-out" sheet. If automated technologies are employed, the logging-out process may be done electronically. Again, all controlled substances must be accounted for, per DEA mandates. Errors in restocking, dispensing, or diversion are just a few reasons why accountability of controlled substances is so essential. Procedures for controlled-substance distribution may vary slightly from one health system to another, but they all adhere closely to the standard principles and requirements.

Controlled substances in Schedules III, IV, and V can be ordered along with the pharmacy's regular order. However, they are invoiced separately because of their controlled status. Controlled substances are shipped to the pharmacy in a tote that is separated from the noncontrolled drugs. Although a pharmacy technician may oversee the receiving of all other medications, a licensed pharmacist should verify incoming controlled substances.

Schedule II

Schedule II drugs (also called C-II drugs) have very specific ordering, receiving, storage, dispensing, inventory, record-keeping, return, waste, and disposal requirements mandated by federal law. C-II drugs, due to their high potential for abuse, have much stricter ordering regulations, set forth by the Drug Enforcement Agency (DEA). The DEA, a division of the U.S. Department of Justice, requires a special form (DEA Form 222) for procurement of C-II medications from a supplier.

Only a pharmacy with a DEA number is allowed to order and dispense Schedule II medications, just as only a prescriber with a DEA number can prescribe them. Although a purchasing and inventory technician may actually fill out the DEA Form 222, the person with power of attorney, typically the pharmacist in charge, must sign it and is the only person permitted to sign a DEA Form 222. In most instances, it is a pharmacist who has the authority to sign the DEA Form 222. The DEA's Controlled Substance Ordering System (CSOS) allows for electronic orders of controlled substances without requiring a paper form DEA 222.

DEA Form 222 contains ten lines on three copies (the original, which is brown, copy 2, which is green, and copy 3, which is blue). After the form is filled out by the pharmacy, the brown and green copies are sent to the supplier, while the blue copy is kept by the pharmacy for its records. The supplier fills the order, keeps the original brown copy, and sends the green copy to the DEA for drug-tracking purposes. The DEA can track a C-II drug from its manufacturing site to the supplier, to the pharmacy, and to the patient. Each dose must be accounted for at all times and at every stage of the distribution process.

Filling out a DEA Form 222 is a precise undertaking; if a mistake is made, a new form must be completed. There can be no cross-outs or changes of any kind on a DEA Form 222. These important guidelines must be followed while filling the DEA Form 222:

- Only pen or typewriter may be used.
- Only one drug may be ordered per line.
- The signature on the DEA Form 222 must match with that on the DEA license or power of attorney form.
- The third copy must be kept for 2 years and must be kept separate from other records and/or forms.

There should be no changes, erasures, or cross-outs. Incorrect forms must be marked *VOID* and kept with other DEA Form 222s. When the C-II drugs are delivered, the person receiving the delivery must be 18 years old, and the date received must be written on the pharmacy's copy. Federal law requires all Form 222s to be kept on file for 2 years. State law may require a longer holding period. Pharmacies are also required to keep separate C-II inventory logs as well as separate storage of C-II prescriptions or dispensing records.

Expired C-II drugs cannot be returned to the manufacturer or wholesaler for credit. Expired C-II drugs must be destroyed, often by a specially licensed company, and recorded on the separate DEA Form 41. DEA Form 41, "Registrants Inventory of Drug Surrendered," is used to inventory and record any C-II drug that must be destroyed. If there is a suspected theft or loss of a controlled substance, DEA Form 160, "Report of Theft or Loss of Controlled Substances," must be completed. Technicians work closely with a pharmacist when handling any C-II drug and C-II paperwork.

Investigational Drugs

Some hospitals or institutional pharmacies, particularly those that may be considered to be a research or teaching facility, may handle investigational medications. Only a licensed physician may initiate the request for such a drug. The first step is to obtain permission from the manufacturer. Without a manufacture's permission, investigational drugs cannot be made available to patients. Investigational drugs are tracked with a perpetual inventory system that is usually maintained by pharmacy technicians. The manufacturer or the sponsor of the study provides instructions that cover the receiving, storage, and return of investigational drugs.

Investigational drugs that have expired or become unstable should not be thrown away but kept, clearly marked, and handled according to instructions from the manufacturer or sponsor of the study. Most facilities will have a separate storage area for investigational drugs as well as a protocol for who may handle investigational drugs. In some large health-system pharmacies, pharmacy technicians are specifically trained for handling and documenting investigational drugs.

Compounded Drugs

Compounded drugs or medications manufactured in a pharmacy usually have strict storage requirements and short expiration dates. Technicians must monitor the production levels, storage, and waste of these materials. The technician must be aware of the employer's policy on the disposal of expired compounded medications and must follow that policy.

Other Inventory Issues

Some medications that have special ordering procedures may require a pharmacy representative to call the manufacturer or wholesaler to provide specific information pertaining to the medication or its use. A few examples are Enbrel injection and Thalomid tablets. Sometimes these specially ordered products are not kept in stock at the wholesaler's warehouse, but are *drop-shipped* from the manufacturer. *Drop-shipped* simply means that the order is billed or charged by the wholesaler, but shipped from a different location, such as from the manufacturer.

Medication availability is also a primary concern for purchasing and inventory technicians. In order to stay abreast of situations such as drug shortages, the pharmacy buyer should be well aware of all that is going on within the pharmacy inventory and the wholesaler.

The inventory technician may find a drug that is *temporarily out of stock*. This means that the supplier does not have the medication and expects a shipment from the manufacturer within a short time. If a medication is out of stock, the pharmacy can wait until the drug is received from the wholesaler or, if it is needed immediately, the pharmacy can "borrow" the medication from another pharmacy and "repay" the pharmacy when a shipment is received.

A *manufacturer back order* happens when the wholesaler is out of the product and none is available from the manufacturer. A back order may last a few days, weeks, or even months. A back order might result from a shutdown of manufacturing, a recall, or even a raw material shortage. When an out of stock or back order occurs, it is the responsibility of the inventory technician and the pharmacist to decide if an alternate manufacturer or an alternate drug should be ordered.

Medication Storage

Medication storage is a very important part of controlling inventory. It is necessary to provide the correct environment for medications and components until they are needed, so that they maintain their potency and stability. If proper environmental control is not maintained, the medications may not be safe and effective for patient use. Factors that affect the environment include:

- Temperature
- Light
- Humidity
- Ventilation
- Sanitation
- Segregation

In a retail pharmacy, medications are stored primarily on the pharmacy inventory shelves. In a hospital setting, medications may be stored in several different areas throughout the institution or outpatient pharmacy including:

- Pharmacy shelves (in both central and satellite pharmacies)
- Refrigerators

- Nursing units and automated dispensing systems
- Clinics and treatment rooms
- Emergency, operating, and recovery rooms

No matter where drugs are located in a facility, the responsibility for all medications falls on the shoulders of the pharmacy staff, particularly those who work with inventory management and control. Storage areas must be secure and accessible only to designated and authorized personnel. Whenever possible, records should be kept of who has accessed the medication storage areas. Areas such as automated dispensing systems, after-hours cabinets, and locked cabinets containing controlled substances are prime areas for such access monitoring.

Segregation of pharmacy supplies and medications should be a high priority. External-use products should be stored separate from internal-use products, just as nasal and inhalation products should be kept separate from otic and ophthalmic preparations. This segregation is required by the Joint Commission to help prevent medication errors and improper use of medications.

Some of the main segregated areas of the pharmacy include:

- Oral tablets, capsules, and powders
- Oral liquids, including solutions, elixirs, syrups, and undiluted antibiotic suspensions
- Topicals, including creams, ointments, and patches
- Ophthalmic medications
- Otic medications
- Orally inhaled medications
- Nasal products
- Rectal suppositories and topical rectal preparations
- Vaginal products
- Injectable
- Cytotoxic medications
- Other hazardous chemicals

In general, most pharmacy inventory is stored alphabetically by drug generic name in the appropriate area of the pharmacy. For example, atenolol tablets are stored in the A section of tablets, capsules, and powders. Also located in that same area, next to the atenolol, will be the trade name Tenormin tablet if that is also a stock item. However, some pharmacies may store inventory alphabetically by trade name. In such a pharmacy, Tenormin tablets would be stored in the T section, and the atenolol would be stored right next to them. This storage method is quickly fading away due to the fact that vast majority of products are now available in generic form. In other pharmacies, the Tenormin might be shelved in the T section and the atenolol in the A section. This method is typically used only in retail pharmacies.

Storage temperature can greatly affect the stability and potency of a medication. Pharmaceuticals are labeled to show the required temperature range for their proper storage. The most common temperature storage requirements are as follows:

- Room temperature (59–86°F or 15–30°C):

  Most tablets, powders, capsules, and liquids
- Refrigerator (36–46°F or 2–8°C):

  Insulin (long-term storage)

  Hematopoietic agents such as Neupogen and Epogen

  Vaccines such as hepatitis A and B, tetanus, pneumococcal, and polio

  Tuberculin skin tests

  Antibiotic injectables that are ready to use, such as Bicillin LA and CR

Suppositories such as Phenergan

Tablets such as Volmax, Alkeran, and several new antiviral medications

Oral liquids such as EES ready-to-use suspension and Orapred

Some ophthalmic preparations such as Viroptic solution

Controlled substances such as Ativan injection

- Freezer (less than 32°F or 0°C)

Each refrigerator should have its own temperature records, and personnel in each department should check the temperature of the refrigerator at least daily. This daily check should be documented in writing and initialed by the responsible personnel.

Safe Handling of Cytotoxic and Hazardous Materials

Cytotoxic and hazardous materials used in the pharmacy require special handling to preserve the safety of both the product and the personnel. The federal Occupational Safety and Health Administration (OSHA) sets standards that govern the special handling and storage of cytotoxic, antineoplastic, or chemotherapy agents as well as other chemicals such as bleach, alcohol, and acids.

OSHA defines a hazardous agent as one that could be either a health hazard or a physical hazard. If there is evidence that either acute or chronic health effects could result if personnel were exposed to the chemical itself, then it should be considered hazardous. Some agents in this category are:

- Carcinogens
- Toxins
- Irritants
- Corrosives
- Other agents that could damage the lungs, eyes, ears, skin, or mucous membranes

A physical hazard is one that could cause physical damage in the workplace. Examples of these types of chemicals are:

- Combustible liquids
- Compressed gases
- Explosives
- Flammables

OSHA standards require that personnel who may be exposed to potentially dangerous drugs and chemicals must complete an orientation and training process that covers all policies and procedures followed by the facility. Personnel should receive "Worker Right to Know" information with this orientation and training.

OSHA requires documentation such as Material Safety Data Sheets (MSDS) for all hazardous materials and chemicals to be stored in the pharmacy. Along with the MSDS, proper warning labels to identify hazardous chemicals are also required.

The MSDS are designed to inform personnel (both employees and emergency responders) about proper procedures for handling a particular substance. These sheets are not meant for consumers but for those who work around and with these chemicals and other hazardous substances on a day-to-day basis. The MSDS should be kept readily available and easily accessible to anyone who may need them at any time. Generally, a binder is kept on the premises that contains MSDS for all chemicals and other hazardous substances that are used or stored in the area. As new items become part of the pharmacy inventory, an MSDS should accompany their arrival and become part of the MSDS file on hand.

The MSDS include information on the following:

- Chemical name and Chemical Abstract Service (CAS) number
- Flammability
- Reactivity
- Flash point
- Department of Transportation (DOT) warnings
- Stability
- National Fire Protection Association (NFPA) classification

Some physical data about the chemical is also listed on the MSDS, including

- Boiling point
- Specific gravity
- Melting point
- Vapor pressure and density

Storage areas for these products should be designed to prevent damage, breakage, spillage, or leakage. Bins and shelves should have frontal barriers to prevent containers from dropping to the floor and breaking or spilling. Hazardous medications to be stored under refrigeration must be kept separate from other medications. They also should be kept in a fashion designed to prevent breakage and contain leakage should a break occur. Hazardous drugs should never be placed in dumbwaiters or pneumatic tubes for transport because mechanical stress on the product could result in contamination of all the areas involved.

As a precaution, pregnant women should not handle cytotoxic or hazardous agents. However, even though dangerous and hazardous substances might be used and stored within the area where you work, the pharmacy workplace need not be hazardous to your health. Safety should be everyone's concern, and all personnel should have the proper training to ensure that the work area is safe for all. The National Institute for Occupational Safety and Health (NIOSH) has established additional industry guidelines and recommendations for handling/preparing hazardous drugs, along with the American Society of Health-System Pharmacists (ASHP), and the International Society of Oncology Pharmacy Practitioners (ISOPP).

Medication Distribution

In an inpatient facility the pharmacy department is in control and responsible for all medications throughout the facility. Medication distribution areas include the unit-dose area, floor stock, and IV admixtures.

When a medication order is received by the pharmacy, it is entered into the computer and the pharmacy technician fills the order in the unit-dose area. In the pharmacy's unit-dose area, all medications are individually packaged, and most packages contain one unit of medication. Unit-dose packages are individually labeled with the drug name, strength, dosage form, lot number, expiration date, and manufacturer name.

The technician fills medications for each new order as they arrive and for the entire patient population during patient cassette fill. In retail pharmacies, most routine and maintenance prescriptions are dispensed for 30 days or more. In a hospital pharmacy, patient medications are generally dispensed as a 24–48 hour supply. This means that the pharmacy fills all the medications needed for each patient every 24–48 hours, depending on the facility's filling policies, using unit-dose medications.

Medication distribution in an inpatient facility includes more than just delivering patient-specific medication to the appropriate area. In a hospital, non–patient-specific medication is also distributed by the pharmacy. This type of medication includes floor stock, emergency medications in crash/code carts, and medications stored in automated dispensing systems and after-hours or night cabinets.

Floor Stock

Floor stock medications are drugs that are kept outside the pharmacy and are not intended specifically for any one patient. When one of these medications is needed, it can be retrieved from floor stock instead of getting it from the pharmacy. Although these medications are stored outside the pharmacy, the pharmacy is still responsible for the storage, control, processing, and billing of floor stock medications. Although some health systems still utilize floor stock, many have concerted to automated dispensing cabinets (ADC). ADCs not only allow for greater control and documentation, but also allow patient or department billing to be handled much more efficiently and accurately.

Automated Dispensing Cabinets

The profession of pharmacy has gradually evolved into providing pharmaceutical care. Changes that occurred during this evolution have caused health-care systems to seek cost-reducing measures and more effective patient/medication safety. As a result, automated dispensing systems and devices are common in today's pharmacies.

The purpose of automation is to enhance patient care and relieve the pharmacist from some of the medication distribution process. Pharmacy technicians are the primary personnel involved in working with, maintaining, and stocking automated dispensing systems. Automated devices such as Pyxis, Omnicell, MedCarousel, and Acu-Dose are most often used in hospital settings. ScriptPro- and Parata-automated dispensing systems are most likely to be found in retail pharmacies. The manufacturers of these different systems also produce accompanying software that can be interfaced with the existing pharmacy software, which makes it much easier to adapt to the new technologies.

Automated systems are intended for use in the distribution of both individual patient prescriptions in retail and unit-dose medication orders in hospitals. Some specific features of hospital-automated dispensing cabinets include the following:

- Medications are contained and administered from unit-dose packaging.
- Medications are provided or dispensed in ready-to-use form when possible.
- Medications are accessible only at the time it is to be administered for patient use.
- A profile of all medications concurrently being used is maintained in pharmacy records for each specific patient.
- Decreased risk for medication error
- Decreased risk for diversion
- Greater tracking and documentation abilities

Crash or Code Carts

A crash or code cart is a wheeled cart that contains the medication, equipment, and supplies that must be readily available for patient resuscitation during cardiac arrest and other medical emergencies. Medical facilities have crash carts in all patient-care areas. When a patient stops breathing, goes into cardiac arrest, or otherwise "crashes," a "Code Blue" is called and the medical personnel wheels the cart to the patient and begins resuscitative measures.

The health system's pharmacy department is responsible for maintaining the crash carts in all areas throughout the facility, due in part to the medications that are stored in them. This includes making sure all required medications are present, that no drugs are expired, and package integrity is intact. Medication can be included on the cart in trays that fit inside the drawers or in tackle boxes that sit on top of the cart.

The pharmacy is responsible for maintaining crash cart drugs and IV solutions, and the technician is responsible for its inventory. All other equipment and supplies are the responsibility of the respective departments. Technicians conduct crash cart inventories during their monthly nursing station inspections or after the crash cart has been used. In most facilities, after the crash cart is opened or used, the medication trays or boxes are brought to the pharmacy and exchanged for new, sealed trays.

In other facilities, the technician must go to the patient-care area to inventory the medication and replace or exchange any drug that has been used or has expired. All medication replaced or exchanged in a crash cart must be checked by the pharmacist.

Pediatric and adult crash carts must be available whenever there is a potential for a child to be treated under a "Code Blue" situation. Pediatric drug dosages and adult drug dosages are two very different identities. A child that accidentally receives an adult dose, especially under an already heightened situation, may become further compromised. It is for this reason state, local, and Joint Commission standards mandate both pediatric and adult crash carts be available. In most facilities these carts will be stored beside one another but have a distinction that separates one from the other.

Most drugs carried in crash carts are in injectable form. Injectable drugs stored in a crash cart need to be used during emergency situations. It is for this reason that most crash carts are filled with prefilled syringes. Prefilled syringes do not require personnel to spend precious time opening syringes and needles and drawing up medications. Although some emergency medications are not available in a prefilled form, the majority of emergency medications such as sodium bicarbonate or epinephrine are available, and this not only is a convenience, but also allows staff to stay focused on the patient's immediate needs.

SUMMARY

Control and management of pharmacy inventory is just one more avenue where the skill of a certified pharmacy technician comes into play. Pharmacy technicians should remember that a pharmacy's inventory is responsible for its profitability. Several factors go into deciding a pharmacy's inventory, and while pharmacy technicians may not be directly responsible for the development of the inventory, they can be responsible for its maintenance.

Shortages, recalls, and back orders are all issues pharmacies must deal with today, but pharmacy technicians that are preceptive to the inventory needs of their pharmacy will reduce the risk of the pharmacy's inability to fill a patient's prescription due to low or back ordered stock. Patients that are unable to receive their medications in a timely manner may be exposed to greater health risks. The first responsibility of the practice of pharmacy is to protect the patient, and having medications available when they are needed is essential for the health and well-being of the patient.

CHAPTER REVIEW QUESTIONS

1. A POS system, which stands for _____, acts like a computerized _____.
   a. Positive output sales, balance sheet
   b. Point-of-sale, tablet
   c. Point-of-sale, balance sheet
   d. Positive output sales, tablet

2. A purchase order must contain the following information: name of drug, dosage form, quantity, as well as _____ and _____.
   a. NDC, drug concentration or strength
   b. Strength of drug, name of manufacturer
   c. NDC, name of manufacturer
   d. Quantity, name of manufacturer

3. Drugs are delivered from the wholesaler in
   a. Totes that have the drug name and quantity on the outside.
   b. Unmarked totes.
   c. Unmarked totes that are color coded.
   d. Totes that are color coded.

4. The FDA has _____ classes of drug recalls, _____ being the highest or most urgent.
   a. 4, I
   b. 5, II
   c. 3, I
   d. 4, III

5. There are five specific classifications for controlled substances, I–V. The DEA requires a _____ form to be completed anytime one of these classifications is purchased.
   a. DEA 555
   b. DEA 106
   c. DEA 202
   d. DEA 222

6. The term *prime vendor* refers to _____.
   a. A wholesale that every pharmacy uses in a local area
   b. An insurance-preferred vendor
   c. A wholesaler from whom a pharmacy purchases 80–90% of its stock
   d. A wholesaler with the best prices

7. In a retail setting the _____ generally makes decision on formulary stock.
   a. The lead pharmacy technician
   b. The pharmacist in charge
   c. The corporate head
   d. The pharmacist with the most seniority

8. The _____ is the amount of drug left on a shelf that will trigger a reorder, whereas the _____ is the quantity of a particular drug product that should be on the shelf at any given time.
   a. Maximum order level, limited order point
   b. Limited order point, minimum order level
   c. Minimum order level, limited order point
   d. Minimum order level, maximum order level

9. A purchase order (PO) sent directly to the manufacturer is known as a
   a. Compromised order.
   b. Indirect purchase order.
   c. Wholesaler requested order.
   d. Direct purchase order.

10. When receiving controlled substances from the wholesaler they will be packed in
    a. Red totes with no invoice.
    b. Separate totes with a separate invoice.
    c. Red totes with a separate invoice.
    d. None of these

Pharmacy Billing and Reimbursement

LEARNING OBJECTIVES

Learning objectives for this chapter will include:

- Understanding what is meant by third-party payer and reimbursement systems.

- Understanding reimbursement policies for insurances plans such as Health Maintenance Organization (HMO), Preferred Provider Organization (PPO), Centers for Medicare and Medicaid Services, as well as private care plans.

- Definition and explanation of adjudication.

The Third-Party Payer: Understanding Reimbursement Systems

As we have already discussed, pharmacy technicians may work in various aspects of the pharmacy profession, but the two main environments will be within a retail or community pharmacy, and a hospital or institutional pharmacy. Pharmacy technicians that work in retail pharmacy are not typically exposed to some of the same duties as the hospital or institutional pharmacy technicians. Conversely, the hospital or institutional pharmacy technicians are not exposed to some of the duties of a retail or community pharmacy technician.

One task that may not be a duty of the hospital or institutional technician, but most definitely will be a duty for the retail or community technician, is dealing with third-party payers. A definition for the term *third-party payer* can be explained like this: any company public or private that pays health insurance benefits or claims on behalf of a third-party, that is, a patient. The third party refers to the patient or the one who is insured and receiving health insurance benefits from a third-party administrator.

The third-party administrator is the insurance company responsible for paying the claims associated with the third party. In other words, the third-party administrator is patient's insurance company. For example, John works in a well-known department store in his town. He has worked there for several years and is very happy with his employment. One of the reasons John is happy with his employment is the insurance benefit. Each year John's employer allows him to pick from several insurance companies. One company is a Health Maintenance Organization (HMO), another is Preferred Provider Organization (PPO), and the last one is a small private company.

As you might suspect, all of these terms can become quite confusing, but they really are not as difficult to understand as they might seem. While a retail-based pharmacy technician, as we stated earlier, will have the most contact with third-party payers, it is still important for hospital or institutional-based pharmacy technicians to understand these concepts.

HMO, PPO, and CMS are all acronyms that become very familiar to a pharmacy technician working in a retail or community pharmacy setting. Health insurance continues to make headlines and, as a result, continues to change at a breakneck pace. Keeping up with all the changes associated with third-party payer, or providers as they are also commonly known, can be a daunting task. Perhaps one of the best places to start is by understanding the acronyms.

Health Maintenance Organization

What is an HMO? Health Maintenance Organizations are insurance companies that provide health insurance benefits to their customers through an approved network of physicians, specialist, health-care systems, and pharmacies. Patients that have health insurance benefits from an HMO must select a Primary Care Physician (PCP) when signing up for their benefits.

PCPs are health-care providers, physicians, physician assistants, or nurse practitioners that are listed and approved to provide care for the HMO's customers. This is also known as an in-network provider. Patients may choose to see a provider outside of the defined network, but will most likely be responsible for paying a higher co-pay. A co-pay is a set fee the patient has agreed to pay for seeing a provider listed within their approved network.

In an HMO, patients must have their PCP request a prior authorization or referral, before the patient receives any specialized services, such as testing, surgical procedures, or care from a specialized field of medicine, that is, endocrinologist or dermatologist. In most HMO situations patients will also be required to have their prescriptions filled at a pharmacy within the network as well in order to only be responsible for their predetermined co-pay.

Preferred Provider Organization

Preferred Provider Organizations (PPOs) are similar to HMOs in that the patient must still select a primary care physician, but the choice of provider is often more extensive. Patients under a PPO may choose a provider within their network or outside of the network with the understanding that patients may have additional costs for their office visits. Additionally, patients that are serviced under a PPO generally do not have referrals to see specialists or have a routine outpatient procedure, such as annual physicals.

Medicare and Medicaid

Medicare

Medicare is a health-care plan that is funded under the federal government. Medicare was established to provide health-care benefits for the elderly, those over the age of 65, as well as those younger than 65 that may have a disability that would prevent them being able to retain employment and receive benefits from an employer. Medicare also aids those with end-stage renal failure by providing them with health-care and prescription services.

There are four different parts to Medicare, each one with a different purpose:

- Medicare Part A—provides patients with hospital benefits, for example a hospital admission due to a severe illness or surgery
- Medicare Part B—provides patient with health-care provider services, such as an annual office visit to their primary care provider
- Medicare Part C or Medicare Advantage—works in much the same way as a PPO
- Medicare Part D—provides the patient with prescription services

All Medicare services are overseen by the federal government under the authorization and authority of the Centers for Medicare and Medicaid Service (CMS), a division of the U.S. Department of Health and Human Services.

Medicaid

Medicaid, while established as a division of the Centers for Medicare and Medicaid Services (CMS), is actually a state run health insurance plan for low-income families and individuals who are unable to afford a typical health insurance plan.

While each state institutes its own criteria for Medicaid eligibility, the federal government works in conjunction with the state to oversee the funding of Medicaid programs. Medicaid programs, unlike Medicare, do not have an age requirement for eligibility.

Mail Order Pharmacy

Many times HMOs as well as PPOs will offer their patients service from a mail order pharmacy. Mail order pharmacies provide services to patients across the United States from a central location. The mail order pharmacy may have several locations, but services to the patient will be provided from the mail order pharmacy closest to the patient's home.

One of the benefits of a mail order pharmacy is that the patient are able to receive a 3-month or 90-day supply of their medication, rather than a 30-day supply. Of course, this will not apply to CII drugs as they can never be filled for more than a 30-day supply and must be filled by a local pharmacy.

Worker's Compensation Claims

Along with the previous mentioned insurance plans, pharmacy technicians may need to process drug insurance claims from worker's compensation. Worker's compensation is a federal mandated program that is run by each state. The program was set up to provide those who may have become injured on the job with health insurance benefits. Under worker's compensation the employer is responsible for any health-care expenses an employee may have suffered due to an on-the-job injury. Not only does this include any provider or hospital service, but prescriptions services as well.

Co-Pays

Most insurance plans will have a set amount patients must pay out of pocket for their health services and drug prescription services. This predetermined fee is known as a co-pay. Co-pays alleviate some of the cost associated with health-care services and drug prescription costs. No matter what the actual cost of the drug might be, patients will only be responsible for their predetermined co-pay.

Patient Data Information

We have learned in previous chapters how important accurate patient profiles are when providing pharmacy services, such as Drug Utilization Review (DUR). The same can be said when providing patient information to insurance companies for prescription drug claims.

Patient information must be accurate and complete when sending a prescription drug claim to an insurer. If any of the patient's information is misleading or inaccurate, the claim will be "kicked back" to the pharmacy. Health insurance plans can reject drug prescription claims for inaccurate patient information, such as

- Patient date of birth
- Marital status
- Account information
- Address verification

When these types of claim issues arise, the pharmacy technician must contact the patient to verify the needed information. Of course, avoiding this issue is best handled by verifying patient information each time the patient drops off or has a prescription filled at the pharmacy. By simply asking the patients if there have been any changes to their information, issues with prescription drug claims can be greatly reduced.

Fraud

Health insurance fraud is a very serious offense that is not taken lightly by state and federal agencies. The Healthcare Fraud and Abuse Control Program, established under the Health Insurance Portability and Accountability Act, makes all forms of insurance fraud a federal crime.

Insurance fraud includes such acts as providing false information on insurance claims, incentives that might be paid from government health-care plans, or falsely reporting charges; for example, stating the charge for a prescription was $25.00 when in fact the charge to the patient was only $15.00.

Penalties for insurance fraud can include loss of license or registration, loss of employment, fines, and even incarceration. The penalties may also extend to the pharmacist as well, especially since it has been established that the pharmacist is responsible for the operations of the pharmacy.

Computer Systems and Adjudication

Computers have reduced the workload for many professionals, and practice of pharmacy is no exception. Prior to the widespread use of computers and software systems, prescription drug claims were handled through a process of multiple paper claims. Not only was this labor intensive, but time consuming as well. Today prescription insurance claims and patient billing are handled electronically through a network of secure computer system and software processes.

Adjudication is the process of transmitting prescription information to a third-party payer for payment. Adjudication is done in real time, meaning the claim is being processed and approved by the insurer while the pharmacy technician is filling the prescription and the pharmacist is verifying the prescription order.

Insurance and prescription drug plans can be a daunting task. Pharmacy technicians are often responsible for processing prescription drug claims and patient billing procedures. Understanding the difference between insurance plans allows the pharmacy technician to better understand how claim processes are conducted, as well as assist the patients with questions they may have concerning their prescription drug claims. Insurance and prescription drug plans are on a continuous road of change. Pharmacy technicians that stay informed of these changes are best equipped to deal with any issues or problems that may develop. Being able to prevent or resolve prescription drug claim issues not only frees up the pharmacist time, but also provides the patient with a more pleasant and efficient pharmacy experience.

CHAPTER REVIEW QUESTIONS

1. Medicare is a health plan that falls under the direction of the _____.
   a. Centers for Medicaid Services
   b. Health and Welfare systems of states
   c. Centers for Medicare and Medicaid Service
   d. Health and Welfare System of America

2. PPOs and HMOs are health insurance systems that may require a patient to _____.
   a. Obtain a referral for certain health-care services
   b. Take a physical prior to insuring the patient
   c. Maintain a zero balance on their plan
   d. Have prescription filled a only one particular pharmacy

3. Penalties for insurance fraud may include
   a. Loss of employment, fines, and suspension.
   b. Loss of degree, fines, and loss of employment.
   c. Loss of employment, fines, and incarceration.
   d. Incarceration, suspension, and fines.

4. Adjudication is the process of
   a. Making something wrong right again.
   b. Correcting a mistake made on a prescription.
   c. Making up for lost wages.
   d. Transmitting information to a third-party payer.

5. A third-party payer may reject a claim for any of the following:
   a. Patient date of birth, marital status, address verification
   b. Patient date of birth, marital status, wrong type of computer system
   c. Wrong type of computer system, address verification, marital status
   d. Wrong type of computer system, wrong date, marital status

6. A network approved provider for an HMO is also known as
   a. Primary Care Physician—PCP
   b. Patient Care Maintenance—PCM
   c. Mandatory Care Provider—MCP
   d. Maintenance Care Provider—MCP

7. There are four different parts to Medicare, Medicare A, B, C, and D. Medicare _____ is the prescription drug plan.
   a. Medicare A
   b. Medicare B and D
   c. None of these are correct
   d. Medicare D

8. Under a Worker's Compensation claim the employer is responsible for
   a. Charges incurred through hospital expenses only.
   b. Charges only after the therapy is completed
   c. Any health expenses related to the injury.
   d. Any health expenses related to the injury, with the exception of prescription fee.

9. A predetermined fee a patient must pay out of pocket is known as a
   a. Small expense fee.
   b. Co-pay.
   c. Administrative fee.
   d. Pharmacy co-op fee.

10. Laws regarding health insurance fraud were established under the _____.
    a. Health Insurance Accounts and Portability Act
    b. Health Insurance Fraud and Liability Act
    c. Affordable Care Act
    d. Health Insurance Portability and Accountability Act

10 Pharmacy Information Systems Usage and Applications

Learning objectives for this chapter will include:

- Usage of Computer Physician Order Entry (CPOE).

- Usage of Electronic Medical Records (EMR).

- Maintaining pharmacy databases, applications, and documentation.

- Usage of Automated Dispensing Cabinets (ADC).

There can be no denying the fact that the use of technology has affected every corner of the world as well as every aspect of our lives. From smartphones that read text messages and give us voice directions to highly evolved computer systems that store hundreds of thousands of bits of information, technology has certainly claimed its place in the day-to-day operations of our working environment. The use of technology in the practice of pharmacy has been no less dramatic.

Over the last decade the practice of pharmacy, and ultimately the practice of medicine, has gone from using handwritten prescriber orders to a system that allows the prescriber to directly input a patient's orders into the health systems computer. Computerized Physician Order Entry (CPOE) has not only made the patient order entry more streamlined and efficient, but also a much safer experience for the patient as well.

CPOE is now the standard for health-care systems across the United States. The process of CPOE is a simple one, but also one that must be implemented with care. While the prescriber is responsible for inputting the patient order into the system, the health system's pharmacy will largely be responsible for assuring the formulary information linked to the computer system is correct.

According to the Institute of Medicine's report, *"To Err is Human,"* medication errors alone are responsible for more than 7000, deaths each year. This report, which was originally published in 2000, forced the health-care profession to take a hard long look at the process that was causing such unimaginable statistics. Administration of the wrong drug, drug-to-drug interactions, overlooked drug allergies, illegible handwriting, and decimal points incorrectly placed were just a few of the reasons that contributed to these statistics. It was clear that a better system of checks and balance was needed, and the answer was Computerized Physician Order Entry.

As stated earlier, pharmacy plays a large role in the implementation and maintenance of CPOE systems. A health system's formulary is maintained by the health system's pharmacy. Ordering drug products, inventorying drug stock, and making changes based upon formularies are just a few of the tasks delegated to pharmacy. CPOE systems are linked directly to a health system's formulary. If the information about the formulary is incorrect, then the risk of error goes up exponentially.

Process of CPOE

When a new drug is adopted into a health system's formulary, the pharmacy is responsible for making sure the item can be correctly identified within the computer system. This means the pharmacy must input all information about the new drug into the systems interface. The process begins by first identifying the drug product, and assuring it is the item to be added. Pharmacy technicians are very often required to complete this type of task.

- Verify the drug ordered is the drug to be input into the system.
- Input all drug information into the computer.
  - Drug name, brand, and generic if applicable
  - Drug strength
  - Quantity of drug—for example, Lisinopril 10 mg 100 count bottle
  - Manufacture
  - Drug NDC (national drug code)

Once all the information has been correctly identified and verified, the pharmacy technician will then scan the item's bar code to ensure the item input into the computer systems links to the information in the system. If any of this information is incorrect, it may cause several issues.

- The incorrect drug may be linked to the bar code.
- Nursing staff may not be able to scan drug orders or medications at the patient's bedside.
- Prescribers may not be able to choose the correct drug product.
- Pharmacy staff may not be able to verify restocks in Automatic Dispensing Cabinets (ADC).
- When restocking pharmacy shelves, pharmacy staff may not be able to verify the correct drug product.

All of these issues have the potential to create a medication error and that wholly defeats the purpose of the implementation of systems like CPOE. It is for this reason accuracy when adding new formulary items or creating a formulary that will be linked to CPOE is critical. As with all processes, pharmacy accuracy is a requirement of safe patient medication practices. CPOE can be extremely effective, but only when those completing the tasks are aware of the extreme need for accuracy during the formulary building process.

Once the formulary information is correctly associated with the drug's bar code and NDC number, the prescriber will be able to choose the correct drug for the patient. Another safeguard of CPOE is safety alerts. CPOE systems help link all of the patient's information into one central field for the prescriber and other health professional to view on screen, whereas with a paper system, the health-care professional would need to obtain reports from various departments, pharmacy, lab, and nursing before an informed decision could be made. This also meant that there was a higher risk for error, simply because there was a greater risk of information being missed. A good example might be patient drug allergies.

A system of checks and balances within the CPOE software allows prescribers, pharmacists, and other health-care professionals to see drug-to-drug interaction, allergy to drug information, duplication of therapy, or other information that may help prevent an adverse drug event. However, CPOE is not an errorless system since alerts are able to overridden by certain users.

Pharmacy technicians should be particularly aware of this idiosyncrasy of CPOE. When inputting of patient information or orders into a computer system using CPOE, pharmacy technicians should never take it upon themselves to override drug alerts. If a drug alert does appear, the pharmacy technician should immediately alert the pharmacist. Once the pharmacist views the alert and verifies the information, the pharmacy technician may proceed with the order, but only after the pharmacist has been able to make a clinical decision about the drug alert.

Bar Code Scanning

The use of bar code scanning in the practice of pharmacy has been critical to the development of safe medication practices. Bar code scanning directly links systems like CPOE. Nurses are able to scan a patient's Electronic Medical Record (EMR) and then the patient's drug order to verify that the medication they are about to give is correct. Of course, as we have mentioned several times, if this information is incorrect, medication errors may occur.

Bar code scanning is also used to link patient information to insurance companies, or to a pharmacy's patient information database. Wholesalers and pharmacies use bar code scanning to reorder drug stock or to alert staff about low stock. However, bar code scanning can only be as effective as their users.

Just like CPOE, bar code scanning may go overlooked, especially if a workload seems particularly heavy, or if there is a system error that doesn't allow the bar code to function properly. Pharmacy technician should never forgo the use of an implanted process such as bar code scanning. It is a safety measure that should be followed through regardless of the workload.

When using bar code scanning, pharmacy technicians must ensure to

- Verify drug information when inputing new products into the system.
  - NDC number
  - Drug name—brand and generic
  - Drug strength
  - Drug quantity—example Benadryl 25 mg capsules #100 per bottle
  - Drug manufacture

If this information is incorrect in the system, it will not link with the item's bar code or the wrong bar code will be linked to the wrong item. Always verify information, and it is also a good practice to have a verified check from another coworker or the pharmacist.

As with CPOE, bar code scanning is a useful tool, but only when the system information is accurate. Not only can it make for a safer experience for the patient, but also it allows the pharmacy to work more efficiently as a health-care team. Restock and reordering processes are handled much more accurately and efficiently. Patient profile information is more easily transmitted to insurance companies, and inventory controls become much more cost effective, which in turn all provides a better and safer experience for the patient.

Automated Dispensing Cabinets

Automated dispensing cabinets (ADCs) are another shining example of technology at work within the health-care field. ADCs can be implemented in virtually every area of a health-care system, from surgical suites to emergency departments. Some common names of ADCs include Pyxis, Omnicell, Medselect, MedDispense, and AcuDose Rx. Regardless of the name, the purpose and use of these machines are all the same: to provide a safe and effective medication therapy for the patient.

An automated dispensing cabinet is a secure cabinet linked to a health-system computer that allows medications to be dispensed to the patient in a cost-effective and time-saving manner. As with any instrument that deals with the process of procuring and storing medication, ADCs are the responsibility of the pharmacy and the pharmacy staff. All medications that are stored in an ADC are linked from the pharmacy's formulary to the ADC, much in the same way they are linked to the CPOE.

When a prescriber orders a drug product for a patient, the order is sent electronically to the pharmacy for verification. Once the order has been verified, the drug label can be printed and the order is filled. When ADCs are used within a patient area, such as a nursing unit or surgical suite, the drug order is verified and sent electronically to the patient's profile on the ADC. When nurses or other health-care providers are ready to administer the order, they access the ADC screen, find the patient by name or medical record number, and select the drug to be administered. Once the correct drug has been selected, the drawer of the ADC where the drug is stored will open and the nurse may retrieve the drug for administration.

Again, if the drug information is not correct, the wrong drug may be dispensed or may not be really available. Some ADCs have individual drug pockets that will open upon selection and others have drawers that open with a flashing light that indicate the correct drug to be dispensed. Controlled substances, such as morphine, may also be stored in ADCs but are typically stored in individual pockets that only allow for a single drug item to be dispensed, and require a count back when a product is dispensed from the drawer.

Not only do ADCs allow for a safer drug experience for the patient by decreasing errors, but also they allow for a faster administration in emergency situations, such as in an emergency department or surgical suite, and decrease drug diversion. Drug diversion is simply the theft of drug products. Controlled substances are most commonly used in drug diversion. Health-care professionals are exposed to controlled substances on a daily basis and drug diversion involving nursing, pharmacy, and other health-care staff is unfortunately becoming an increasing issue. ADCs help to alleviate a large part of this problem, because a record of all transactions, restocks, patient order administrations, and new stock is readily available within the system.

Pharmacy is solely responsible for the stock and restock of ADCs as well as investigation of any issues related to suspected drug diversion. Pharmacy technicians are often the personnel responsible for maintaining ADCs as well as investigating drug diversion claims. It is essential that record-keeping process for ADCs be implemented on a daily basis. ADCs that have poor record-keeping process also make for poor investigative tools when dealing with issues of drug diversion. Remember, the pharmacy is ultimately responsible for all issues related to the purchase, sale, and issue of controlled substances. State boards of pharmacies and the DEA will look the pharmacy department for answers relating to drug diversion and incomplete or inaccurate record keeping will only add to these issues.

Keeping all this in mind, pharmacy technicians tasked with the maintenance of ADCs should address any issues related to stock counts or patient administration records immediately. The trail is easier to follow if it is investigated earlier rather than later. Paper trails can be not only time consuming, but also difficult to follow, which only complicates the issues at hand.

Electronic Medical Records

CPOE, Bar Code Scanning, and ADCs are all linked electronically to one another. Electronic Medical Records (EMRs) may also be linked to these systems. EMRs are used to provide health-care professionals with instant access to a patient's medical history. They include such information as

- Patient demographics
  - Name
  - Date of Birth
  - Address
  - Phone numbers
- Patient medical history
  - Past surgical procedures
  - Hospital stays
  - Illnesses

- ■ Testing—current and past
- ■ Medication—current and past
- Insurance and billing information
- Patient medical record number

All of this information is essential in order for the health-care worker to provide the best possible course of treatment for the patient. Pharmacy uses EMRs to review patient medication orders and to develop course of treatment. Although the information may be readily available, it is important to remember it is highly protected information and should always remain secure and protected.

Under the Health Insurance Portability and Accountability Act (HIPAA), health-care professional may not share or unnecessarily obtain information concerning a patient's medical history. This is an issue that is taken quite seriously and violations of HIPAA can carry suspension, dismissal from employment, fines, and even incarceration. As health-care professionals, pharmacy technicians are expected to maintain the security and privacy of the patients they serve. It is never right to access a patient's medical record based on your own personal curiosity, and certainly never because the patient is a relative or neighbor. Complete patient care is protection of all aspects, including patient information.

SUMMARY

Finally, pharmacy technicians should keep in mind that technology, while effective and largely more efficient than the earlier paper process, is only as effective and efficient as the information that it helps to store. If drug information such as NDC numbers or bar code information is not input accurately into an electronic system, patients will not be any safer than they were with the paper process.

Pharmacy technicians are often tasked with maintaining electronic systems.

With the need for more pharmacist based clinical intervention, the pharmacy technician will be required to be the keeper of the electronic systems mentioned within this chapter, and ultimately be key to the safety and efficiency of patient drug therapies.

CHAPTER REVIEW QUESTIONS

1. CPOE systems have built-in alert systems when there is a potential for drug error. When the pharmacy technician is alerted to such an error, they should
   a. Alert their IT department.
   b. Call the prescriber.
   c. Alert the pharmacist.
   d. Override because it's a system glitch.

2. CPOE is linked to the drug product's
   a. Color.
   b. NDC number and bar code.
   c. Manufacturer's computer system.
   d. Patient's home phone number.

3. According to the Health Institute's "To Err is Human" report, more than _____ deaths each year are drug error related.
   a. 10 thousand
   b. 7 million
   c. 10 million
   d. 7 thousand

4. If a drug product is entered into a CPOE system incorrectly, nursing staff may be
   a. Unable to scan the order and drug at the patient's bedside.
   b. unable to file a patient report.
   c. Incapable of providing complete patient care.
   d. Unable to clock out on time.

5. In health-care systems, bar code scanning is typically linked to a patient's _____.
   a. Previous administration records
   b. Insurance record and billing
   c. Food choices
   d. Electronic Medical Record

6. Maintenance of automated dispensing cabinets, or ADCs, is the responsibility of
   a. The IT department, because they are linked to computer systems.
   b. Drug manufacturers, because they store medication.
   c. The pharmacy department.
   d. The nursing department.

7. Drug diversion is simply the _____.
   a. The permission required to use controlled substances
   b. Stealing of prescription drugs by a health-care professional
   c. Pharmacy term that means the same as restocking
   d. A DEA form used to procure controlled substances

8. The DEA and the state board of pharmacy will ultimately look to the _____ for answers concerning drug diversion.
   a. The local police
   b. The patient to whom the medication was administered
   c. The nurse that administered the medication
   d. The pharmacy department

9. EMR stands for _____.
   a. Emergency Medical Record
   b. Electronic Maintenance Record
   c. Enveloped Medical Record
   d. Electronic Medical Record

10. EMR information is protected by _____.
    a. The Affordable Care Act
    b. The Health Information Profitability and Accountability Act
    c. The Health Information Portability and Profitability Act
    d. None of these

11 Review of Pharmacy Calculations

Learning objectives for this chapter will include:

- Recognizing and converting the various systems of measurement.
- Calculating ratios and proportions.
- Performing dosage calculations.
- Solving concentration and dilution problems.
- Calculating milliequivalents.
- Calculating flow rates.
- Solving alligations.
- Performing business calculations.

Introduction

Pharmacy calculations are often a large portion of the national pharmacy technician certification exams, and most students are very intimidated by math. However, it is imperative that pharmacy technicians be comfortable performing pharmacy calculations, because almost every aspect of pharmacy involves some sort of calculation. Therefore, to be successful in the certification exam and in practice, pharmacy technicians must master pharmaceutical calculations.

Systems of Measurement

As a pharmacy technician, you will rely on three systems of measurement to perform specific pharmacy calculations: the metric system, the household system, and the apothecary system. The metric system is the most widely recognized and utilized system for measurement in health care, but technicians must still be able to work with all the three systems.

Tables 11-1 through 11-4 provide a review of the common metric prefixes and equivalents when working with the three systems of measurement.

Ratios and Proportions

Most pharmacy calculations can be solved either using an algebraic equation or using ratios and proportions. The ratio-and-proportion technique establishes two fractions that are equal to each other, using "given" and "needed" information in the problem.

Table 11-1 Metric System Prefixes with Standard Measures

	UNIT	ABBREVIATION	EQUIVALENTS
Weight	gram	g or gm	1 g = 1000 mg = 1,000,000 mcg
	milligram	mg	1 mg = 1000 mcg = 0.001 g
	microgram	mcg	1 mcg = 0.001 mg = 0.000001 g
	kilogram	kg	1 kg = 1000 g
Volume	liter	L or l	1 L = 1000 mL
	milliliter	mL or ml	1 mL = 1 cc = 0.001 L
	cubic centimeter	cc	1 cc = 1 mL = 0.001 L
Length	meter	m	1 m = 100 cm = 1000 mm
	centimeter	cm	1 cm = 0.01 m = 10 nm
	millimeter	mm	1 mm = 0.001 m = 0.1 cm

Table 11-2 Household Measure Equivalents

3 teaspoons	=	1 tablespoon
2 tablespoons	=	1 fluid ounce
8 fluid ounces	=	1 cup
2 cups	=	1 pint
2 pints	=	1 quart
4 quarts	=	1 gallon

Table 11-3 Household-to-Metric Conversions

HOUSEHOLD MEASURE		METRIC EQUIVALENT
1 teaspoon	=	5 mL
1 tablespoon	=	15 mL
1 fluid ounce	=	30 mL
1 pint	=	473 mL
1 gallon	=	3785 mL
1 cup	=	240 mL
1 ounce	=	28.35 g
1 pound	=	454 g
1 pound	=	16 oz

Once the ratios and proportions are determined, you can solve for the unknown x. When setting up ratios and proportions, determine what you "know" about the problem and set it equal to what is "needed or unknown," which is x. Always ensure that all units of measure are equivalent.

$$\text{What you know} = \text{What you need}$$
$$(\text{drug strength}) = (\text{patient dose})$$

Table 11-4 Apothecary-to-Metric Conversions

APOTHECARY MEASURE		METRIC EQUIVALENT
16.23 minims	=	1 mL
1 fluid dram	=	4 mL
1 fluid ounce	=	30 mL
1 ounce	=	8 drams
1 dram	=	60 grains
6 fluid ounces	=	180 mL
8 fluid ounces	=	240 mL
16 fluid ounces	=	500 mL
32 fluid ounces	=	1000 mL
1 grain	=	65 mg
1 ounce	=	480 grains
15 grains	=	1 g
1 pound	=	16 oz
2.2 pounds	=	1 kg

EXAMPLE: How much Amoxil, 250 mg/5 ml, should a patient take for each dose of the following prescription? Amoxicillin, 375 mg po qid.

First, set up the problem. Be sure that all units of measure are the same on each side of the equation:

$$\text{What you know} = \text{What you need}$$

$$\frac{250 \text{ mg}}{5 \text{ ml}} = \frac{375 \text{ mg}}{x \text{ ml}}$$

Now, solve for x and cross-multiply:

$$250\,(x) = 375\,(5)$$
$$250x = 1875$$

Divide by 250 to get x by itself:

$$\frac{250x}{250} = \frac{1875}{250}$$
$$x = 7.5$$

Answer: $x = 7.5$ ml or 1½ tsp

Following are some examples of how ratios and proportions can be used in pharmacy calculations.

example 11.1

Convert 2.5 oz to grams.

We know that 1 oz = 30 g, so we can set up the following ratios and proportions:

$$\frac{1\,\text{oz}}{30\,\text{g}} = \frac{2.5\,\text{oz}}{x\,\text{g}}$$

$$x = 7.5$$

Cross-multiply and divide by x:

$$1x = 75$$
$$x = 75\,\text{g}$$

Answer: 2.5 oz is equivalent to 75 g.

IMPORTANT

Concentrations of many medications are expressed as a percent strength, such as Bactroban 2%. The percent strength represents how many grams of active ingredient are in 100 mL (liquid preparations) or 100 g (solid preparations). In other words, Bactroban 2% ointment would contain 2 g of drug per 100 g.

---

example 11.2

How many grams of drug are contained in 1 L of a 25% solution?

By definition, a 25% solution contains 25 g of drug per 100 mL; therefore, we can set up the following ratios and proportions:

$$\frac{25\,\text{g}}{100\,\text{mL}} = \frac{x}{1000\,\text{mL}}$$

Cross-multiply:

$$100x = 25{,}000$$

Divide both sides by 100:

$$\frac{100x}{100} = \frac{25{,}000}{100}$$
$$x = 250$$

Answer: $x = 250$ g. Therefore, 1 L of a 25% solution contains 250 g of drug.

example 11.3

How many *milligrams* of drug are there in 500 g of a 30% ointment?

By definition, a 30% ointment contains 30 g of drug per 100 g of ointment. Therefore, we can set up the following ratios and proportions:

$$\frac{30\,\text{g}}{100\,\text{g}} = \frac{x}{500\,\text{g}}$$

Cross-multiply:

$$100x = 15{,}000$$

Divide both sides by 100:

$$\frac{100x}{100} = \frac{15{,}000}{100}$$
$$x = 150$$

$x = 150$ g. However, the question asked for *milligrams*, so the answer must be converted to milligrams:

Cross-multiply:

$$\frac{1\,\text{g}}{150\,\text{g}} = \frac{1000\,\text{mg}}{x}$$
$$1x = 150{,}000$$

Divide both sides by 1:

$$\frac{1\,x}{1} = \frac{150{,}000}{1}$$
$$x = 150{,}000$$

Thus, $x = 150{,}000$ mg.

Answer: Therefore, 500 g of a 30% ointment contains 150,000 mg of drug.

Dosage Calculations

Dosage calculations, which can include determining the number of doses, dispensing quantities, or ingredient quantities, are all performed using ratios and proportions.

example 11.4

Rx: Amoxicillin, 125 mg/5 mL, #150 mL, Sig: 1 tsp po tid. How many doses will be dispensed in all? What is the prescription day's supply?

We know that tid means three times per day; therefore, we can set up the following ratios and proportions:

$$\frac{1\,\text{tsp}}{5\,\text{mL}} = \frac{x\,\text{tsp}}{150\,\text{mL}}$$

Cross-multiply:

$$5x = 150$$

Divide both sides by 5:

$$\frac{5x}{5} = \frac{150}{5}$$

Answer: $x = 30$ tsp. Therefore, this order contains 30 tsp, or 30 doses in total.

Next, how long will the prescription last if the patient takes the drug tid?

$$\frac{3\,\text{doses}}{1\,\text{day}} = \frac{30\,\text{doses}}{x\,\text{days}}$$

Cross-multiply:

$$3x = 30$$

Divide both sides by 3:

$$\frac{3\,x}{3} = \frac{30}{3}$$

Answer: $x = 10$ days. Therefore, this order will last for 10 days.

example 11.5

Rx: Amoxicillin, 125 mg/5 mL, #150 mL, Sig: 1 tsp po tid. How many grams of amoxicillin are there in 150 mL?

There are 125 mg per teaspoon, so we can set up the following ratios and proportions:

$$\frac{125 \text{ mg}}{5 \text{ mL}} = \frac{x}{150 \text{ mL}}$$

Cross-multiply:

$$5x = 18{,}750$$

Divide both sides by 5:

$$\frac{5x}{5} = \frac{18{,}750}{5}$$

$$x = 3750 \text{ mg}$$

Answer: Because $x = 3750$ mg, this order contains 3.75 g or 3750 mg of amoxicillin.

example 11.6

Rx: Hydroxyzine, 20 mg IV, q4–6h prn itching. How many milliliters of 25-mg/ml hydroxyzine are needed for each dose?

We know the drug strength is 25 mg/ml, and we need to know how many milliliters are needed for a 20-mg dose, so the proportion is

$$\frac{25 \text{ mg}}{\text{mL}} = \frac{20 \text{ mg}}{x \text{ ml}}$$

Cross-multiply:

$$25(x) = 20(1)$$

Divide both sides by 25:

$$\frac{25x}{25} = \frac{20}{25}$$

Answer: Because $x = 0.8$, we need 0.8 ml of 25-mg/ml hydroxyzine for a 20-mg dose.

$$x = 0.8$$

Pediatric Dosing

Children and infants often require special considerations when calculating appropriate dosages. Common methods of calculating pediatric dosages are by body weight (mg/kg), by Fried's rule for infants, or by Clark's or Young's rule for children. When calculating by mg/kg, you will first need to convert the patient's weight from pounds to kilograms.

FORMULA

Weight Conversion

$$1 \text{ kg} = 2.2 \text{ lb}$$

Pediatric Dosing Based on Body Weight

example 11.7

A child weighs 45 lb; what is her weight in kilograms?

Using the weight conversion formula, you can set up the ratios and proportions:

$$\frac{1 \text{ kg}}{2.2 \text{ lb}} = \frac{x}{45 \text{ lb}}$$

Cross-multiply:

$$45 = 2.2(x)$$

Divide both sides by 2.2:

$$x = 20.45$$

Answer: This patient weighs 20.45 kg.

example 11.8

For the same patient as in Example 11.7, what is an appropriate dose for the following prescription? Rx: Ventolin syrup, 0.2 mg/kg/day in three divided doses.

Using the weight conversion from Example 11.7, set up the equation and solve:

$$0.2 \text{ mg} \times 20.45 \text{ kg} = 4.09$$

So, this patient should receive 4.09 mg/day. Divide by 3 to calculate how much the patient will take for each dose.

Answer: Therefore, each dose will have approximately 1.36 mg.

example 11.9

Rx: Amoxicillin, 30 mg/kg/day divided q12h × 10 days. How much will the patient take with each dose, and how much should be dispensed for a 10-day supply? The drug available is amoxicillin, 125 mg/5 ml susp, and the patient weighs 27.5 lb.

First, convert the patient's weight from pounds to kilograms:

$$\frac{2.2 \text{ lb}}{1 \text{ kg}} = \frac{27.5 \text{ lb}}{x \text{ kg}}$$

Cross-multiply:

$$2.2 \,(x) = 27.5 \,(1)$$

Divide both sides by 2.2:

$$\frac{2.2 \, x}{2.2} = \frac{27.5}{2.2}$$

$$x = 13.64$$

The patient's weight is 12.5 kg.

Next, you need 30 mg/kg per day divided q12h:

$$30 \text{ mg} \times 12.5 \text{ kg} = 375 \text{ mg per day}$$

$$\frac{375 \text{ mg}}{2 \text{ doses per day}} = 187.5 \text{ mg per dose}$$

Next, to determine how much should be given for each dose, set up a proportion:

$$\frac{125 \text{ mg}}{5 \text{ ml}} = \frac{187.5 \text{ mg}}{x}$$

Cross-multiply:

$$125 \, (x) = 187.5(5)$$

Divide both sides by 125:

$$\frac{125}{125} = \frac{937.5}{125}$$

$$x = 7.5$$

Answer: The patient dose is 7.5 ml.

To determine the amount to dispense for the prescription:

$$7.5 \text{ ml} \times 2 \text{ doses per day} \times 10 \text{ days} = 150 \text{ ml}$$

Pediatric Dosing Using Fried's, Clark's, and Young's Rules

FORMULA

Fried's Rule for Infants

$$\frac{\text{Age (in months)} \times \text{Adult dose}}{150} = \text{Dose for infant}$$

example 11.10

The recommended adult dose for penicillin is 250 mg po q6h. What would the dose be for a 9-month-old infant?

Use Fried's rule:

$$\frac{9 \text{ months} \times 250 \text{ mg}}{150} = \text{Infant's dose}$$

$$\text{Infant's dose} = 15 \text{ mg}$$

Answer: The answer is 15 mg. Therefore, the penicillin dose for a 9-month-old infant is 15 mg every 6 hr.

FORMULA

Clark's Rule

$$\frac{\text{Weight (pounds)} \times \text{Adult dose}}{150} = \text{Dose for child}$$

example 11.11

The recommended adult dose for erythromycin ethylsuccinate is 400 mg every 6 hr. What is the dose for a child who weighs 40 kg?

First, to use Clark's rule, the weight has to be in pounds, so convert 40 kg to pounds:

$$\frac{1 \text{ kg}}{2.2 \text{ lb}} = \frac{40 \text{ kg}}{x \text{ lb}}$$

Cross-multiply:

$$2.2(40) = 1(x)$$

Divide both sides by 2.2:

$$\frac{40}{2.2} = \frac{1x}{2.2}$$

The patient weighs 88 lb.

$$x = 88$$

Now, plug weight into the Clark's rule formula:

$$\frac{88 \times 400}{150} = \text{child's dose}$$

$$\frac{35,200}{150} = 234.666 \approx 234.67 \text{ mg}$$

Answer: Therefore, the dose for a child weighing 40 kg is 234.67 mg.

FORMULA

Young's Rule

$$\frac{\text{Age (in years)} \times \text{Adult dose}}{\text{Age} + 12} = \text{Dose for child}$$

---

example 11.12

The recommended adult dose for amoxicillin is 500 mg po q6h. What would the dose be for an 8-year-old child?

Use Young's rule:

$$\frac{8 \times 500 \text{ mg}}{8 + 12} = \text{Child's dose}$$

$$\frac{4000}{20} = 200$$

Answer: The dose for an 8-year-old child is 200 mg.

Concentrations

Concentration calculations are used to determine the percent strength or the amount of active ingredient in a particular preparation. *Percent* means parts per 100. The *percent strength* is the amount of the desired ingredient in the final product.

When solids are dissolved in liquids, the solid is considered the *solute* and the liquid is considered the *solvent*. When a liquid is mixed with another liquid, the liquid that occurs in the smaller quantity is the *solute* and the larger quantity of liquid is the *solvent*. Percentage concentrations of pharmaceuticals may be classified in one of the following three types:

$$W/W\% = \frac{gm}{100\ gm} = \text{Number of grams of the drug in 100 g of the final product}$$

$$W/V\% = \frac{gm}{100\ ml} = \text{Number of grams of the drug in 100 ml of the final product}$$

$$V/V\% = \frac{ml}{100\ ml} = \text{Number of milliliters of the drug in 100 ml of the final product}$$

EXAMPLES:

1. How many grams of dextrose are there in 500 ml of D50W?
   D50W means that there are 50 g of dextrose in 100 ml of final product.
   Therefore,

$$\frac{50\ gm}{100\ ml} = \frac{x\ gm}{500\ ml} \rightarrow 100x = 50 \times 500 \rightarrow x = \frac{25,000}{100} \rightarrow x = 250\ gm$$

2. How many grams of NaCl are there in 1 L of normal saline?
   Normal saline is 0.9% sodium chloride (NaCl), so there are 0.9 g of NaCl in 100 ml of normal saline.

$$\frac{0.9\ gm}{100\ ml} = \frac{x\ gm}{1000\ ml} \rightarrow 100x = 0.9 \times 1000 \rightarrow x = \frac{900}{100} \rightarrow x = 9\ gm$$

example 11.13

If there are 8 g of active ingredient in 240 g of an ointment, what is the W/W%?

$$\frac{8\ g}{240} = \frac{x\ g}{100}$$

Solve for *x* by cross-multiplying:

$$240(x) = 8(100)$$

Divide both sides by 240:

$$\frac{240x}{240} = \frac{800}{240}$$

$$x = 3.33$$

Answer: There are 3.33 g of active ingredient in every 100 g of ointment. Therefore, by definition, the percent strength is 3.3%.

example 11.14

If there are 10 g of active ingredient in 500 ml of sodium chloride, what is the W/V%?

$$\frac{10\ g}{500\ ml} = \frac{x\ g}{100\ ml}$$

Solve for *x* by cross-multiplying:

$$500(x) = 10(100)$$

Divide both sides by 500:

$$\frac{500x}{500} = \frac{1000}{500}$$

$$x = 2$$

Answer: There are 2 g of active ingredient in every 100 ml of sodium chloride. Therefore, by definition, the percent strength of the solution is 2%.

---

example 11.15

If 40 mL of active ingredient is diluted to 1 L, what is the V/V%?

$$\frac{40 \text{ mL}}{1000 \text{ mL}} = \frac{x \text{ mL}}{100 \text{ mL}}$$

Solve for x by cross-multiplying:

$$1000(x) = 40(100)$$

Divide both sides by 1000:

$$\frac{1000x}{1000} = \frac{4000}{1000}$$

$$x = 4$$

Answer: There are 4 mL of active ingredient in every 100 mL of solution. Therefore, by definition, the percent strength is 4%.

---

example 11.16

If 1 pint of a solution contains 50 g of active ingredient, what is the percent strength (W/V)?

$$\frac{50 \text{ gm}}{473 \text{ ml}} = \frac{x \text{ gm}}{100 \text{ ml}}$$

Solve for x by cross-multiplying:

$$473(x) = 50(100)$$

Divide both sides by 473:

$$\frac{473}{473} = \frac{5000}{473}$$

$$x = 10.57$$

Answer: There are 10.57 g of active ingredient in every 100 ml of solution. Therefore, by definition, the percent strength is 10.57%.

---

example 11.17

If you mix 30 g of 65% hydrocortisone (HC) with 60 g of 13% HC, what is the percent strength (W/W) of the final product?

First, we need to determine how many grams of HC are there in each individual component.

65% HC:

$$\frac{65\ gm}{100\ gm} = \frac{x\ gm}{30\ gm}$$

Solve for x by cross-multiplying:

$$100(x) = 65(30)$$

Divide both sides by 100:

$$\frac{100x}{100} = \frac{1950}{100}$$

$$x = 19.5$$

Answer: There are 19.5 g of HC in 30 g of 65% hydrocortisone.

13% HC:

$$\frac{13\ gm}{100\ gm} = \frac{x\ gm}{60\ gm}$$

Solve for x by cross-multiplying:

$$100(x) = 60(13)$$

Divide both sides by 100:

$$\frac{100x}{100} = \frac{780}{100}$$

$$x = 7.8$$

Answer: There are 7.8 g of HC in 60 g of 13% hydrocortisone.

Therefore, if we mix 30 g of 65% HC and 60 g of 13% HC, we will have 90 g of product containing 27.3 g of hydrocortisone (19.5 + 7.8).

To determine the final concentration:

$$\frac{x\ gm}{100\ gm} = \frac{27.3\ gm}{90\ gm}$$

Solve for x by cross-multiplying:

$$90(x) = 27.3(100)$$

Divide both sides by 90:

$$\frac{90x}{90} = \frac{2730}{90}$$

$$x = 30.3$$

Answer: $x = 30.3$, so the final concentration of the 90 g is 30.3%.

Dilutions

Oftentimes a pharmacy has to dilute a concentrated stock solution with distilled or sterile water to compound a less concentrated solution for a prescription. Pharmacies may also dilute a concentrated solid preparation (cream, unguent, paste, etc.) with an inactive ingredient (aquaphor, vaseline, lanolin, etc.) to prepare a less concentrated solid preparation. The following formulas can be used for diluting stock solutions or preparations:

Initial volume $\times$ Initial strength = Final volume $\times$ Final strength

$$V_1 \times S_1 = V_2 \times S_2$$

Initial quantity $\times$ Initial strength = Final quantity $\times$ Final strength

$$Q_1 \times S_1 = Q_2 \times S_2$$

Initial volume (V_1) or quantity (Q_1) = Volume/weight of solution #1 (stock solution)

Initial strength (S_1) = Strength of solution #1 (stock solution)

Final volume (V_2) or quantity (Q_2) = Volume/weight of solution #2 (desired solution)

Final strength (S_2) = Strength of solution #2 (desired solution)

EXAMPLES:

1. How many milliliters of 70% alcohol can be made from 1 pint of 91% alcohol?

$$V_1 \times S_1 = V_2 \times S_2$$

$$473 \text{ ml} \times 91\% = x \text{ ml} \times 70\% \rightarrow 43{,}043 = 70x = \frac{43{,}043}{70} = x \rightarrow x = 614.9 \text{ ml}$$

2. How much water will be needed for the previous problem?

Total volume prepared (70%) = 614.9 ml

Volume of stock solution used (91%) = −473 ml

Volume of distilled water needed = 141.9 ml

Therefore, if you dilute 1 pint of 91% alcohol with 141.9 ml of distilled water, you will obtain 614.9 ml of 70% alcohol solution.

3. How many grams of 2.5% hydrocortisone (HC) cream should be mixed with an ointment base to prepare 500 gm of 1% HC?

$$Q_1 \times S_1 = Q_2 \times S_2$$

$$x \text{ gm} \times 2.5\% = 500 \text{ ml} \times 1\% \rightarrow 2.5x = 500 \rightarrow x = \frac{500}{2.5} \rightarrow x = 200 \text{ gm}$$

4. How much of the ointment base will be needed for the previous problem?

Total amount prepared (1%) =   500 gm

Amount of stock prepared used (2.5%) = −200 gm

Volume of distilled water needed =   300 gm

Therefore, you will need to mix 200 g of 2.5% HC with 300 g of ointment base to prepare 500 g of 1% HC.

IMPORTANT

When diluting concentrated stock solutions or preparations, the volume or weight and the strength have to be in the same unit of measure on each side of the equals sign.

EXAMPLE: You need to prepare 473 ml of a 200-mg/ml sorbitol solution. You have only a 70% sorbitol solution available.

Note that the strengths of the desired solution and the stock solution are not in the same unit. The strengths have to be converted to the same unit of measure before they can be plugged into the formula. You can either change 200 mg/ml to percent *or* change 70% to mg/ml.

example 11.18

How much of 25% HCl stock solution is required to make 1 oz of 10% HCl solution?

Use the formula $V_1 \times S_1 = V_2 \times S_2$.

$$x \times 25 = 30 \times 10$$
$$25x = 300$$

Divide both sides by 25:

$$\frac{25x}{25} = \frac{300}{25}$$
$$x = 12$$

Answer: Therefore, 12 mL of the 25% stock solution is needed to make 30 mL of the desired solution.

Milliequivalents

Milliequivalents (mEq) is a unit of measure that is commonly used in compounding total parenteral nutrition (TPN). These units may look intimidating, but you can treat them like any other unit of measure and make calculations using ratios and proportions.

example 11.19

Electrolyte	Stock Vial	Rx Order	How Many mL?
NaCl	4 mEq/mL	40 mEq	_____

Using the information provided, set up the ratios and proportions to solve:

$$\frac{4 \text{ mEq}}{1 \text{ ml}} = \frac{40 \text{ mEq}}{x \text{ ml}}$$

Cross-multiply:

$$40 = 4x$$

Divide both sides by 4:

$$x = 10$$

So, 10 mL of 4-mEq/ml NaCl should be added to the TPN.

Intravenous Flow Rates

Intravenous (IV) flow rates are commonly expressed in either ml/hr or gtt/min. When the rate is expressed in ml/hr, it is called the IV rate, which is the speed at which an IV solution is infused into a patient. When the rate is expressed in gtt/min it is called the drip rate, which is the speed at which the IV administration set is calibrated to in order to achieve the IV rate. For example, if a patient has an IV ordered at 100 ml/hr, the nurse has to calculate the drip rate so she can calibrate the IV administration set appropriately to set an IV rate of 100 ml/hr.

FORMULA

IV Rate

$$\frac{\text{Volume to be infused (ml)}}{\text{Infusion time (hr)}} = \text{ml/hr}$$

EXAMPLE: Rx: D5W 1 L q6h. What is the IV rate?

$$\frac{1000 \text{ ml}}{6} = 166.67 = 167 \text{ ml/hr}$$

IMPORTANT

IV rates should always be rounded to the nearest whole number (ml), because decimals cannot be input into the IV administration pump.

IV Frequency or Schedule

The frequency or schedule of an IV is the time it takes to infuse a specific volume of solution. An IV's frequency/schedule is usually expressed in hours. Do not follow standard rounding rules. Always round an IV's frequency/schedule down to the nearest whole number in hours, as this will ensure that the patient gets enough IV solution.

FORMULA

IV Frequency or Schedule

$$\frac{\text{Total volume to be infused}}{\text{IV rate}} = \text{q\_\_\_\_hr}$$

EXAMPLE: Rx: NS 1 L to be infused @ 145 ml/hr. What is the frequency of a 1-L IV bag?

$$\frac{2000 \text{ mL}}{145 \text{ ml/hr}} = 13.79 = \text{q 13 hr}$$

IV Drip Rates

An IV drip rate is used by the caregiver to calibrate the IV administration set to ensure the correct infusion of IV solution. Each IV administration set is labeled with a drop factor (gtt/ml). The drop factor determines how many drops per milliliter are delivered in that particular IV set. Not all IV sets have the same drop factor. Be sure you know the correct drop factor before beginning.

FORMULA

IV Drip Rate

$$\frac{\text{Volume to be infused (ml)}}{\text{Infusion time (min)}} \times \text{IV set drop factor} = \text{Drops/min}$$

example 11.20

Rx: D5W, 400 mL to run over 4 hr. IV drop factor: 10 gtt/mL. Determine the rate of infusion in gtt/min.

$$\frac{400 \text{ mL}}{240 \text{ min}} \times \frac{10 \text{ gtt}}{\text{ml}} = \text{gtt/min}$$

Cancel like units before solving:

$$\frac{400 \text{ m̶L̶}}{240 \text{ min}} \times \frac{10 \text{ gtt}}{\text{m̶l̶}} = \text{gtt/min}$$

Multiply across (400×10) and divide by 240 to get the answer.

Answer: $16.67 \approx 17$ gtt/min.

example 11.21

Rx: NS 2 L IV q24h. IV drop factor: 60 gtt/mL.

$$\frac{2000 \text{ mL}}{1440 \text{ min}} \times \frac{60 \text{ gtt}}{\text{ml}} = \text{gtt/min}$$

Cancel like units before solving:

$$\frac{2000 \text{ m̶L̶}}{1440 \text{ min}} \times \frac{60 \text{ gtt}}{\text{m̶l̶}} = \text{gtt/min}$$

Multiply across (2000×60) and divide by 1440 to get the answer.

Answer: $83.33 \approx 83$ gtt/min.

Alligations

Alligations are used when mixing together two different strengths of the same active ingredient, so that the strength of the final product is the one that is desired. You can solve alligation problems easily by using the alligation grid shown below. First, input the amount of the higher strength, the lower strength, and the desired strength. Then take the difference on the diagonals (which should always be a positive number) to determine the number or part needed. To finish solving the alligation, read across the grid as you would a book, from left to right. The number or parts of the higher strength needed should be listed as a fraction of the total number of parts needed—which is solved by simply adding the numbers in the right column.

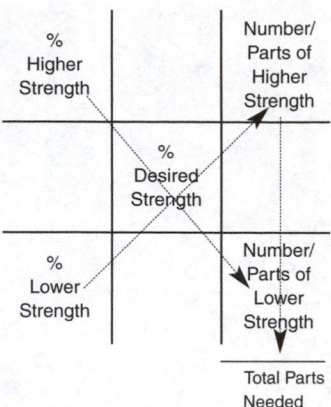

If you are using a solvent or diluent such as water, cream/ointment base, or normal saline (assuming that sodium chloride is not the active ingredient), use a percent strength of zero since it contains no active ingredient.

example 11.22

Rx: Hydrocortisone 5% cream, 120 g. You have in stock 2% hydrocortisone cream and 10% hydrocortisone cream. How much of each should be used to make 120 g of 5% hydrocortisone cream?

Set up an alligation grid:

% Higher Strength 10		Number/ Parts of Higher Strength 3
	% Desired Strength 5	
% Lower Strength 2		Number/ Parts of Lower Strength 5
		Total Parts Needed: 8

To make this order you should use three parts (out of eight total parts) of the 10% cream and five parts (out of eight total parts) of the 2% cream. Because we know the proportion required and the total amount needed, we can calculate the actual amount required of each product by multiplying the total quantity by the proportion needed:

$$\text{Quantity of 10\% HC needed: } 120 \text{ g} \times 3/8 = 45 \text{ g}$$
$$\text{Quantity of 2\% HC needed: } 120 \text{ g} \times 5/8 = 75 \text{ g}$$

Therefore, if you mix 45 g of 10% HC cream with 75 g of 2% HC cream, the resulting 120 g of HC cream will have a strength of 5%.

example 11.23

Rx: Clotrimazole 0.5% ointment. How much 10% clotrimazole powder and ointment base should be mixed together to prepare 240 g of ointment?

Set up an alligation grid:

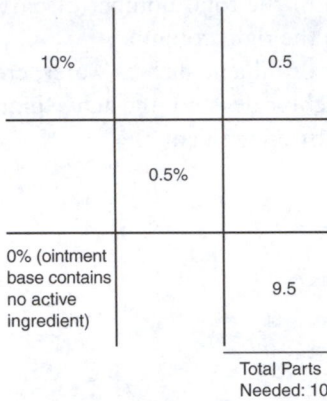

To make this order you should use 0.5 parts (out of 10 total parts) of the 10% and 9.5 parts (out of 10 total parts) of the ointment base cream. Because we know the proportion required and the total amount needed, we can calculate the actual amount required of each product by multiplying the total quantity with the proportion needed:

$$\text{Quantity of 10\% clotrimazole needed: } 240 \text{ g} \times 0.5/10 = 12 \text{ g}$$
$$\text{Quantity of 2\% clotrimazole needed: } 240 \text{ g} \times 9.5/10 = 228 \text{ g}$$

Therefore, if you mix 12 g of 10% clotrimazole powder with 228 g of ointment base, the resulting 240 g of clotrimazole cream will be at a strength of 0.5%.

Business Math

Although pharmacy technicians do not have to be accountants, they must have a basic understanding of the accounting and business calculations that are used in many practice settings. Following are the most common business math calculation formulas used in pharmacy.

FORMULA

Selling Price, Cost, and Markup

$$\text{Selling price} = \text{Cost} + \text{Markup}$$

FORMULA

Calculating Markup Percentage

$$\text{Markup percentage} = \frac{(\text{Selling price} - \text{Cost})}{\text{Cost}} \times 100$$

FORMULA

Calculating Gross Profit

Selling price − Invoice cost = Gross profit

FORMULA

Calculating Gross Profit Percentage

$$\frac{(Price - Cost)}{Cost} \times 100 = Gross\ profit\ percentage$$

FORMULA

Calculating Net Profit

Net profit = Selling price − (Cost + Overhead)

---

example 11.24

A blood pressure monitor costs the pharmacy $18.65, and the store adds a 20% markup to all medical devices. What is the selling price of the monitor?

$$Selling\ price = \$18.65 + (\$18.65 \times 20\%)$$
$$= \$18.65 + \$3.73$$

Therefore, selling price = $22.38

example 11.25

A bottle of 81-mg aspirin is priced at $2.89; the invoice cost is $1.98. What is the amount of the markup, and what is the markup percentage?

$$\$2.89 = \$1.98 + markup$$

Subtract $1.98 from both sides:

$$\$0.82 = markup$$

To determine the markup percentage, use the other formula:

$$Markup\ \% = (\$2.89 - \$1.98)/\$1.98 \times 100$$
$$= \$0.82/\$1.98 \times 100$$

Therefore, markup % = 41.4%

Practice Problems

To practice the calculations from this chapter, please take the Math Practice Tests in chapters 13, 14, and 15.

SUMMARY

Many pharmacy technicians find pharmacy calculations to be the most difficult aspect of pharmacy practice; however, a very large part of pharmacy practice and of the national certification exam focuses on calculations. It is important to remember that no matter how intimidating these pharmacy calculations may seem at first glance, most can be solved either by using simple ratios and proportions or by using an algebraic formula. It is important for pharmacy technicians to master these calculations, not only for the national exam, but also to function successfully on the job and, most important, for patient safety.

CHAPTER REVIEW QUESTIONS

1. Rx: Albuterol, 1.5 tsp po bid. Disp: 120 ml. How many milligrams of albuterol will be taken per day?
   a. 6 mg
   b. 12 mg
   c. 10 mg
   d. 20 mg

2. Rx: Amoxicillin/potassium clavulanate, 45 mg/kg/day in three divided doses. The patient weighs 54 lb. How many milligrams will the patient receive for each dose?
   a. 2430 mg
   b. 368.25 mg
   c. 810 mg
   d. 1105 mg

3. 480 ml = _____ tsp.
   a. 32
   b. 48
   c. 64
   d. 96

4. 3.5 gallons = _____ ml.
   a. 3785
   b. 14,000
   c. 13,320
   d. 13,249

5. Rx: D5 1/2 NS 1 L IV q8h. What is the IV rate?
   a. 80 ml/hr
   b. 120 ml/hr
   c. 125 ml/hr
   d. 75 ml/hr
   e. 90 ml/hr

6. Rx: 1/2 NS IV @ 75 ml/hr. What is the frequency of a 1-L IV bag?
   a. q12h
   b. q13h
   c. q14h
   d. q24h

7.

Electrolyte	Stock Vial	Rx Order	How Many mL?
KCl	2 mEq/mL	90 mEq	_____

   a. 60 mL
   b. 15 mL
   c. 10 mL
   d. 30 mL
   e. 45 mL

8. How many milliliters of 2.7% NaCl will be needed to be added to distilled water to make 1 L of normal saline?
   a. 333 mL
   b. 667 mL
   c. 500 mL
   d. 250 mL

9. PenVK 500,000 units in 50 mL is to be administered over 30 minutes. The IV is set at a drop factor of 20 gtt/ml. What is the infusion rate in drops per minute?
   a. 1.6 gtt/min
   b. 3.3 gtt/min
   c. 16 gtt/min
   d. 33 gtt/min
   e. 333 gtt/min

10. What is the markup percentage on a box of latex gloves that is invoiced at $3.39 and sold for $5.36?
    a. 42%
    b. 73%
    c. 58%
    d. 27%

Top 200 Drugs

Please note that duplicates indicate different manufacturers.

RANK	DRUG NAMES BASED ON TOTAL DOLLARS	DRUG NAMES BASED ON PRESCRIPTION COUNT
1	Nexium	HYCD/APAP
2	Abilify	Levothyroxine Sodium
3	Crestor	HYCD/APAP
4	Advair Diskus	Lisinopril
5	Cymbalta	HYCD/APAP
6	Humira	Simvastatin
7	Enbrel	Azithromycin
8	Remicade	Proair HFA
9	Copaxone	Crestor
10	Neulasta	Levothyroxine Sodium
11	Singulair	Synthroid
12	Rituxan	Nexium
13	Plavix	Atorvastatin Ca
14	Atripla	Ibuprofen (Rx)
15	SPIRIVA Handihaler	Trazodone HCl
16	OxyContin	Metoprolol Tartrate
17	Januvia	Azithromycin
18	Avastin	Warfarin Sodium
19	Lantus	Cymbalta
20	Truvada	Fluticasone Propionate
21	Lantus SoloSTAR	Singulair
22	Epogen	Hydrochlorothiazide
23	Diovan	Ventolin HFA
24	Lyrica	Advair Diskus
25	Lipitor	Pravastatin Sodium
26	Celebrex	Amoxicillin
27	Herceptin	Amlodipine Besylate
28	Gleevec	Omeprazole (Rx)

(continued)

RANK	DRUG NAMES BASED ON TOTAL DOLLARS	DRUG NAMES BASED ON PRESCRIPTION COUNT
29	Namenda	Omeprazole (Rx)
30	Actos	Amoxicillin
31	Avonex	Lisinopril/HCTZ
32	Lucentis	Metoprolol
33	Vyvanse	Hydrochlorothiazide
34	Suboxone	Amlodipine Besylate
35	Seroquel	Diovan
36	Zetia	Alprazolam
37	Methylphenidate ER	Metformin HCl
38	AndroGel	Metformin HCl
39	Incivek	Simvastatin
40	Diovan HCT	Fluconazole
41	Lidoderm	Oxycodone/APAP
42	Atorvastatin Calcium	Omeprazole (Rx)
43	Symbicort	Omeprazole (Rx)
44	Rebif	SMX/TMP
45	NovoLog	Lorazepam
46	Seroquel XR	Meloxicam
47	Tricor	Prednisone
48	Alimta	Clonazepam
49	Eloxatin	Tramadol HCl
50	Levemir	Furosemide
51	Combivent	Sertraline HCl
52	Viagra	Plavix
53	Proair HFA	Gabapentin
54	Procrit	Fluoxetine HCl
55	Niaspan	Simvastatin
56	Nasonex	Vitamin D
57	NovoLog FlexPen	Lisinopril
58	Lovaza	Atorvastatin
59	Humalog	Calcium
60	Flovent HFA	Fluticasone
61	Neupogen	Propionate
62	Reyataz	Simvastatin
63	Vytorin	Citalopram HBR
64	Isentress	Lantus
65	Budesonide	Ibuprofen (Rx)
66	Janumet	Amoxicillin/Clavulanate Potassium

RANK	DRUG NAMES BASED ON TOTAL DOLLARS	DRUG NAMES BASED ON PRESCRIPTION COUNT
67	Aranesp	Vyvanse
68	Cialis	Metoprolol
69	Aciphex	Ciprofloxacin HCl
70	Adderall XR	Lipitor
71	Restasis	Escitalopram
72	Pradaxa	Metformin HCl
73	Gilenya	SPIRIVA Handihaler
74	Prezista	Alprazolam
75	Betaseron	Celebrex
76	Orencia	Zolpidem Tartrate
77	Varivax	Alprazolam
78	Vesicare	Sertraline HCl
79	Victoza 3-Pak	Lyrica
80	Dexilant	Citalopram HBR
81	Lexapro	Atenolol
82	Synagis	Tramadol HCl
83	Benicar	Nasonex
84	Lunesta	Simvastatin
85	Evista	Carvedilol
86	Prevnar 13	Cephalexin
87	Enoxaparin Sodium	Tramadol HCl
88	Synthroid	Warfarin Sodium
89	Renvela	Venlafaxine HCl ER
90	Atorvastatin Calcium	Cyclobenzaprine
91	Xeloda	Abilify
92	Zyvox	Lisinopril
93	Ventolin HFA	Furosemide
94	Velcade	Zolpidem
95	Xolair	Januvia
96	Sensipar	Metformin HCl
97	Erbitux	Lisinopril
98	Humalog Kwikpen	Lisinopril
99	Stelara	Naproxen
100	Xgeva	Methylphenidate ER
101	Benicar HCT	Cyclobenzaprine
102	Sandostatin LAR	Diovan HCT
103	Mirena	Prednisone

(*continued*)

RANK	DRUG NAMES BASED ON TOTAL DOLLARS	DRUG NAMES BASED ON PRESCRIPTION COUNT
104	Zostavax	Cyclobenzaprine
105	Focalin XR	Viagra
106	Tarceva	Metoprolol Succinate
107	Cubicin	Lantus Solostar
108	Detrol LA	Potassium Cl
109	Zometa	Zetia
110	Treanda	Furosemide
111	Colcrys	Suboxone
112	Solodyn	Namenda
113	Escitalopram Oxalate	Clonazepam
114	Gardasil	Zolpidem
115	Pristiq	Lorazepam
116	Pegasys Convenience Pack	Amoxicillin
117	Invega Sustenna	Cialis
118	Strattera	Prednisone
119	Trilipix	Amphetamine Salts
120	Revlimid	Methylprednisolone
121	Asacol	Pantoprazole Sodium
122	Bystolic	Diazepam
123	Viread	Allopurinol
124	Enoxaparin Sodium	Furosemide
125	Loestrin 24 Fe	Amoxicillin Trihydrate/Clavulanate Potassium
126	Yervoy	Lorazepam
127	Avodart	Gabapentin
128	Lexiscan	Escitalopram Oxalate
129	Lovenox	Ranitidine HCl
130	Epzicom	Atenolol
131	Exelon	Omeprazole
132	Amphetamin Salt ER	Digoxin
133	Gamunex-C	Bystolic
134	NuvaRing	Amitriptyline
135	Amphetamin Salt ER	Flovent HFA
136	Escitalopram Oxal	Pravastatin
137	Provigil	Loestrin 24 Fe
138	Norvir	Risperidone
139	Epipen 2-Pak	OxyContin
140	Forteo	Simvastatin

RANK	DRUG NAMES BASED ON TOTAL DOLLARS	DRUG NAMES BASED ON PRESCRIPTION COUNT
141	Risperdal Consta	Simvastatin
142	Premarin	Carvedilol
143	Zytiga	Paroxetine HCl
144	Welchol	Triamterene/HCTZ
145	Metoprolol Succinate	Potassium Cl
146	Onglyza	Doxycycline Hyclate
147	Xifaxan	Bupropion
148	Byetta	Doxycycline Hyclate
149	Aggrenox	Lovastatin
150	Opana Er	APAP/Codeine
151	Aloxi	Ciprofloxacin
152	Privigen	Klor-Con M20
153	Lumigan	Lexapro
154	Intuniv	Tricor
155	Travatan Z	Temazepam
156	Pulmozyme	Albuterol
157	Pneumovax 23	Gabapentin
158	Zyprexa	Cyclobenzaprin HCl
159	HYCD/APAP	Famotidine
160	Angiomax	Triamcinolone Acetonide
161	Lialda	Alprazolam
162	Cimzia	Alendronate Sodium
163	Geodon	Oxycodone HCl
164	Actonel	Amoxicillin
165	Prograf	Triamterene/HCTZ
166	Fentanyl	Atorvastatin Calcium
167	Ortho-Tri-Cyclen Lo 28	Alprazolam
168	NovoLog FlexPen Mix	Clindamycin
169	Ranexa	Tamsulosin HCl
170	Qvar	Levothyroxine Sodium
171	Afinitor	Atenolol
172	Invega	Lisinopril
173	Tysabri	Ranitidine HCl
174	Temodar	Benicar
175	Nuvigil	Symbicort
176	Sprycel	Mupirocin
177	Tasigna	Niaspan

(continued)

RANK	DRUG NAMES BASED ON TOTAL DOLLARS	DRUG NAMES BASED ON PRESCRIPTION COUNT
178	Adacel	Lovaza
179	Valcyte	Prednisone
180	Exforge	Premarin
181	Nutropin AQ	Nuvaring
182	Zosyn	Dexilant
183	Amphetamine Salts	Metoprolol
184	Effient	Cheratussin AC
185	Claravis	Hydrochlorothiazide
186	Advair HFA	Metoprolol Tartrate
187	Chantix	Levoxyl
188	Reclast	Penicillin VK
189	Vidaza	Metronidazole
190	Abraxane	Amlodipine Besylate
191	Gammagard Liquid	HYCD/APAP
192	Tamiflu	Azithromycin
193	Complera	Naproxen
194	Maxalt	Allopurinol
195	Ciprodex	Actos
196	Activase	Diazepam
197	Vimpat	Bupropion HCl XL
198	Simponi	Losartan Potassium
199	Synvisc-One	Lidoderm
200	Sutent	Gabapentin

Practice Certification Exam I

This practice exam has been designed to simulate the certification exam in both the number and style of questions as well as the content. You should be able to complete this exam within 2 hr.

1. Of the following choices, which pair of drugs are H$_2$ antagonists?
   a. Zantac and Prevacid
   b. Prinivil and Tagamet
   c. Pepcid and Zantac
   d. Vasotec and Motrin

2. The drug enalapril would be categorized into which of the following classification groups?
   a. beta-blocker
   b. ACE inhibitor
   c. NSAID
   d. antiemetic

3. The retail price of a prescription is based on average wholesale price (AWP) plus a dispensing fee. Using the following fee table, calculate the retail price of a prescription for 30 tablets if a bottle of 100 tablets has an AWP of $76.78.

AWP	DISPENSING FEE
$0–$5.00	$4.75
$5.01–$10.00	$5.75
$10.01–$20.00	$6.75
$20.00 and up	$7.75

   a. $30.78
   b. $13.72
   c. $23.03
   d. $32.91

4. Of the following prescription drugs, which cannot be prescribed with refills?
   a. nifedipine
   b. lorazepam
   c. methylphenidate
   d. hydrocodone/acetaminophen

5. A technician answers the phone and the patient calling states that, after taking a medication she received from the pharmacy a few hours earlier, she is not feeling well and would like to know the side effects of the medication. The technician should:

   a. tell the patient the side effects of the medication, since they are commonly known to all pharmacy personnel

   b. put the patient on hold and notify the pharmacist of the situation

   c. ask the patient to hold while he looks up the side effects in a reference book

   d. tell the patient to lie down and maybe the side effects will wear off soon

6. A local dermatologist has special-ordered 60 g of 1.5% hydrocortisone cream for a patient. The pharmacy has in stock a 2.5% hydrocortisone cream and a 1% hydrocortisone cream. How much of each will the technician need to prepare this compound correctly?

   a. 40 g of 2.5% and 20 g of 1%

   b. 40 g of 1% and 20 g of 2.5%

   c. 30 g of each strength

   d. 45 g of 1% and 15 g of 2.5%

7. Who must initiate an order for an investigational drug for patient use?

   a. a pharmacy director

   b. a pharmacist

   c. a technician

   d. a physician

8. How many 500-mg metronidazole tablets will be needed to compound 150 ml of 3% metronidazole suspension?

   a. 7

   b. 9

   c. 10

   d. 18

9. A medication given to reduce a fever is called:

   a. an analgesic

   b. an antitussive

   c. an anthelmintic

   d. an antipyretic

10. Medications that are prepackaged into unit-dose or unit-of-use containers must have the following information included on the package labeling:

    a. patient's name, dispensing date, name of medication, and directions for use

    b. medication name and strength, lot number, and expiration date

    c. medication name and strength, lot number, and directions for use

    d. directions for use, medication name and strength, and expiration date

11. A patient brings the following prescription into your pharmacy: Amoxil 400 mg po tid for 10 days. Your pharmacy has in stock an Amoxil oral suspension 250 mg/5 ml. What is the exact volume of medication you will need to correctly and completely fill the prescription for the patient?

    a. 150 ml

    b. 168 ml

    c. 240 ml

    d. 200 ml

12. When mixing cytotoxic agents for intravenous use, what type of syringe is required?

    a. glass

    b. Luer-Loc

    c. slip-tip

    d. reusable

13. Calculate the flow rate in drops per minute if a physician orders D5W/NS 1400 ml over 12 hr using an administration set that delivers 40 gtt/ml.

    a. 87 gtt/min

    b. 68 gtt/min

    c. 78 gtt/min

    d. 117 gtt/min

14. Inventory turnover rate refers to:

    a. how often employees quit and new employees are hired to replace them

    b. how long it takes the pharmacy to process a new prescription

    c. how many times a year shelves are inspected for expired medications

    d. how often medications are used and reordered

15. The portion of the retail price of a prescription that the patient must pay is known as the:

    a. deductible

    b. co-payment

    c. average wholesale price

    d. none of the above

16. How many capsules will it take to completely fill the following prescription: Cephalexin 500 mg, i po tid × 14 days?

    a. 14 capsules

    b. 21 capsules

    c. 28 capsules

    d. 42 capsules

17. Although state laws differ on record retention, federal law requires that prescription records be kept for _____ year(s).

    a. 1

    b. 5

    c. 2

    d. 7

18. Prescription medications are often referred to as _____ drugs because of the federal law that requires the packaging to display the following message: "Rx Only."
    a. controlled
    b. legend
    c. prescription
    d. none of the above

19. Stock rotation is the task of making sure that:
    a. the shortest expiration date is in the back
    b. the longest expiration date is in the front
    c. the shortest expiration date is in the front
    d. a and b

20. Which of the following is classified as a beta-blocker?
    a. allopurinol
    b. enalapril
    c. propranolol
    d. verapamil

21. A patient in the hospital needs KCl 8 mEq IV stat. The pharmacy stocks KCl 2 mEq/ml in a 10-mL multidose vial. What is the correct volume to be drawn up?
    a. 2.5 mL
    b. 4 mL
    c. 0.4 mL
    d. 0.04 mL

22. What document is used by the pharmacy to pay the wholesaler for a drug order?
    a. packing slip
    b. invoice
    c. purchase order
    d. DEA Form 222c

23. Diphenhydramine is the generic name for which of these drugs?
    a. Benadryl
    b. Dramamine
    c. Bentyl
    d. Soma

24. The pharmacy receives a prescription for 4 oz of 5% ointment. The pharmacy stocks the ointment in strengths of 2% and 10%. To prepare the prescription, how much of each stock ointment is needed?
    a. 50 g of 2% and 70 g of 10%
    b. 12 g of 2% and 108 g of 10%
    c. 75 g of 2% and 45 g of 10%
    d. 45 g of 2% and 75 g of 10%

25. What is the correct temperature for storing an item in the refrigerator?
    a. 2–8°C
    b. less than 36°F

26. 300 mL of a Cipro 5% suspension contains how many grams of active ingredient?
    a. 1.5 g
    b. 15 g
    c. 3 g
    d. 30 g

27. The term used to refer to protection of a patient's identity and health information is:
    a. motility
    b. compatibility
    c. mortality
    d. confidentiality

28. According to federal law, what is the maximum number of refills permitted for a Schedule III controlled substance?
    a. six refills within one year
    b. three refills within 90 days
    c. five refills within six months
    d. no refills are allowed

29. In the NDC number 69907-3110-01, what does section "3110" identify?
    a. manufacturer
    b. drug product
    c. package size
    d. number of tablets in the bottle

30. To what class of controlled substances does Lortab belong?
    a. II
    b. III
    c. IV
    d. V

31. The trade name for glipizide is:
    a. Diabinese
    b. Micronase
    c. Glucophage
    d. Glucotrol

32. What is the total volume of D5W needed for a 24-hr period if the infusion runs at a rate of 125 ml/hr?
    a. 3000 mL
    b. 1000 mL
    c. 2400 mL
    d. 1250 mL

33. The recommended dose for gentamicin injection is 5 mg/kg/day in three divided doses. If a patient weighs 164 lb, how many milligrams should that patient receive for each dose?
    a. 25 mg
    b. 75 mg
    c. 124 mg
    d. 373 mg

c. 15–30°C
d. 59–86°F

34. Which of the following drugs is classed as an H_2 antagonist?
    a. clonidine
    b. ranitidine
    c. loratadine
    d. clemastine

35. If a patient calls in for refills on Prinivil and Diabeta, which of the following combinations of medications need to be filled for the patient?
    a. lisinopril and glipizide
    b. enalapril and glyburide
    c. enalapril and glipizide
    d. lisinopril and glyburide

36. How much neomycin powder must be added to fluocinolone cream to dispense an order for 60 g of fluocinolone cream with 0.5% neomycin?
    a. 120 mg
    b. 240 mg
    c. 300 mg
    d. 600 mg

37. Which of the sig codes given refers to the following directions: Take two tablets by mouth every 4–6 hr as needed?
    a. 2 tabs q4–6h prn
    b. 2 tabs po q4–6h prn
    c. 2 tabs po q4–6h
    d. a or c

38. The pharmacy receives an order for 10% ointment, but it stocks only 5% and 15%. In what ratio would the two stock ointments need to be mixed in order to compound the prescription order correctly?
    a. 1:1
    b. 1:2
    c. 2:1
    d. 1:3

39. Which of the following drugs is most likely to cause photosensitivity?
    a. nifedipine
    b. naproxen
    c. tetracycline
    d. glyburide

40. After reconstitution, how many 250-mg doses of Claforan can be withdrawn from a 2-g vial?
    a. 2 doses
    b. 4 doses
    c. 6 doses
    d. 8 doses

41. A medication that should be protected from exposure to light is:
    a. promethazine
    b. tetracycline

    c. erythromycin
    d. nitroglycerin

42. The blower on the laminar airflow workbench should remain on at all times. If it is turned off for any reason, it should remain on for at least _____ before being used to prepare IV admixtures and other products.
    a. 15 min
    b. 1 hr
    c. 30 min
    d. 45 min

43. Which of the following needle sizes has the largest bore?
    a. 18 gauge
    b. 27 gauge
    c. 23 gauge
    d. 29 gauge

44. When metronidazole is dispensed for a patient, which auxiliary label should be affixed to the dispensing container?
    a. no alcohol
    b. no dairy products
    c. take with food or milk
    d. may cause drowsiness

45. If 500 mL of a 15% solution is diluted to 1500 mL, how would you label the final strength of the solution?
    a. 20%
    b. 5%
    c. 0.05%
    d. 0.20%

46. KCl supplements are most often used in combination with:
    a. labetalol
    b. lisinopril
    c. naproxen
    d. furosemide

47. A prescription reading "iii gtt a.s. tid prn pain" should have which set of directions printed on the dispensing label?
    a. Instill 3 drops in the left eye three times daily as needed for pain.
    b. Instill 3 drops in the left ear three times daily as needed for pain.
    c. Instill 3 drops in the right ear two times daily as needed for pain.
    d. Instill 3 drops in the right eye three times daily as needed for pain.

48. A patient with a penicillin allergy is most likely to exhibit a sensitivity to:
    a. tetracycline
    b. erythromycin

c. cefaclor
d. gentamicin

49. A Tylenol #3 tablet contains 30 mg of codeine. The amount of codeine is also equivalent to:

a. $\frac{1}{4}$ gr

b. $\frac{1}{2}$ gr

c. 1 gr
d. 2 gr

50. An IV infusion order is written for 1 L of D5W/0.45% NS to run over 12 hr. The set that will be used delivers 15 gtt/ml. What is the flow rate in gtt/min?

a. 7 gtt/min
b. 21 gtt/min
c. 25 gtt/min
d. 125 gtt/min

51. Zovirax and Epivir are both classed as _____ agents.

a. antimalarial
b. tuberculosis
c. antiviral
d. antifungal

52. A physician writes an order for a patient to receive KCl 40 mEq/1 L NS @ 80 ml/hr. What amount of KCl will the patient receive per hour?

a. 6.8 mEq
b. 3.2 mEq
c. 2.3 mEq
d. 8.6 mEq

53. Na is the chemical symbol for which of the following elements?

a. sodium
b. nitrogen
c. hydrochloride
d. potassium

54. When withdrawing medication from an ampule, what size filter needle will be sufficient to filter out any tiny glass fragments that might have fallen into the solution?

a. 0.2 micron
b. 0.5 micron
c. 2 micron
d. 5 micron

55. Which of the following conditions is the drug rifampin used to treat?

a. influenza
b. tuberculosis

c. nail fungus
d. urinary tract infection

56. When measuring liquid in a graduated cylinder, where is the volume of liquid read?

a. top surface of the liquid
b. top of the meniscus
c. center of the meniscus
d. bottom of the meniscus

57. How many grams of 2% silver nitrate ointment will deliver 1 g of the active ingredient?

a. 4 g
b. 50 g
c. 25 g
d. 20 g

58. The federal law enacted in 1970 that requires the use of child-resistant safety caps on all dispensing containers unless otherwise desired by the patient is known as the:

a. Controlled Substances Act
b. Poison Prevention Act
c. Pure Food and Drug Act
d. Harrison Narcotic Act

59. Into what size bottle will a prescription for 180 mL of cough syrup best fit?

a. 2 oz
b. 4 oz
c. 6 oz
d. 8 oz

60. To ensure that it is working properly, the laminar airflow workbench should be inspected by qualified personnel at least:

a. every six months
b. every year
c. every three years
d. every five years

61. If a patient should receive a medication at 15 mg/kg/day in three equally divided doses, what will be the approximate dose if the patient weighs 142 lb?

a. 968 mg
b. 323 mg
c. 2904 mg
d. 284 mg

62. If one of your pharmacy's patients has had an adverse drug reaction, _____ should be used to report it.

a. the HCFA form
b. the MedWatch form
c. DEA Form 222c
d. the Universal Claim Form

63. A pharmacy wants to make a 30% profit on an item that costs $4.50. What would the retail selling price have to be in order to make such a profit?
    a. $6.23
    b. $7.10
    c. $5.85
    d. $6.40

64. Which statement is true concerning the drug tetracycline?
    a. It should be given with food or milk for best absorption.
    b. It should not be given with milk products or antacids for best absorption.
    c. It should be given with milk because it is upsetting to the stomach.
    d. Exposure to sunlight will not affect a patient taking this medication.

65. Under what schedule of controlled substances does the drug temazepam fall?
    a. II
    b. III
    c. IV
    d. V

66. When storing an item at a controlled room temperature, the temperature of the room should be:
    a. 2–8°C
    b. 36–46°F
    c. higher than 30°C
    d. 15–30°C

67. A list of medications that a physician may prescribe from within a given institutional setting is called:
    a. an MSDS
    b. a formulary
    c. a closed panel of drugs
    d. an open system

68. Which of the following is considered PHI under HIPAA regulations?
    a. patient address
    b. patient date of birth
    c. patient name
    d. all the above

69. If a vial slips from your hand while you are preparing an IV admixture and breaks on the floor or other surface, a spill kit must be used to clean the area if the vial contained which of the following medications?
    a. ceftriaxone
    b. potassium chloride
    c. amphotericin b
    d. vinblastine

70. During cleaning of the laminar airflow workbench while preparing IV admixtures, which of the following statements is true?
    a. The work surface should be cleaned first using a continuous side-to-side motion.
    b. 70% isopropyl alcohol should be sprayed onto the HEPA filter to ensure its cleanliness.
    c. The sides should be cleaned from top to bottom, working outward from the filter.
    d. The sides should be cleaned from top to bottom, working toward the filter.

71. What volume of 5% aluminum acetate solution will be needed if 120 mL of 0.05% solution is extemporaneously compounded for a prescription?
    a. 12 mL
    b. 1.2 mL
    c. 8.3 mL
    d. 0.83 mL

72. How many 1-L bags will be needed if D5W is to run at 60 ml/hr for 20 hr?
    a. one bag
    b. two bags
    c. three bags
    d. four or more bags

73. What document is used by the wholesaler to pull the pharmacy's order from its shelves?
    a. packing slip
    b. invoice
    c. purchase order
    d. DEA Form 222c

74. A pharmacy has 20 mL of a 1:200 solution in stock. If the pharmacist has asked the technician to dilute the solution to 500 mL, what will be the strength of the final product?
    a. 2%
    b. 2.5%
    c. 25%
    d. 0.02%

75. When an antibiotic injection is given in a small volume of solution that is connected to the main line of IV fluids the patient receives, it is commonly known as an:
    a. IV bag
    b. IV injection
    c. IV piggyback
    d. IV push

76. The largest gelatin capsule used for extemporaneous compounding is:
    a. 000
    b. 0
    c. 10
    d. 5

77. All manipulations in the laminar airflow work-bench should take place at least _____ from within the front edge of the hood.
    a. 4 in.
    b. 6 in.
    c. 8 in.
    d. 10 in.

78. In an inpatient setting, the pharmacy must receive a direct copy of a physician's order before filling an initial dose. Which of the following is not considered a direct copy?
    a. fax
    b. photocopy
    c. computer-generated transfer
    d. phone call acknowledging the verbal order

79. Which of the following drugs is classified as a calcium channel blocker?
    a. amlodipine
    b. atenolol
    c. enalapril
    d. nitroglycerin

80. When using a manual inventory system, items that need to be ordered are written down by all pharmacy personnel. This writing of a list of items that need to be ordered is referred to as:
    a. a purchase order
    b. an invoice
    c. a want book
    d. an MAR

81. Which of the following DEA numbers would not be valid for Dr. Ann Cosgrove?
    a. AC6782329
    b. AC3081421
    c. AC1355672
    d. BC3421234

82. Of all drug recall classes, a _____ recall would not likely cause harm to the patient, because it is the least severe.
    a. Class I
    b. Class II
    c. Class III
    d. Class IV

83. The form used for ordering Schedule II narcotics is known as:
    a. DEA Form 240
    b. DEA Form 222
    c. DEA Form 121
    d. DEA Form 200

84. Which of the following drugs requires special pharmacy handling and ordering?
    a. controlled substances
    b. chemotherapy drugs
    c. investigational drugs
    d. all the above

85. The Orange Book is most often used to find _____.
    a. generic equivalents
    b. direct prices
    c. therapeutic equivalents
    d. manufacturer's standards

86. Nursing station inspections of available pharmaceuticals are primarily the responsibility of the:
    a. nurse
    b. pharmacist
    c. pharmacy director
    d. pharmacy technician

87. Which of the following pairs of medications could cause a major drug–drug interaction if taken together by a patient?
    a. hydrocodone and naproxen
    b. warfarin and aspirin
    c. penicillin and trimethoprim
    d. glyburide and metformin

88. A patient takes NPH insulin according to the following dosage regimen: 35 units sq every morning and 15 units every evening. How many 10 mL vials of insulin U-100 (100 units/mL) will the patient need for a 30-day supply?
    a. one vial
    b. two vials
    c. three vials
    d. four or more vials

89. Which of the following medications should always be dispensed in a glass container?
    a. aminophylline
    b. dopamine
    c. potassium
    d. nitroglycerin

90. Ampicillin powder for injection should be reconstituted with and diluted in _____ for best stability.
    a. D5W
    b. 0.9% sodium chloride
    c. Lactated Ringers
    d. 0.45% sodium chloride

14 Practice Certification Exam II

T his practice exam has been designed to simulate the certification exam in both the number and style of questions as well as the content. You should be able to complete this exam within 2 hr.

1. Mixing ingredients in order to provide a prescription for a specific patient or a small group of patients is known as:
   a. manufacturing
   b. compressing
   c. compounding
   d. adjudication

2. The device used to compound three-in-one total parenteral nutrition solutions is the:
   a. PhaSeal
   b. Automix
   c. Pyxis
   d. MedCarousel

3. A solid dosage form containing active and inactive ingredients and prepared by either compression or molding methods is a:
   a. capsule
   b. tablet
   c. emulsion
   d. paste

4. A method used to identify an employee's individual strengths and weaknesses and provide the employer with information relative to the employee's capacity for retention and promotion is the:
   a. personnel checklist
   b. process validation
   c. employee performance appraisal
   d. employee handbook

5. Mixing calcium gluconate and sodium phosphate together in the same syringe will cause:
   a. precipitation
   b. incompatibility
   c. intolerance
   d. injunction

6. A preparation of finely divided undissolved drugs dispersed in a liquid vehicle is:
   a. an elixir
   b. a solution
   c. a syrup
   d. a suspension

7. A _____ is a system in which the item is deducted from inventory as it is sold or dispensed.
   a. turnover
   b. Pyxis
   c. Baker cell
   d. POS system

8. Which of the following OTC drugs is contraindicated for a patient taking warfarin?
   a. diphenhydramine
   b. loratidine
   c. psyllium
   d. aspirin

9. Atenolol is to Tenormin as Ramipril is to _____.
   a. Accupril
   b. Lyrica
   c. Aciphex
   d. Altace

10. Effective communication in pharmacy practice can be hindered by:
    a. visual impairment
    b. auditory loss
    c. speech impairment
    d. all of the above

11. Which of the following laws requires pharmacists to counsel Medicaid patients?
    a. Controlled Substances Act
    b. Omnibus Budget Reconciliation Act of 1990
    c. Medicare Part D
    d. Health Insurance Portability and Accountability Act

12. A solid dosage form in which the drug substance is enclosed either in a hard or soft soluble container or a shell of a suitable form of gelatin is a:
    a. capsule
    b. pill
    c. tablet
    d. suppository

13. What is the generic name for Effexor?
    a. vardenafil
    b. venlafaxine
    c. verapamil
    d. valacyclovir

14. The only drug approved to treat high blood pressure during pregnancy is:
    a. lidocaine
    b. clonidine
    c. metoprolol
    d. methyldopa

15. The only antihypertensive drug available as a transdermal delivery system is:
    a. nicotine
    b. clonidine
    c. nitroglycerin
    d. lidocaine

16. From the following information, calculate the amount in grams of cetyl ester wax needed to make 1 lb of cold cream:

cetyl ester wax	12.5 parts
white wax	12.0 parts
mineral oil	56.0 parts
sodium borate	0.5 parts
water	19.0 parts

    a. 56.75 g
    b. 12.5 g
    c. 60 g
    d. 0.125 g

17. The drug of choice for emergency IV therapy for arrhythmias is:
    a. lidocaine
    b. sodium bicarbonate
    c. dopamine
    d. adrenalin

18. The most important drug in managing atrial flutter and fibrillation is:
    a. digitalis
    b. amlodipine
    c. doxazosin
    d. quinine

19. A substance or a mixture of substances added to a tablet to facilitate its breakup or disintegration after administration is a:
    a. terminator
    b. disintegrator
    c. binder
    d. diluent

20. The antagonist to warfarin is:
    a. heparin
    b. phytonadione
    c. methyldopa
    d. penicillin VK

21. The _____ provides guidelines for the recall of devices that could cause serious adverse effects.
    a. Safe Medical Devices Act
    b. Kefauver–Harris Amendment
    c. Durham–Humphrey Amendment
    d. Medical Device Amendment

22. Schedule II drugs are ordered using:
    a. DEA Form 224a
    b. DEA Form 222
    c. DEA Form 363a
    d. DEA Form 510a

23. An imbalance between oxygen supply and oxygen demand in cardiac muscle may produce a condition known as:
    a. congestive heart failure
    b. heartburn
    c. myocardial infarction
    d. angina pectoris

24. From the following information, calculate in kilograms the quantity of miconazole needed to prepare 12 kg of powder:

zinc oxide	1 part
calamine	2 parts
miconazole	1.5 parts
bismuth subgalate	3 parts
talc powder	8 parts

    a. 15.5 kg
    b. 0.097 kg
    c. 1.16 kg
    d. 1.5 kg

25. Patients on thiazide diuretics are frequently told to take supplements of or eat foods that are high in which element?
    a. calcium
    b. sodium
    c. chlorine
    d. potassium

26. When entering a prescription into the computer, the technician uses T1T3 for the directions "Take 1 tablet by mouth 3 times daily." T1T3 is an example of a:
    a. pharmaceutical abbreviation
    b. national drug code
    c. bar code
    d. sig code

27. If state and federal guidelines are different on how long a pharmacy should retain its records, the pharmacy should:
    a. always follow the federal guidelines
    b. always follow the state guidelines
    c. follow the guideline that requires the records to be kept for the shortest period of time
    d. follow the guideline that requires the records to be kept for the longest period of time

28. A pharmacy technician dilutes a 1-g vial of cefazolin with 9.6 ml of sterile water. The resulting solution has a concentration of 100 mg/ml. How much solution should be drawn up for a 500-mg dose?
    a. 4.8 ml
    b. 3 ml
    c. 10 ml
    d. 5 ml

29. How much sucralfate 1 gm/10 ml is required for a dose of 600 mg?
    a. 0.06 ml
    b. 0.6 ml
    c. 6 ml
    d. 60 ml

30. In pharmacies, how can controlled substances be stored?
    a. Controlled substances can be stored in an unlocked cabinet.
    b. Controlled substances can be stored in a securely locked, substantially constructed cabinet.
    c. Controlled substances (Schedule III through V) can be stored on the pharmacy shelves among noncontrolled substances in a manner designed to deter theft.
    d. either b or c

31. _____ is a drug agent extracted from cattle lung.
    a. Proventil HFA
    b. Survanta
    c. Bonine
    d. Serevent

32. Patients taking _____ should always be warned NOT to consume alcohol.
    a. metronidazole
    b. tetracycline
    c. albuterol
    d. prednisone

33. The _____ was a direct result of the thalidomide disaster and made manufacturers more accountable for their products.
    a. Comprehensive Drug Abuse Prevention and Control Act
    b. Medical Device Amendment
    c. Durham–Humphrey Amendment
    d. Kefauver–Harris Amendment

34. Patients should be advised not to drink milk or eat dairy products while taking:
    a. calcium carbonate
    b. tetracycline
    c. penicillin
    d. calciferol

35. Patients should be advised to drink plenty of water and to avoid the sun while taking:
    a. TMP-SMZ
    b. cephalexin
    c. propranolol
    d. warfarin

36. Which of the following auxiliary labels is needed on a prescription for tetracycline?
    a. take with food or milk
    b. may cause drowsiness
    c. do not drink alcohol
    d. may cause photosensitivity

37. _____ are a class of pharmaceutical agents that kill or inhibit the growth of infection-causing microorganisms.
    a. Anesthetics
    b. Antilipidemics
    c. Antibiotics
    d. Antihistamines

38. When a drug recall is issued, which of the following information is listed on the recall along with the drug name and strength?
    a. NDC
    b. lot number
    c. expiration date
    d. distribution date

39. When liquid medications are repackaged into oral syringes, the syringe must:
    a. not be amber in color
    b. be sterile
    c. not be able to accept a needle
    d. be made of glass

40. The agency that oversees the Controlled Substances Act is the:
    a. State Board of Pharmacy
    b. American Society of Health System Pharmacists
    c. Food and Drug Administration
    d. Drug Enforcement Agency

41. If a medication is taken "p.c.," it will be taken:
    a. before meals
    b. around the clock
    c. after meals
    d. with meals

42. All of the following are true statements except:
    a. All controlled substances must be inventoried on the day the pharmacy first dispenses controlled substances.
    b. The inventory of Schedule II medications requires an exact count or measure, while other schedules may be estimated.

    c. Prescriptions are the primary records for the acquisition of controlled substances by a pharmacy.
    d. The beginning inventory plus all acquisitions minus dispensing by prescriptions or to other practitioners should equal the current inventory count.

43. A patient weighs 165 lb. How many kilograms does the patient weigh?
    a. 165,000 kg
    b. 75 kg
    c. 363 kg
    d. 330 kg

44. Which of the following vitamins is a fat-soluble vitamin?
    a. thiamine
    b. pyridoxine
    c. cyanocobalamin
    d. phytonadione

45. If an insurance company pays only for a 14-day supply and the prescription is for "i-ii po q4-6h," what is the maximum number of tablets that can be dispensed?
    a. 56
    b. 84
    c. 168
    d. 224

46. Which of the following dosage forms will best mask the bad taste of a drug?
    a. suspension
    b. sublingual tablet
    c. chewable tablet
    d. gel-cap

47. The pharmacy receives an order for lidocaine 2 g in 250 ml of D5W to be infused at 1.5 mg/min. What is the flow rate in ml/hr?
    a. 11 ml/hr
    b. 22 ml/hr
    c. 33 ml/hr
    d. 44 ml/hr

48. Another term used to describe insulin-dependent diabetes is:
    a. non–insulin-dependent diabetes
    b. Type I diabetes
    c. Type II diabetes
    d. diabetes insipidus

49. A _____ drug is active against both gram-positive and gram-negative bacteria.
    a. neg-gram
    b. bacteriostatic
    c. broad-spectrum
    d. narrow-spectrum

50. Oral contraceptives interact with:
    a. antibiotics
    b. anticonvulsants
    c. antifungals
    d. all of the above

51. The pharmacy stocks potassium chloride in 20-mEq vials. The concentration of each vial is 2 mEq/ml. How many milliliters are needed for a 30-mEq dose?
    a. 2 ml
    b. 15 ml
    c. 20 ml
    d. 30 ml

52. The maximum allowable cost that an insurer will pay per tablet or dispensing unit for a given product is the:
    a. co-payment
    b. deductible
    c. U&C
    d. MAC

53. Estrogen is contraindicated with:
    a. migraines
    b. smokers
    c. thrombosis history
    d. all of the above

54. What is the percentage strength of a solution if 1 gallon contains 150 g of active ingredient?
    a. 0.396%
    b. 1%
    c. 1.5%
    d. 3.96%

55. The Anabolic Steroids Act of 1990 placed anabolic steroids into which controlled-substance category?
    a. C-II
    b. C-III
    c. C-IV
    d. C-V

56. The _____ requires that most prescription drugs be dispensed in a childproof container.
    a. Poison Prevention Act
    b. Safe Medical Devices Act
    c. Prescription Drug Marketing Act
    d. Medical Device Amendment

57. _____ should be taken with 8 oz of water before the first food of the day, and the patient must avoid lying down for at least 30 min after taking it.
    a. Miacalcin
    b. Didronel
    c. Fosamax
    d. Hydrocortisone

58. Digoxin is classified as:
    a. an antihypertensive
    b. a calcium channel blocker
    c. an ACE inhibitor
    d. a cardiac glycoside

59. If a patient is allergic to opioids, he should avoid taking:
    a. acetaminophen
    b. morphine
    c. aspirin
    d. penicillin

60. Which of the following is used to induce labor contractions?
    a. epinephrine
    b. serotonin
    c. dopamine
    d. oxytocin

61. A medication that is used to manage high blood pressure is an:
    a. antitussive
    b. antihypertensive
    c. antipyretic
    d. antibiotic

62. The _____ prohibits the sale of drug samples and reimportation of prescriptions and establishes fair pricing guidelines.
    a. Orphan Drug Act
    b. Prescription Drug Marketing Act
    c. Durham–Humphrey Amendment
    d. Kefauver–Harris Amendment

63. A decrease in susceptibility to a drug's effects from continued use is known as:
    a. addiction
    b. synergism
    c. sensitivity
    d. tolerance

64. A substance with a high potential for abuse that has no currently accepted medical use in the United States and for which there is a lack of accepted safety for use would be classified as:
    a. C-I
    b. C-II
    c. C-III
    d. C-IV

65. Which of the following DEA numbers is valid?
    a. Dr. Russ   AR123456879
    b. Dr. Black   AB56897
    c. Dr. Jones   AJ1234563
    d. Dr. Smith   CS2468217

66. Which of the following would provide the technician with the most up-to-date and complete information on how to place an inventory order?
    a. MSDS
    b. OSHA guidelines
    c. Pyxis User Manual
    d. Policy & Procedures Manual

67. The rate at which inventory is used is called:
    a. sales journal
    b. sales volume
    c. turnover
    d. net profit

68. Low blood glucose is known as:
    a. glucosuria
    b. hypoglycemia
    c. polyuria
    d. hyperglycemia

69. Certain controlled substances do not bear the federal caution legend and may be sold without a prescription. These products have small quantities of controlled substances included in them and may be sold if certain requirements are met and the proper records are kept. The restrictions on the sale include the following except:
    a. The sale must be made by the pharmacist or a certified pharmacy technician.
    b. The purchaser must be at least 18 and must either be known to the pharmacist or have substantial identification.
    c. Not more than 8 oz or more than 48 dosage units of any substance containing opium in any 48-hr period may be furnished to the purchaser. Not more than 4 oz or 24 dosage units of any other controlled substance may be sold in any 48-hr period.
    d. Pharmacists must maintain a record of the sale in a bound book.

70. Which of the following is the agent of choice for accidental poisonings, when induction of vomiting is required?
    a. activated charcoal
    b. demulcents
    c. syrup of ipecac
    d. diphenhydramine elixir

71. Sources of insulin include all of the following except:
    a. cow
    b. horse
    c. pig
    d. human

72. According to federal law, written prescriptions must contain all of the following information except the:
    a. patient's phone number
    b. physician's phone number
    c. drug name and strength
    d. date written

73. A possible cross-sensitivity to _____ is possible for a patient with a severe allergy to penicillin.
    a. cephalosporins
    b. sulfonamides
    c. macrolides
    d. antihypertensives

74. Convert the ratio strength of 1:5000 to a percent strength.
    a. 0.0002%
    b. 0.002%
    c. 0.02%
    d. 2%

75. Upon discovery of an expired drug, the pharmacy technician should:
    a. rotate the drug to the front of the stock
    b. destroy the drug
    c. follow the pharmacy P&P regarding expired drugs
    d. call the FDA for disposal of the drug

76. A _____-micron filter is commonly used to filter solutions withdrawn from ampoules.
    a. 0.2
    b. 0.5
    c. 2
    d. 5

77. The _____ is a document that contains the goals, policies, and procedures relevant to the employee and the job the employee is assuming.
    a. employee handbook
    b. corporate prospectus
    c. planogram
    d. administration handbook

78. The _____ is used to record the balances that private patients, government agencies, insurance companies, managed-care contractors, and insurers owe the pharmacy.
    a. balance sheet
    b. accounts receivable ledger
    c. cash disbursements journal
    d. sales journal

79. Control of the amount, type, and quality of health care provided to patients within a benefit program is referred to as:
    a. health insurance
    b. managed care
    c. benefit plans
    d. pharmaceutical care

80. The bolded section of the National Drug Code 0001-009-012 indentifies the:
    a. drug's manufacturer
    b. the drug's name, strength, and dosage form
    c. the package size
    d. both a and c

81. 1 pint = _____ ml
    a. 30
    b. 473
    c. 946
    d. 3785

82. The provision of drug therapy intended to achieve outcomes that improve the patient's quality of life as it is related to the cure or prevention of a disease, elimination or reduction of a patient's symptoms, or arresting or slowing of a disease process is:
    a. pharmaceutical care
    b. managed care
    c. socialized medicine
    d. practice of pharmacy

83. The FDA recall of a product that will cause serious or fatal consequences is classified as:
    a. Class I
    b. Class II
    c. Class III
    d. Class IV

84. Devices:
    a. do not have any restrictions.
    b. are defined as instruments, apparatuses, implements, machines, and so on.
    c. may be restricted to sale only on the written or oral order of a practitioner licensed to administer such a device.
    d. both b and c

85. The principle that states that patients have the right to full disclosure of all relevant aspects of care and must give explicit consent to treatment before treatment is initiated is:
    a. confidentiality
    b. fidelity
    c. informed consent
    d. moral reasoning

86. _____ is a company that buys from the manufacturer and sells to hospitals, pharmacies, and other pharmaceutical dispensers.
    a. The Food and Drug Administration
    b. A wholesaler
    c. A retailer
    d. A mass merchandiser

87. Drugs that are not intended to be sold by a pharmacy, but are intended to promote the sale of that particular drug, are known as:
    a. legend drugs
    b. sample drugs
    c. investigational drugs
    d. over-the-counter drugs

88. The _____ created the legend class of drugs.
    a. Comprehensive Drug Abuse Prevention and Control Act
    b. Medical Device Amendment
    c. Durham–Humphrey Amendment
    d. Kefauver–Harris Amendment

89. A prescription is written for 1 lb of 3% salicylic acid in white petrolatum. How many milligrams of salicylic acid are needed?
    a. 13,620 mg
    b. 13.62 mg
    c. 1362 mg
    d. 48 mg

90. The _____ is used to record what the pharmacy owes its suppliers and other creditors.
    a. accounts payable ledger
    b. accounts receivable ledger
    c. purchases journal
    d. cash receipts journal

Practice Certification Exam III

This practice test has been designed to simulate the certification exam in both number and style of questions as well as the content. You should be able to complete this exam within 2 hr.

1. Certification is:
   a. the process of granting recognition or vouching for conformance with a standard
   b. the process by which a nongovernmental agency or association grants recognition to an individual who has met certain predetermined qualifications specified by that agency or association
   c. the general process of formally recognizing professional or technical competence
   d. the process of making a list or being enrolled in an existing list

2. Which route of medication administration is used to inject drugs into muscle?
   a. sub-q
   b. IV
   c. ID
   d. IM

3. A connection between two or more computer systems that allows for the transfer of data is:
   a. an interface
   b. a terminal
   c. a bar code
   d. a window

4. A policies and procedures manual may provide guidance in each of the following areas except:
   a. personal orientation, training, and evaluation
   b. correct aseptic (sterile) technique
   c. activities of technicians outside the workplace
   d. position or job descriptions

5. An ongoing systematic process for monitoring, evaluating, and improving the quality of pharmacy services is:
   a. peer review
   b. quality assurance
   c. process validation
   d. job performance evaluation

6. Sterile products should be prepared at least
   _____ inches from the front edge of
   the laminar airflow hood.
   a. 6
   b. 10
   c. 2
   d. 3

7. If you add 4.5 ml of diluent to a 1.5-g vial for a
   final concentration of 250 mg/ml, what is the total
   volume in the vial after reconstitution?
   a. 4.5 ml
   b. 5 ml
   c. 5.5 ml
   d. 6 ml

8. All of the following are required on a prescription
   label except:
   a. name and address of the pharmacy
   b. name of the prescriber
   c. serial number of the prescription
   d. telephone number of the patient

9. A prescription can be refilled:
   a. only once
   b. as many times as the pharmacist deems
      necessary
   c. as many times as the prescriber indicates
      on the prescription within a specified time
      period
   d. only at the location where it was originally
      filled

10. What would the check digit be for the following
    DEA number: AB369145_?
    a. 3
    b. 8
    c. 4
    d. 0

11. Which of the following best describes controlled
    substances in Schedule I?
    a. drugs with no accepted medical use in the
       United States
    b. drugs with a low to moderate potential for
       physical dependence
    c. drugs with no potential for abuse
    d. drugs that are available without a prescription

12. A 500-mL quantity of D10W contains how many
    grams of dextrose?
    a. 100 g
    b. 10 g
    c. 50 g
    d. 20 g

13. The Poison Prevention Packaging Act of 1970
    mandated all of the following except:

a. Prescription drugs may be exempt if the prescriber or consumer requests noncompliant
   packaging.
b. Household cleaners must be packaged in
   childproof containers.
c. A limited number of prescription drugs are
   exempt (such as sublingual nitroglycerin).
d. The special packaging requirements are
   extended to nonprescription drugs.

14. Sublingual tablets are:
    a. placed under the tongue
    b. dissolved in a liquid and release bubbles
    c. placed inside the cheek
    d. chewed before swallowing

15. The Omnibus Budget Reconciliation Act of 1990
    (OBRA 90) requires pharmacists to perform
    the following functions for patients receiving
    Medicaid:
    a. drug therapy review
    b. counseling
    c. financial consultation
    d. both a and b

16. The generic name for Xanax is:
    a. acyclovir
    b. allopurinol
    c. alprazolam
    d. aminodarone

17. Which statement concerning Synthroid is correct?
    a. The drug strength is measured in micrograms.
    b. The usual dose is 50–100 g/day.
    c. The drug is given 3 times a day.
    d. It is used to treat diabetes.

18. Prescription drugs are also known as:
    a. legend drugs
    b. new drugs
    c. over-the-counter drugs
    d. investigational drugs

19. Which of the following IV solutions is considered
    isotonic?
    a. D5 1/2 NS
    b. Sodium chloride 3%
    c. D10W
    d. NS

20. All of the following are true concerning patient
    participation in an investigational drug study
    except:
    a. The patient must sign an informed consent.
    b. Participation is voluntary.
    c. The patient may withdraw from the study at
       any time.
    d. The patient must be paid.

21. You receive a prescription for Ceclor suspension 125 mg/5 mL, 1.5 tsp tid × 10 days. The correct quantity to dispense is
    a. 125 mL
    b. 150 mL with one refill
    c. 200 mL
    d. 225 mL

22. Rx: Cortisporin gtts, use ud. Upon receiving the prescription, the technician should:
    a. fill the prescription with generic ophthalmic drops
    b. tell the patient that the prescriber must be contacted to verify ROA
    c. affix a "for the eye" auxiliary label to the container
    d. tell the patient to wash hands before administering so the drops will remain sterile

23. Which of the following drugs are commonly used to treat ulcers?
    a. digoxin and captopril
    b. prednisone and dexamethasone
    c. quinidine and quinine
    d. Tagamet and Zantac

24. Rx: Ceftriaxone 750 mg IVPB q12h. The home-care technician needs to prepare a 7-day supply. How many 1-g vials will be needed?
    a. 15
    b. 6
    c. 10
    d. 11

25. What is the powder volume if a vial's final volume is 50 ml after adding 34.6 ml of diluent?
    a. 34.6 ml
    b. 15.6 ml
    c. 50 ml
    d. 15.4 ml

26. When filling a prescription for Tylenol with codeine 30 mg, a technician should do all the following except:
    a. file the prescription as a Schedule III controlled substance
    b. affix an auxiliary label cautioning against performing tasks requiring alertness or driving
    c. verify that the patient is not allergic to Tylenol or codeine
    d. inform the patient that this medication is a potent anti-inflammatory agent

27. How many grams of active ingredient are in 16 oz of a 25% solution?
    a. 4
    b. 5.2

c. 25
d. 120

28. A computer insurance error message "patient not found" or "invalid ID number" indicates that:
    a. the patient must pay cash.
    b. the patient does not appear to be enrolled in the insurance program; check for errors such as misspelling of the patient's name
    c. the patient does not have any condition that requires treatment
    d. the pharmacy must return the prescription to the patient

29. When filling an inpatient's medication drawer, the technician notices that the fill list contains both enalapril and lisinopril. The technician should:
    a. fill only one drug
    b. notify the pharmacist
    c. call the doctor
    d. tell the nurse to give the medications at least 4 hr apart

30. Of the following insulins, which could be added to an IV infusion?
    a. Novolog Mix 50/50
    b. Humulin NPH
    c. Humulin R
    d. Humulin 70/30

31. The portion of the prescription costs that the patient must pay in a given time period before the third-party insurer will begin paying is called a:
    a. fee-for-service
    b. co-payment
    c. deductible
    d. co-insurance

32. If a pediatric patient is to receive ampicillin oral suspension, which of the following is not necessary?
    a. Ensure that the patient is not allergic to PCN.
    b. Affix an expiration date to the label after reconstitution.
    c. Affix a "shake well before using" label.
    d. Use aseptic technique to reconstitute the medication.

33. Which of the following resources could not be used to determine whether a parenteral medication must be filtered?
    a. the package insert
    b. *Handbook on Injectable Drugs*
    c. the IV pharmacist
    d. *American Drug Index*

34. The offer to counsel under OBRA 90 may be made:
    a. in writing
    b. orally
    c. by a technician
    d. all of the above

35. If you believe someone has presented a fraudulent prescription at your pharmacy, the appropriate action is to:
    a. discreetly call the police
    b. discreetly call the prescriber
    c. discreetly notify the pharmacist
    d. discreetly ask the customer how he got the prescription

36. You receive an order for etoposide. In preparing this drug, you should not:
    a. wear protective apparel
    b. dispose of extra drug according to policy
    c. prepare it in a biological safety cabinet
    d. prepare the drug in a horizontal laminar flow hood

37. While a mother is waiting for her child's antibiotic prescription, she asks the technician what to give the child for fever. The technician should:
    a. suggest aspirin; it's the least expensive antipyretic
    b. inform the pharmacist that the mother would like help choosing a nonprescription product
    c. offer to sell the mother acetaminophen
    d. suggest over-the-counter diphenhydramine

38. Rx: Vanceril (beclomethasone) inhaler; dispense #1; sig: ii puffs inhaled bid. In filling the prescription, the technician should:
    a. inform the patient that this drug is a corticosteroid that has many serious side effects
    b. include the following specific directions on the label: "Inhale 2 puffs into each nostril three times a day"
    c. provide the patient the package insert included with the inhaler
    d. tell the patient to use this inhaler only when he really needs it

39. When selling an over-the-counter nasal decongestant spray (phenylephrine), which question can the technician answer without referring the customer to the pharmacist?
    a. Can I take this drug with my blood pressure medicine?
    b. I keep using this spray, but my nose seems to get stuffier. Should I use it more often?
    c. Is a less expensive generic available?
    d. I've had this cold for four weeks. Do you think I should see the doctor?

40. Rx: Amoxicillin suspension 5 mL po tid × 10 days. Upon review, you realize that the prescriber did not indicate the drug concentration. You should:
    a. dispense the capsules instead
    b. alert the pharmacist to the problem
    c. ask the patient which concentration he prefers
    d. prepare the prescription with the 250-mg/ml concentration because it is most frequently ordered

41. Which of the following could contribute to a medication error?
    a. failure to rotate stock appropriately
    b. preparing more than one prescription at a time
    c. not reading the drug product label carefully
    d. all the above

42. When accepting a prescription for warfarin from a patient, the technician should:
    a. notify the pharmacist if the patient is also buying aspirin; there is an interaction between these medications
    b. tell the patient to take the warfarin in the morning and the aspirin in the afternoon
    c. tell the patient to take an iron supplement because this drug thins the blood
    d. tell the patient to eat foods that are high in vitamin K

43. The risk of a decimal point error is reduced by writing "seven milligrams" as:
    a. 0.7 g
    b. 7 mg
    c. 7.0 mg
    d. 0.70 g

44. Which of the following drugs is stored in the pharmacy refrigerator?
    a. nystatin vaginal tablets
    b. Viroptic ophthalmic drops
    c. tetanus toxoid vaccine
    d. all the above

45. A patient calls the pharmacy asking why his heart medication is white instead of the usual yellow color. Upon investigation, it is discovered that the prescription was filled with digoxin 0.25 mg instead of the 0.125-mg strength. Which of the following is the most appropriate action to take?
    a. Tell the patient to cut the tablets in half and take one-half tablet daily.
    b. Ask the patient to bring the prescription back to the pharmacy so that you can secretly exchange it for the correct dose.
    c. Explain the situation to the pharmacist, correct the error, and document the error per procedures.

d. Prepare a new prescription with the 0.125-mg strength and inform the patient that pharmacists are solely responsible for the accuracy of prescriptions.

46. Which of the following is not ordered on DEA Form 222?

a. morphine
b. hydromorphone
c. diazepam
d. secobarbital

47. Which of the following is not required on a unit-dose prepackaged label?

a. drug strength
b. lot number
c. patient room number
d. expiration date

48. A physician calls the pharmacy asking about the maximum dose of a new medication. The technician answering the phone remembers hearing the pharmacist answer this question earlier that same day. How should the technician handle this call?

a. Inform the physician that the maximum dose is 500 mg twice daily, because that was the dose the pharmacist gave earlier that day.
b. Ask another technician and relay the information to the physician.
c. Look up the answer to the question in *Facts and Comparisons* and inform the physician.
d. Refer the question to the pharmacist.

49. A prescription with the directions to be given o.u. should be administered to:

a. both eyes
b. the left eye
c. the right ear
d. the left ear

50. The usual dose of milk of magnesia is 30 cc. This is equivalent to:

a. 3 tbsp
b. 3 tsp
c. 1 tsp
d. 2 tbsp

51. Which vaccine has to be stored frozen before use?

a. oral polio
b. injectable polio
c. influenza
d. pneumococcal

52. If a product is labeled to expire August 2012, what is the last date it should be used by?

a. August 01, 2012
b. September 01, 2012
c. July 31, 2012
d. August 31, 2012

53. A patient's dose of NPH U-100 insulin is 35 units qam. How much should be drawn up and administered by the nurse each morning?

a. 0.035 ml
b. 0.35 ml
c. 3.5 ml
d. 35 ml

54. A technician reading a medication order for a patient notices an abbreviation with which he is not familiar. Which of the following is not an acceptable way to clarify the meaning of the abbreviation?

a. Call the prescriber.
b. Ask the pharmacist.
c. Refer to the lists of approved abbreviations in the policy and procedures manual.
d. Ask the senior technician.

55. Which agent is not used for the treatment of tuberculosis?

a. pyrazinamide
b. rifampin
c. ethambutol
d. vinblastine

56. Federal refill limitations for a Schedule III controlled-substance prescription are:

a. maximum of five refills and within the six-month period after initial filling of the prescription
b. maximum of five refills and not more than one year after date of issuance
c. maximum of ten refills and within six months of the date the prescription was written
d. maximum of five refills and within six months of the date the prescription was written

57. Which cytotoxic drug does not require refrigeration?

a. vinblastine
b. cyclophosphamide
c. asparaginase
d. carmustine

58. The set of procedures for preparation of sterile products that is designed to prevent contamination is called:

a. eutectic mixing
b. filtration
c. trituration
d. aseptic technique

59. An example of a drug used as an anticonvulsant is:

a. aspirin
b. chlorpromazine
c. carbamazepine
d. lithium

60. Which of the following statements about quality is true?

    a. Quality control is a process of checks and balances.
    b. Quality is defined by what our customers perceive.
    c. Quality improvement is an important part of meeting regulatory agency (such as JCAHO) requirements.
    d. All of the above

61. Triazolam is most commonly ordered:

    a. TID prn
    b. BID
    c. QAM
    d. QHS prn

62. Rx: Cortisporin solution ii gtts a.u. Which of the following medications should be dispensed?

    a. otic solution
    b. ophthalmic solution
    c. topical ointment
    d. ophthalmic ointment

63. Convert 1:1000 to a percent strength.

    a. 0.001%
    b. 0.01%
    c. 0.1%
    d. 1%

64. Rx: Ovral-28 i tab po daily. Disp: 3 month supply with 3 refills. If the patient's insurance pays for only a one-month supply, the technician should fill a one-month supply and adjust the refills to:

    a. 4
    b. 11
    c. 12
    d. the refills must remain at 3

65. If a patient is noted to have experienced an allergic reaction to a medication, the technician should:

    a. tell the patient that the doctor made a mistake, and refuse to fill the prescription
    b. tell the patient to take the medication anyway, since it is a doctor's order
    c. ask the patient the type of allergic reaction experienced, note the patient's response, and alert the pharmacist
    d. call the prescriber for a new prescription

66. If a prescription is written for a trade drug and is marked (according to state law) that a substitution is not allowed:

    a. a generic drug can still be dispensed if the trade is not available
    b. the specific brand-name drug must be dispensed
    c. send the patient back to the physician's office for clarification
    d. fill with a generic drug but notate that it has been substituted for the brand

67. 360 ml = _____ tablespoons.

    a. 6
    b. 12
    c. 24
    d. 36

68. Three fluid ounces is equal to _____ mL.

    a. 120
    b. 90
    c. 100
    d. 150

69. Order: D5 1/2 NS 2L over 10 hr. What is the IV rate?

    a. 80 ml/hr
    b. 100 ml/hr
    c. 125 ml/hr
    d. 200 ml/hr

70. Fentanyl has a concentration of 0.5 mg/mL. How many milliliters do you need for a 950-mcg dose?

    a. 190 mL
    b. 0.19 mL
    c. 19 mL
    d. 1.9 mL

71. According to most insurance coverage, if a prescription is written for a brand-name product and "may substitute" is marked on it:

    a. the brand-name drug must be dispensed
    b. the generic drug must be dispensed
    c. the generic drug can be dispensed if the patient and the pharmacist agree
    d. the prescription is written incorrectly

72. The last step in processing a new prescription is:

    a. computer data entry
    b. prescription filling
    c. dispensing
    d. counseling by a pharmacist

73. During prescription computer entry, the technician is responsible for all the following except:

    a. entering accurate patient demographic information
    b. entering any allergies the patient reports
    c. handling insurance claims messaging
    d. handling drug interaction messaging

74. Rx: Penicillin 125 mg/5 ml oral susp, 250 mg po tid × 10 days. How many milliliters will be dispensed?

    a. 300 mL
    b. 150 mL
    c. 100 mL
    d. 120 mL

75. When receiving a drug–drug, drug–disease state, or drug–allergy interaction computer message, the technician should:

    a. inform the patient that the prescription cannot be filled
    b. alert the doctor to the mistake
    c. ignore the message if the patient has previously had the prescription filled
    d. alert the pharmacist to the problem

76. All of the following drugs are antidotes except:

    a. activated charcoal
    b. Digibind
    c. cefazolin
    d. naloxone

77. Which of the following is not required on a prescription label?

    a. the prescription number
    b. directions on how to take the medication
    c. the prescribing physician's name
    d. the physician's DEA number

78. The sterile parts of a syringe that may never be touched are the:

    a. plunger and barrel
    b. tip and plunger
    c. barrel and hub
    d. tip and hub

79. Why are vertical laminar airflow hoods required when preparing chemotherapy medication?

    a. They provide optimal preparer protection.
    b. Contaminated air is not blown toward the preparer.
    c. Vertical airflow hoods are not required when mixing chemotherapy drugs.
    d. Both a and b

80. Which of the following medications must be protected from light?

    a. amphotericin B
    b. heparin

    c. tobramycin
    d. lanoxin

81. Rx: Metronidazole 500 mg po qid × 7 days. How many 0.25-g tablets are needed to fill the prescription?

    a. 14
    b. 28
    c. 42
    d. 56

82. All of the following medications must be stored in the refrigerator, except:

    a. tetanus toxoid
    b. insulin
    c. tobramycin
    d. amoxicillin

83. Which of the following conditions is not commonly treated in the home-care environment?

    a. sepsis
    b. osteomyelitis
    c. chronic pain
    d. malnutrition

84. All of the following drugs are laxatives except:

    a. bisacodyl tablets
    b. Citrucel powder
    c. FiberCon tablets
    d. Pancrease capsules

85. Which of the following drugs is available as an injection, topical cream, and ophthalmic solution?

    a. tobramycin
    b. furosemide
    c. gentamicin
    d. nystatin

86. Which of the following drugs is not available in an oral form and an injectable form?

    a. ranitidine
    b. furosemide
    c. prochlorperazine
    d. ibuprofen

87. Order: Tobramycin 130. How many milliliters of tobramycin 80 mg/2 ml are needed for one dose?

    a. 0.325 mL
    b. 3.25 mL
    c. 1.625 mL
    d. 1.7 mL

88. A 1000-mL bag of D5W is to infuse over 8 hr using an IV set with a drop factor of 10 gtt/ml. What is the flow rate in gtt/min?

    a. 12.5 gtt/min
    b. 21 gtt/min
    c. 22 gtt/min
    d. 125 gtt/min

89. Federal law allows _____ refills of Schedule II narcotic prescriptions.

    a. 6
    b. 1
    c. 0
    d. 12

90. All of the following medications must be prepared in a vertical laminar airflow hood except:

    a. cisplatin
    b. cyclophosphamide
    c. cefotaxime
    d. etoposide

Practice Certification Exam IV

This practice exam has been designed to simulate the certification exam in both number and style of questions as well as the content. You should be able to complete this exam within 2 hr.

1. When ordering Schedule II controlled substances, who signs the order form?
   a. the narcotic technician
   b. the pharmacist on duty
   c. the pharmacy manager
   d. the pharmacy person with power of attorney

2. Compounding equipment used in the IV room must be cleaned at least:
   a. once a week
   b. once a day
   c. once an hour
   d. once a year

3. Examples of dispersions include:
   a. syrups and elixirs
   b. tinctures, fluid extracts
   c. aromatic waters, diluted acids
   d. suspensions, emulsions

4. What is the maximum number of products that can be ordered on a DEA Form 222?
   a. 1
   b. 5
   c. 8
   d. 10

5. In addition to the dosage form, the term *delivery system* refers to:
   a. use of the drug as a therapeutic, pharmacodynamic, diagnostic, prophylactic, or destructive agent
   b. the chemical composition of the drug
   c. restrictions placed on the ordering, storage, and dispensing of the drug because of its classification
   d. physical characteristics of the dosage form that determine the method of administration and the site of action of the drug

6. A customer comes into your retail pharmacy with a prescription, and his address has changed. As a technician, you should:
   a. let the pharmacist handle the situation
   b. input him into the computer system as a new patient and create a new profile
   c. update his patient profile with the new information
   d. ignore the information, because the address is not needed to fill the prescription

7. Good manufacturing practices are regulated by the:
   a. Texas State Board of Pharmacy
   b. FDA
   c. DEA
   d. Manufacturers of America

8. Which of the following would most likely not be found in a pharmacy policy and procedures manual?
   a. hiring practices
   b. management of dangerous drugs
   c. inventory control of pharmaceuticals
   d. good compounding practices

9. How many milliliters of a 250-mg/5-ml liquid are needed for a 0.75-g dose?
   a. 1.5 ml
   b. 7.5 ml
   c. 10 ml
   d. 15 ml

10. A person with a thiamine deficiency has an inadequate supply of:
    a. vitamin B-12
    b. vitamin B-6
    c. vitamin D
    d. vitamin B-1

11. A 500-mg/250-ml dopamine IV is infusing at 1000 mcg per minute. What is the flow rate in ml/hr?
    a. 10 ml/hr
    b. 20 ml/hr
    c. 30 ml/hr
    d. 50 ml/hr

12. Which of the following is not a factor that affects how a prescriber doses a medication?
    a. weight
    b. insurance
    c. age
    d. physical condition

13. Which of the following dosage forms deteriorates and loses potency faster than tablets?
    a. suppositories
    b. oral inhalers
    c. liquids
    d. capsules

14. Repackaging large, non-patient-specific quantities of medications to be used over long periods of time is an example of _____ repackaging.
    a. extemporaneous
    b. batch
    c. patient-specific
    d. unit dose

15. Of the following equipment, which would least likely be used to compound a prescription for an oral suspension?
    a. mortar
    b. compounding slab
    c. graduated cylinder
    d. pestle

16. You receive a rejected insurance claim stating "refill too early." Which of the following could be the potential reason for the rejected claim?
    a. wrong patient code
    b. wrong quantity dispensed
    c. wrong days' supply
    d. patient does not have current coverage

17. A PRN medication is one that is:
    a. given continuously around the clock
    b. given at set time intervals
    c. given only in response to a specific parameter
    d. given rectally

18. Which of the following medications is contraindicated in pregnant women?
    a. indomethacin
    b. isotretinoin
    c. ibuprofen
    d. itraconazole

19. Which of the following equipment is used to compound TPNs?
    a. Pyxis
    b. ScriptPro
    c. Automix
    d. Omnicell

20. Which of the following is indicated for active duodenal ulcers?
    a. Ropinirole HCl
    b. Risperidone
    c. Risedronate Sodium
    d. Ranitidine

21. A patient asks what OTC medication she should take for persistent heartburn. The pharmacy technician should:
    a. tell the patient to take Prilosec OTC
    b. tell the patient to talk to her doctor
    c. tell the patient to talk with the pharmacist on duty
    d. tell the patient to go to the emergency room

22. Aluminum hydroxide and diphenhydramine are mixed in a 3:1 ratio. How much of each is required to make 4 oz of suspension?
    a. 100 ml/20 ml
    b. 90 ml/30 ml
    c. 75 ml/25 ml
    d. 60 ml/60 ml

23. Rx: Platinol IV 20 mg/m^2/day for 5 days. If the patient's BSA is 1.52 m^2, how much of the drug must be drawn up for one dose if the concentration of the Platinol vial is 50 mg/50 ml.
    a. 20 ml
    b. 30 ml
    c. 30.4 ml
    d. 50 ml

24. Rx: Lasix 40 mg IV q8h. How many 10-ml furosemide, 10-mg/ml multidose vials should the pharmacy technician send for a 24-hr supply?
    a. 1
    b. 2
    c. 3
    d. 4

25. What is the IV rate (ml/hr) if the patient has 2000 ml of D5W infused every 24 hr?
    a. 38 ml/hr
    b. 48 ml/hr
    c. 83 ml/hr
    d. 84 ml/hr

26. Penicillin suspension is available in a concentration of 250 mg/5 ml. How many teaspoons are required for a 375-mg dose?
    a. ½ tsp
    b. ¾ tsp
    c. 1½ tsp
    d. 1¾ tsp

27. The drug rifampin requires which of the following auxiliary labels?
    a. take with food or milk
    b. may cause discoloration of urine or feces
    c. do not take with aspirin
    d. may cause photosensitivity

28. A 10-ml U-100 insulin vial has a concentration of:
    a. 100 units per 10 ml
    b. 100 units per ml
    c. 100 units per 0.5 ml
    d. 100 units per 100 ml

29. A patient who is currently taking warfarin should not take which of the following controlled-substance medications?
    a. meperidine
    b. Percocet
    c. Dilaudid
    d. Percodan

30. Which of the following routes of administration has the quickest onset of action?
    a. IV
    b. ID
    c. po
    d. pr

31. Of the following information, which is not required on a unit-dose package?
    a. expiration date
    b. patient name
    c. lot number
    d. drug strength

32. The PPI for an oral inhaler prescription is required to be dispensed:
    a. only the first time the prescription is dispensed
    b. once a year
    c. each time the prescription is dispensed
    d. only upon the prescriber's request

33. What is the cost for 60 tablets if the pharmacy's cost is $42.10 per 100 tabs and a 25% markup is applied?
    a. $25.26
    b. $30.31
    c. $52.63
    d. $31.58

34. Which of the following medications is indicated for congestive heart failure?
    a. phenytoin
    b. glyburide
    c. valacyclovir
    d. captopril

35. How many grams of hydrocortisone are in 120 g of hydrocortisone 0.5% ointment?
    a. 0.6 g
    b. 6 g
    c. 60 g
    d. 66 g

36. The concentration of an injectable drug is 30 mg/5 ml. What volume is required for a 38.4-mg dose?
    a. 5.6 ml
    b. 6.4 ml
    c. 7.7 ml
    d. 7.8 ml

37. The recommended dose for cefadroxil is 30 mg/kg/day in two divided doses. How much should be given in each dose for a child who weighs 40 lb?
    a. 1200 mg
    b. 600 mg
    c. 545 mg
    d. 273 mg

38. How many 125-mg doses are in 10 g of drug?
    a. 10 doses
    b. 20 doses
    c. 40 doses
    d. 80 doses

39. The term *gauge* refers to:
    a. the diameter of the needle's shaft
    b. the length of the needle
    c. the size of the needle's lumen
    d. the needle's bevel

40. If a pharmacy technician receives an insurance error message stating an invalid "ICD-9" code, this means that which information is incorrect?
    a. drug strength
    b. drug manufacturer
    c. drug NDC
    d. patient diagnosis

41. Rx: Piroxicam 20 mg ii po bid. How many milligrams will the patient take in a 24-hr period?
    a. 20 mg
    b. 40 mg
    c. 80 mg
    d. 120 mg

42. How many 10-mg morphine tablets are needed to prepare 100 ml of a 1-mg/ml morphine solution?
    a. 1 tablet
    b. 5 tablets
    c. 10 tablets
    d. 20 tablets

43. A chemotherapy spill kit is required to be in close proximity of the preparer when an IV of which of the following drugs is compounded?
    a. famciclovir
    b. acyclovir
    c. cyclophosphamide
    d. morphine sulfate

44. The trade name for oseltamivir phosphate is:
    a. Tenormin
    b. Temovate
    c. Theo-dur
    d. Tamiflu

45. Which of the following sublingual drugs must be dispensed in its original glass container?
    a. isosorbide
    b. nitroglycerin
    c. zolpidem
    d. lorazepam

46. If 30 g of an ointment contains 250 mg of drug, what is the percent strength of the preparation?
    a. 0.1%
    b. 0.38%
    c. 0.48%
    d. 0.83%

47. If a prescriber discontinues a patient's investigational drug, what should the pharmacy do with the remaining drug?
    a. return it to the physician
    b. return it to the patient
    c. destroy the investigational drug
    d. return the drug to the manufacturer

48. If the pharmacy inventory is shelved alphabetically by generic name, under which letter would the drug Pamelor be found?
    a. B
    b. D
    c. N
    d. P

49. To maintain perpetual inventory control, the pharmacy must update records:
    a. whenever inventory is purchased or sold
    b. whenever sales figures are updated
    c. to identify low turnover
    d. to generate orders

50. 0023-022-11. The bolded portion of the NDC identifies the:
    a. drug strength
    b. manufacturer
    c. drug product
    d. package size

51. What is meant by the term *drug inventory rotation*?
    a. Using the drugs with the longest expiration date first
    b. Making sure that drugs with the longest expiration date are placed at the front of the shelf
    c. Making sure that drugs with the shortest expiration date are placed at the front of the shelf
    d. Making sure that drugs with the shortest expiration date are placed at the back of the shelf

52. The purpose of a hospital formulary is to:
    a. provide a listing of drugs approved by the insurance company
    b. provide a listing of the institution's approved drug products
    c. provide a listing of all FDA-approved drugs available
    d. provide the pharmacy technician with a listing of drugs in the pharmacy inventory

53. Tylenol #3 is listed on which schedule of controlled substances?
    a. Schedule I
    b. Schedule II
    c. Schedule III
    d. Schedule IV

54. Which of the following pharmacy records is most likely to be used to track medication that has been recalled?
    a. productivity report
    b. drug utilization report
    c. temperature logs
    d. purchase orders

55. The term *inventory turnover rate* refers to:
    a. the delivery turnaround time from the wholesaler
    b. how often the pharmacy rotates stock
    c. how often the pharmacy uses inventory
    d. how the inventory is ordered

56. The expiration date on a medication bottle states 7/12. When does the medication expire?
    a. July 1, 2012
    b. June 1, 2012
    c. July 31, 2012
    d. July 31, 2013

57. Which of the following drugs must be ordered using DEA Form 222?
    a. diazepam
    b. acetaminophen with codeine tablets
    c. meperidine
    d. guaifenesin with codeine liquid

58. Which of the following medications is indicated for the treatment of diabetes?
    a. Actonel
    b. Actos
    c. Adderall
    d. Advair

59. The term *inventory PAR level* refers to:
    a. the maximum quantity of inventory to be kept on the shelves
    b. the minimum quantity of inventory to be kept on the shelves
    c. the quantity of drug that should be ordered each time
    d. both a and c

60. Which of the following reference sources supplies the same information as is on a package insert?
    a. Red Book
    b. Orange Book
    c. PDR
    d. *Drug Facts and Comparisons*

61. Which of the following is indicated for the treatment of depression?
    a. Patanol
    b. Paxil
    c. Pepcid
    d. Peridex

62. How much 70% sorbitol is needed to prepare 8 fluid ounces of 50% sorbitol?
    a. 5.7 ml
    b. 11.2 ml
    c. 171.4 ml
    d. 336 ml

63. Which of the following topical medications requires special chemotherapy handling?
    a. Hytone 2.5%
    b. Kenalog 2.5%
    c. Efudex 5%
    d. Elidel 1%

64. Using the drug's _____ is the best method for pharmacy technicians to ensure that they are dispensing the correct drug.
    a. expiration date
    b. lot number
    c. wholesaler item number
    d. NDC

65. Pharmacies are required to have which of the following types of pharmacy balance?
    a. electronic
    b. Class A
    c. Class B
    d. Harvard Trip

66. A maintenance medication is not in stock. What is the proper procedure for the technician to follow?
    a. tell the patient he has no choice but to go to a different pharmacy
    b. tell the patient that the prescription cannot be filled
    c. inform the pharmacist and see if she can call the prescriber and ask to substitute a drug that is in stock
    d. ask the patient if you can call an alternate pharmacy of his choice to see if that pharmacy stocks the medication

67. Which of the following drugs would most likely have an "automatic stop order" in a hospital pharmacy?
    a. antitussives
    b. IV infusions
    c. investigational drugs
    d. antibiotics

68. Convert 1:10,000 to a percent strength.
    a. 0.0001%
    b. 0.001%
    c. 0.01%
    d. 0.1%

69. Pharmacy technicians deliver medications to nursing stations and pick up new physician's orders during their:
    a. IV delivery rounds
    b. chemotherapy delivery rounds
    c. floorstock delivery rounds
    d. medication delivery rounds

70. Which of the following would not result if a pharmacy technician filed an inaccurate insurance claim for a prescription?
    a. denied claim
    b. delayed claim
    c. increase in insurance payment to the pharmacy
    d. decrease in insurance payment to the pharmacy

71. A drug product that requires refrigeration should be stored at a temperature between:
    a. −25 and −10°C
    b. 2 and 8°C
    c. 8 and 15°C
    d. 20 and 25°C

72. When there is an incorrect box count, the technician receiving the order should:
    a. not accept any part of the order
    b. accept the order as complete
    c. document the incorrect box count with the delivery person
    d. accept the order and hope the wholesaler sends the balance

73. Which class of recalls can cause severe adverse effects or death?
    a. Class I
    b. Class II
    c. Class III
    d. Class IV

74. Material Safety Data Sheets are required by which of the following?
    a. FDA
    b. HIPAA
    c. USP
    d. OSHA

75. Which of the following drugs is *not* exempt from the Poison Prevention Packaging Act?
    a. oral inhalers
    b. nitroglycerin sl tablets
    c. unit-dose medications used in an institutional setting
    d. diazepam

76. If the refill section is left blank, the pharmacy can:
    a. give the patient as many refills as he wants
    b. assume that no refills were intended to be given
    c. give the patient a 1-year supply
    d. not fill the prescription

77. Which of the following laws requires pharmacists to counsel Medicaid patients?
    a. HIPAA
    b. OSHA
    c. OBRA 90
    d. COBRA

78. If a pharmacy technician discovers that a medication has expired, he or she should:
    a. dispense the drug if it expired within the last week
    b. discard the drug
    c. follow the pharmacy return policies
    d. dispense the drug at a discount price

79. The best source of information on compounding a medication is
    a. *Remington's Pharmaceutical Sciences*
    b. *Facts and Comparisons*
    c. *Pharmaceutical Dosage Forms and Drug Delivery Systems*
    d. *Approved Drug Products with Therapeutic Equivalence Evaluation*

80. The willingness of a patient to take a drug in the amount prescribed is called:
    a. ease of administration
    b. route of administration
    c. dosage
    d. compliance

81. Which of the following is not one of the five rights of medication administration?
    a. right route
    b. right dose
    c. right medication
    d. right doctor

82. How often should pharmaceutical balances and scales be professionally certified for accuracy?
    a. once a month
    b. every 6 months
    c. every year
    d. every 10 years

83. Which of the following is considered a covered entity under HIPAA regulations?
    a. health-care provider
    b. health plan
    c. health-care clearinghouse
    d. all the above

84. Which of the following technologies is used in only a retail or outpatient pharmacy setting?
    a. Pyxis
    b. Omnicell
    c. ScriptPro
    d. AcuDose Rx

85. Where can a technician find information on the pharmacy's best practices for quality drug delivery?
    a. HIPAA notice of disclosure
    b. MSDS book
    c. JCAHO Web site
    d. P&P manual

86. Which of the following would pay for a person's outpatient expenses?
    a. Medicare Part A
    b. Medicare Part B
    c. Medicare Part C
    d. Medicare Part D

87. Which of the following drugs is indicated for the treatment of cold sores?
    a. Valtrex
    b. Zovirax
    c. Atarax
    d. Soriatane

88. The purpose of clinical pharmacy is to:
    a. dispense medications
    b. compound medication
    c. report adverse reactions or interactions to medications
    d. provide information about medication

89. Licensing and general professional oversight of pharmacists and pharmacies is carried out by:
    a. colleges of pharmacy
    b. American Pharmaceutical Society
    c. ASHP
    d. state pharmacy boards

90. A biochemically reactive component in a drug is known as:
    a. an inactive ingredient
    b. an inert ingredient
    c. a diluent
    d. an active ingredient

chapter 17

Practice Certification Exam V

This practice exam has been designed to simulate the certification exam in both number and style of questions as well as the content. You should be able to complete this exam within 2 hr.

1. The portion of the cost of a prescription that a patient with third-party insurance must pay is the:
   a. deductible
   b. U&C
   c. MAC
   d. co-payment

LINE #	PATIENT'S NAME	QUANTITY DISPENSED	QUANTITY RECEIVED	CURRENT BALANCE
1	Beginning Balance			87
2	Barbara Jones	42		44
3	Received from wholesaler		100	144
4	Thomas Watkins	24		120

2. On the above perpetual inventory for a Schedule II controlled substance, which line contains an error?
   a. 1
   b. 2
   c. 3
   d. 4

3. If a patient experiences an adverse reaction to a prescription, the reaction should be reported to:
   a. the Joint Commission
   b. MedWatch
   c. the state board of pharmacy
   d. the drug manufacturer

4. All of the following define the term *drug* except:
   a. an article intended for use in the diagnosis, cure, mitigation, treatment, or prevention of disease in humans or other animals
   b. an article recognized in the USP, the NF, and the Homeopathic Pharmacopoeia of the United States
   c. a device used for a life-sustaining or life-supporting function
   d. an article (other than food) intended to affect the structure or any function of the body

5. All of the following methods for filing prescriptions are allowed except:

   a. a system using three prescription file drawers: one drawer for CII prescriptions, one drawer for CIII, CIV, and CV prescriptions, and one drawer for all others

   b. a system using two prescription file drawers: one drawer for all controlled-substance prescriptions and one drawer for all other prescriptions

   c. a system using five prescription file drawers: one drawer for CII, one drawer for CIII, one drawer for CIV, one drawer for CV, and one drawer for all other prescriptions

   d. a system using two prescription file drawers: one drawer for CII prescriptions and one drawer for all other prescriptions including CIII, CIV, and CV

6. Each of the following is a characteristic desired in an intravenous solution except:

   a. pH of 6
   b. sterility
   c. clarity
   d. pyrogen-free

7. Which of the following information is not required to be on a retail prescription label?

   a. pharmacy name and phone number
   b. prescription number
   c. patient's phone number
   d. prescriber's name

8. An air vent on a vented administration set should be a _____-micron filter vent to be considered a sterilizing filter.

   a. 10
   b. 0.2
   c. 0.5
   d. 5

9. How long will it take a 150-ml IV to infuse at a rate of 50 ml/hr?

   a. 1 hr
   b. 2 hr
   c. 2.5 hr
   d. 3 hr

10. A _____ is a device designed to reduce the risk of airborne contamination during the preparation of an IV admixture by providing an ultraclean environment.

   a. autoclave
   b. automix
   c. laminar airflow hood
   d. HEPA filter

11. _____ is an unintended side effect of a medication that is negative or in some way injurious to a patient's health.

   a. A contraindication
   b. An adverse effect
   c. An indication
   d. A warning

12. The _____ is a form used in institutional settings to prescribe medications.

   a. prescription
   b. medication order
   c. MAR
   d. fill list

13. If an accident occurs involving a hazardous substance that is stored in the pharmacy, what document will provide instructions on actions that need to be taken?

   a. policies and procedure manual
   b. MSDS
   c. employee handbook
   d. OSHA "Right to Know" pamphlet

14. A pharmacy fills three prescriptions using sulfur powder. The first prescription uses 10 g, the second uses 0.5 kg, and the third uses 25 mg. What was the total amount of sulfur used to fill the three prescriptions?

   a. 510.025 g
   b. 35.5 g
   c. 510.25 g
   d. 60.25 g

15. Which organization requires that oral products be stored separate from inhaled products, topical preparations be separated from injectables, and so on?

   a. DEA
   b. PTCB
   c. APHA
   d. Joint Commission

16. An automatic stop order is most likely to be issued for which of the following drugs?

   a. clonidine 0.3-mg tablets
   b. acetaminophen/codeine 325-mg/60-m tablets
   c. amlodipine 5-mg tablets
   d. furosemide 40-mg tablets

17. _____ occurs when a drug is substantially degraded or destroyed by the liver's enzymes before it reaches the circulatory system.

   a. Enzyme induction
   b. Tolerance
   c. A first-pass effect
   d. Metabolism

18. The _____ classified drugs according to their potential for abuse.
    a. Controlled Substances Act
    b. Medical Device Amendment
    c. Comprehensive Drug Abuse Prevention and Control Act
    d. Anabolic Steroid Control Act

19. The abbreviation PR stands for:
    a. per recommendation
    b. previous records
    c. rectally
    d. percent reduction

20. All of the following concerning DEA Form 222 are true except:
    a. It is in triplicate.
    b. Copy 1 and Copy 2 are forwarded to the supplier.
    c. Multiple items may be ordered per line.
    d. There are 10 lines on the form.

21. The _____ is a price that is determined by a survey of the usual and customary prices for a prescription within a given geographic area.
    a. MAC
    b. deductible
    c. U&C
    d. UAC

22. Administrations of large volumes of solution over several hours at a slow, constant rate are known as:
    a. continuous infusion
    b. an infusion pump
    c. intermittent infusion
    d. a piggyback

23. The DEA form used to surrender C-II medications for disposition is:
    a. Form 222
    b. Form 224
    c. Form 41
    d. Form 363

24. Administration of relatively small volumes of solution over a short time at specific intervals is known as:
    a. continuous infusion
    b. TPN
    c. intermittent infusion
    d. enteral nutrition

25. Pastilles are:
    a. placed under the tongue and dissolved
    b. inserted into the vagina
    c. placed into the pouch of the lower eyelid
    d. held in the mouth and sucked

26. Extended-release dosage forms are formulated to:
    a. have longer shelf lives than regularly formulated products
    b. release medication slowly over an extended period of time
    c. increase the number of doses a patient must take in a day
    d. lengthen the amount of time before a prescription must be refilled

27. Which of the following routes of medication administration is not a parenteral route?
    a. subq
    b. pr
    c. I.D.
    d. I.M.

28. Add 1.17 kg, 1.59 g, and 260 mg.
    a. 262.76 g
    b. 1461.35 g
    c. 3.02 g
    d. 1171.85 g

29. Which of the following are one-time-use containers?
    a. an ampoule
    b. an IV piggyback
    c. a unit-dose package
    d. all the above

30. Which of the following units of measure represents the smallest unit of weight?
    a. gram
    b. milligram
    c. kilogram
    d. microgram

31. The word _____ indicates directions for use.
    a. magma
    b. scribe
    c. signa
    d. indication

32. When preparing a TPN solution containing calcium, phosphate, and other ingredients, which of the following statements is true?
    a. The calcium and phosphate should be mixed together in the same syringe before being injected into the TPN solution.
    b. The calcium should be added first, then all other additives, then add the phosphate last.
    c. The phosphate should be added first, then all other additives, then add the calcium last.
    d. The calcium and phosphate should be added last, after all other additives.

33. A system that maintains a continuous record of every item in inventory so that it always shows stock on hand is known as:
    a. perpetual inventory
    b. a POS system
    c. turnover
    d. reorder points

34. A cough-and-cold tablet contains the following amounts of active ingredients:

acetaminophen	325 mg
chlorpheniramine maleate	2 mg
pseudoephedrine hydrochloride	30 mg
dextromethorphan	15 mg
guaifenesin	100 mg

    The pharmacy has 2 kg of acetaminophen, 5 g of chlorpheniramine maleate, and an unlimited supply of the other ingredients. How many tablets can be prepared?
    a. 6153
    b. 2500
    c. 2885
    d. 5000

35. A 0.9% sodium chloride solution is _____.
    a. hypotonic
    b. isotonic
    c. hypertonic
    d. none of the above

36. Capsules are medications enclosed in gelatin. They are available in several sizes. Which of the following sizes is the smallest?
    a. 000
    b. 00
    c. 0
    d. 1

37. A person diagnosed with GERD is likely to be prescribed which of the following medications?
    a. propranolol
    b. ciprofloxin
    c. phenytoin
    d. esomeprazole

38. Which of the following is not true regarding nitroglycerin?
    a. It is indicated for angina pectoris.
    b. It is sensitive to light and moisture, so it should be dispensed in amber glass containers.
    c. It is an exception to the Poison Prevention Act.
    d. It is stable for one year after dispensing.

39. A bulk vial of cefazolin indicates an expiration date of May 2012. Which of the following statements is true regarding the use of this cefazolin vial?

a. The vial may be used for up to one year after the printed expiration date.
b. The vial must be used by May 1, 2012.
c. The vial can be used through the last day of May 2012.
d. The vial may be used for up to six months after the printed expiration date.

40. A patient is receiving Timentin 3.1 g q6h via a CADD Plus pump at home. Which of the following information is mandatory on a label in the home-care setting?
    a. patient address
    b. prescriber's phone number
    c. drug NDC
    d. transcribed directions

41. Which controlled-substance classification includes sedative and hypnotic drugs?
    a. C II
    b. C III
    c. C IV
    d. C V

42. You receive an order to prepare 250 mg of dobutamine in a 100-mL CADD cassette with NS as the diluent. Dobutamine is available as a 12.5-mg/mL solution. How many milliliters of dobutamine do you need to prepare this prescription?
    a. 20 mL
    b. 40 mL
    c. 200 mL
    d. 400 mL

43. How much 10% dextrose can be prepared from 500 ml of 70% dextrose?
    a. 3500 ml
    b. 1400 ml
    c. 7140 ml
    d. 2050 ml

44. The pharmacist asks you to check the compatibility of parenteral phenytoin with sodium chloride 0.9%. Which reference should you select to find this information?
    a. *Handbook of Injectable Drugs*
    b. *Remington's Pharmaceutical Sciences*
    c. *Medication Teaching Manual: The Guide to Patient Drug Information*
    d. *Drug Facts and Comparisons*

45. In which of the following functions may a well-trained technician participate?
    a. documenting investigational drug use
    b. preparing chemotherapeutic agents
    c. purchasing and inventory control
    d. all of the above

46. Checking the temperature of a refrigerator that stores medications on a daily basis is:
    a. an example of a quality-control mechanism used to meet Joint Commission requirements
    b. a method to assure proper storage of medications and avoid waste
    c. a mechanism to satisfy a technician's job duties as set by the pharmacy director
    d. all the above

47. In a hospital pharmacy, the technician can assist the pharmacist in all the following ways except:
    a. dispensing STAT medications without the pharmacist's approval
    b. alerting the pharmacist when a medication order appears to be written in error (for example, overdose)
    c. obtaining a patient's lab results
    d. alerting the pharmacist if a nonformulary drug has been ordered

48. All of the following statements are false except:
    a. A technician needs a license to practice in a central pharmacy and a separate license to practice in a satellite pharmacy.
    b. The technician can dispense medications without a final check by a pharmacist.
    c. A technician can answer questions related to patient-specific drug information.
    d. A technician can retrieve lab data for the pharmacist to use in making clinical judgments on patient care.

49. To be considered a generic equivalent for a trade-named drug product, the substitute must be:
    a. bioequivalent
    b. the same color
    c. made by the same manufacturer
    d. the same shape

50. Cleaning a vertical laminar airflow hood includes using which of the following agents?
    a. isopropyl alcohol
    b. sterile water
    c. povidone-iodine
    d. both a and b

51. You are asked to make fluorouracil 4000 mg in 1000 mL of sodium chloride 0.9%. What auxiliary label should be placed on the prepared admixture?
    a. Protect from light.
    b. Caution: Federal law prohibits the transfer of this drug to any person other than the patient for whom it was prescribed.
    c. Chemotherapy/biohazard.
    d. Administer with food or milk.

52. A pharmacy technician is preparing heparin 25,000 units in 500 ml of dextrose 5% in water. The concentration on the label should read:
    a. 250 units/ml
    b. 125 units/ml
    c. 100 units/ml
    d. 50 units/ml

53. Which of the following statements is (are) true regarding the technician's role in formulary issues?
    a. The technician can screen for orders that are nonformulary and alert the pharmacist.
    b. The technician can alert the purchasing agent when the par level of a formulary item is getting low.
    c. The technician can initially screen orders that are considered expensive or have potential for complication and alert the pharmacist.
    d. all of the above

54. Which of the following are ways in which the technician can participate in quality improvement?
    a. mapping out the work flow of a system or process requiring improvement
    b. collecting data for the evaluation of a process
    c. calling the physician to discuss appropriate drug therapy
    d. both a and b

55. If a patient tells you that his six-month-old child ingested "some" iron tablets, the pharmacy technician is responsible for:
    a. looking up the toxic dose of ferrous sulfate in *Facts and Comparisons*
    b. instructing the parent to buy activated charcoal
    c. telling the parent that "some" iron tablets will not harm the child
    d. instructing the parent to call the local poison control center

56. When giving drug information to the patient, which of the following is the least desirable source?
    a. patient package insert
    b. *USP DI Advice for the Patient*
    c. a manufacturer's "patient education" brochure
    d. a drug package insert

57. At cart fill, you identify an order to refill both cisapride and fluconazole for a patient. You should:
    a. notify the pharmacist of a possible drug interaction
    b. fill the cart, because a drug interaction screening has already been done by the pharmacist
    c. do nothing, because no drug interaction exists between the two agents
    d. call the physician to change the antibiotic

58. *American Drug Index* provides the following information:
    a. brand-to-generic-name cross-referencing
    b. available medication dosage forms
    c. manufacturer name, address, and phone number
    d. all of the above

59. Questions that may be answered by Material Safety Data Sheets include all of the following except:
    a. What precautions must be taken when preparing and dispensing Adriamycin?
    b. What is the dosing of activated charcoal for accidental poisoning?
    c. How should an employee exposed to Adriamycin be treated?
    d. How should a chemotherapy spill be cleaned?

60. All of the following are required when filling and dispensing a prescription for a metaproterenol oral metered-dose inhaler except:
    a. auxiliary label: For oral inhalation only
    b. auxiliary label: Shake well
    c. patient instructions
    d. auxiliary label: Take with food

61. A retail pharmacy is having a sale on an OTC drug. If the item's regular price is $6.80 and it is to be marked down 40%, what will be the selling price of the item?
    a. $2.72
    b. $4.08
    c. $4.80
    d. $2.27

62. The most common and uncomplicated route of administration is:
    a. intravenous
    b. intramuscular
    c. oral
    d. sublingual

63. A troche is also known as:
    a. an effervescent tablet
    b. a lozenge
    c. a granule
    d. a gelatin capsule

64. Which of the following drugs should be stored in the hospital's CII stock?
    a. diazepam
    b. codeine with acetaminophen
    c. phenobarbital
    d. hydromorphone

65. A patient is being provided with TPN, and the following order has been sent to the pharmacy. If the pharmacy stocks magnesium sulfate 10% (0.8 mEq/ml) in a 10-mL vial, what is the volume of drug that should be added if 24 mEq/2 L is ordered?
    a. 2.15 mL
    b. 30 mL
    c. 0.8 mL
    d. 0.3 mL

66. Which of the following vitamins is needed for proper blood clotting?
    a. vitamin A
    b. vitamin D
    c. vitamin E
    d. vitamin K

67. As a pharmacy technician in a home-care environment, you might be responsible for which of the following tasks?
    a. picking and packing medical supplies
    b. delivering supplies to the patient's home
    c. purchasing drugs and medical supplies
    d. all of the above

68. A type of reimbursement whereby a pharmacy receives a predetermined amount of money for a defined group of patients regardless of the number of prescriptions filled is:
    a. fee-for-service
    b. co-payment
    c. capitation
    d. no payment

69. Typical data collected from the patient at the prescription drop off window can include:
    a. weight for children and infants
    b. allergies
    c. emergency phone numbers
    d. all of the above

70. What volume of medication will deliver a dose of 65 mg if the vial label reads 10 mg/5 ml?
    a. 6.5 ml
    b. 13 ml
    c. 32.5 ml
    d. 130 ml

71. Examples of quality-control measures utilized when preparing an IVPB include:
    a. pulling the drug from the shelf and double-checking to ensure that the vial is correct
    b. calculating the correct dose and volume to withdraw from the vial to ensure that the vial is correct
    c. checking the IVPB for particulate matter after injecting the medication
    d. all of the above

72. The _____ is a set amount that must be paid by the patient for each benefit period before the insurer will cover additional expenses.
    a. co-payment
    b. deductible
    c. garnishment
    d. MAC

73. Personal protective equipment should be used properly when handling hazardous medications. This consists of:
    a. gloves
    b. gown
    c. mask
    d. all the above

74. How many tablets will be dispensed for a prescription indicating that a patient is to take 1 tablet po bid for 30 days?
    a. 30
    b. 60
    c. 90
    d. 120

75. Of the following tasks involved in pharmacy practice, which is allowed by law for technicians to perform?
    a. giving or receiving a verbal copy
    b. counseling a patient on the use of his medication
    c. receiving a verbal order from a physician
    d. filling a unit-dose cart

76. Which of the following is equal to 32 tbsp?
    a. 473 ml
    b. 3785 ml
    c. 16 fluid oz
    d. 480 g

77. Amphotericin B should be mixed only in _____ for compatibility.
    a. 0.9% sodium chloride
    b. LR
    c. 0.45% sodium chloride
    d. D5W

78. Which of the following is not an automated dispensing system that might be found in an inpatient pharmacy?
    a. Script-Pro
    b. Omnicell
    c. Pyxis
    d. Baxa Robot

79. After preparing IV doxorubicin, how should the technicians dispose of the used needles?
    a. Dispose of needles in an approved biohazard sharps container without recapping.

    b. Bend needles so they cannot possibly be reused.
    c. Dispose of needles in an approved hazardous sharps container without recapping.
    d. Discard needles into a cardboard box that has been identified for needle waste

80. Which of the following drugs is indicated for the treatment of weight management?
    a. phentermine
    b. phenobarbital
    c. phanazopyridine
    d. paroxetine

81. Of the following information, which would not be found on a prescription label?
    a. dispensing pharmacist's initials
    b. name of medication
    c. prescriber's signature
    d. patient's name

82. _____ is a procedure conducted under controlled conditions in a manner that minimizes the chance of contamination resulting from the introduction of microorganisms.
    a. Pharmaceutical care
    b. Aseptic technique
    c. Sterilization
    d. Autoclaving

83. Maximum and minimum inventory levels for each drug are known as:
    a. reorder points
    b. M&M inventory
    c. POS points
    d. the Maxim system

84. Which of the following would be stored within the topical section of the pharmacy's inventory?
    a. Erythromycin 2% soln
    b. Mylanta liquid
    c. Nystatin 100,000 units/ml susp
    d. Gentamicin 80-mg/2-ml inj

85. Which of the following drugs would not likely be found on an emergency crash cart?
    a. epinephrine injection
    b. cimetidine injection
    c. lidocaine injection
    d. dopamine injection

86. How many 1-liter bags of dextrose 5% will the IV technician need to send for a 24-hr supply if the infusion rate is 125 mL/hr?
    a. 6
    b. 5
    c. 4
    d. 3

87. What is the pharmacy technician's best defense against contamination when preparing patient prescriptions?
    a. spraying with Lysol
    b. proper hand washing
    c. mopping with chlorine bleach
    d. wearing gloves

88. Which of the following medications is not used to treat hypertension?
    a. lisinopril
    b. terazosin
    c. metoprolol
    d. etodolac

89. How many 5-mg tablets are needed to fill the following prescription? Prednisone 5-mg tablets

per sliding scale, 20 mg daily × 2 d, 15 mg daily × 2 d, 5 mg bid × 2 d, 2.5 mg bid × 2 d, 2.5 mg daily × 2 d
    a. 20 tabs
    b. 21 tabs
    c. 22 tabs
    d. 15 tabs

90. Calculate the flow rate for an IV of 1000 mL to run over 8 hr with a set calibrated at 20 gtt/mL.
    a. 42 gtt/min
    b. 17 gtt/min
    c. 125 gtt/min
    d. 50 gtt/min

18 Math Practice Test I

Complete this test to review pharmacy calculations.

1. Rx: Diphenhydramine 0.1% solution, 500 ml. How much diphenhydramine 0.25% solution will be needed to prepare the prescription?
   a. 100 ml
   b. 200 ml
   c. 350 ml
   d. 400 ml

2. Rx: Albuterol oral solution, 3 mg po tid. Disp: 14-day supply. If the pharmacy dispenses albuterol 2-mg/5-ml solution, how much is needed to fill the prescription?
   a. 7.5 ml
   b. 42 ml
   c. 126 ml
   d. 315 ml

3. Rx: Clotrimazole 0.5% ointment, 60 g. How many grams of clotrimazole 1% should be mixed with ointment base to prepare the prescription?
   a. 5 g
   b. 15 g
   c. 30 g
   d. 60 g

4. How much sorbitol 70% must be mixed with sterile water to prepare 1 L of sorbitol 25% solution?
   a. 280 mL
   b. 357 mL
   c. 643 mL
   d. 720 mL

5. 4350 ml = _____ tbsp.
   a. 9
   b. 145
   c. 870
   d. 290

6. How many teaspoons are in 12.5 ml?
   a. 1½
   b. 2
   c. 2¼
   d. 2½

7. Rx: Cimetidine 300-mg tab po qid. Disp: 3-month supply. How many cimetidine 300-mg tabs are needed to fill the prescription?
   a. 120
   b. 180
   c. 240
   d. 360

8. Rx: Cleocin 150-mg capsules, 300 mg po bid. Disp: 100 caps. What is the prescription's days' supply?
   a. 10
   b. 20
   c. 25
   d. 30

9. Dr. William Wiggins is treating Edna Edwards with Amoxil for an ear infection. He writes a prescription for Amoxil 30 mg/kg/day in divided doses q8h for 10 days. Edna is six months old and weighs 26.4 lb. How much will be given to Edna in each dose if the pharmacy dispenses amoxicillin 125-mg/5-ml susp?
   a. 3.75 ml
   b. 4.8 ml
   c. 5 ml
   d. 5.2 ml

10. Rx: Cefazolin 1 g IVPB q8h. The 2-g vial states that after reconstitution with 15.5 ml of sterile water, the concentration of the resulting solution is 1 g/10 ml. What is the powder volume of the vial?
    a. 4.5 ml
    b. 5 ml
    c. 10 ml
    d. 12.5 ml

11. Rx: Heparin IV @ 1400 units/hr. The IV bag contains NS 1 L with 40,000 units of heparin. Calculate the rate in ml/hr.
    a. 29 ml/hr
    b. 30 ml/hr
    c. 35 ml/hr
    d. 40 ml/hr

12. Dr. Betty Brown writes a prescription for Pam Pennison for Ceclor Susp 20 mg/kg/day po divided q8h × 10 days. Pam is five years old and weighs 48 lb. How much will be given to Pam in each dose if the pharmacy dispenses Ceclor 187-mg/5-ml susp?
    a. 2.5 ml
    b. 3.2 ml
    c. 3.9 ml
    d. 8.6 ml

13. If 80 ml of D70W is infused, how many milligrams of dextrose will the patient receive?
    a. 56 mg
    b. 560 mg
    c. 5600 mg
    d. 56,000 mg

14. Rx: Ceftazidime 3 g × 9 doses. How many ceftazidime 10-g vials will the technician need to reconstitute to prepare the 9 doses?
    a. two
    b. three
    c. four
    d. five

15. A 100-ml IV bag has a strength of 30%. How many grams of solute does this represent?
    a. 3 g
    b. 1.5 g
    c. 30 g
    d. 15 g

16. How many grams of active ingredient will you need to prepare 2.5 gallons of a 45.6% solution?
    a. 431.49 g
    b. 4314.9 g
    c. 43,149 g
    d. 50,000 g

17. You have a 500-ml bag of D51/2 NS. How many grams of NaCl does this bag contain?
    a. 7.5 g
    b. 4.5 g
    c. 2.5 g
    d. 2.25 g

18. Doxycycline 100-mg caps cost $23.40/100 caps and the pharmacy applies a 40% markup on cost. What will a patient be charged for 60 caps?
    a. $5.62
    b. $14.04
    c. $19.66
    d. $21.36

19. Rx: Azithromycin 0.5 g IVPB daily. The 500-mg vial states that the concentration after reconstitution is "250 mg/5 ml." How many milliliters will need to be withdrawn to prepare one dose?
    a. 5 ml
    b. 7.5 ml
    c. 10 ml
    d. 25 ml

20. If you are using 258 ml of hydrochloric acid to prepare a total volume of 2 pints, what is the percentage of hydrochloric acid?
    a. 12.9%
    b. 15.6%
    c. 27.3%
    d. 29.8%

21. Order: NS 1 L with 35,000 units of heparin infusing @ 20 ml/hr. Calculate the hourly dosage of heparin.

    a. 350 units/hr
    b. 700 units/hr
    c. 1400 units/hr
    d. 3500 units/hr

22. What is the percent strength of 1 pint of solution containing 56 g of Camphor?

    a. 84.4%
    b. 53.2%
    c. 13.9%
    d. 11.8%

23. Rx: Heparin IV @ 2000 units/hr. The IV bag contains NS 1 L with 40,000 units of heparin. The IV set delivers 15 gtt/ml. Calculate the rate in gtt/min.

    a. 9 gtt/min
    b. 10 gtt/min
    c. 13 gtt/min
    d. 15 gtt/min

24. Digoxin 0.25-mg tabs cost $10.23/100 tabs and the pharmacy applies a 32% markup on cost plus a $4.50 dispensing fee. What will the patient be charged for 90 tabs?

    a. $16.65
    b. $13.71
    c. $12.15
    d. $9.21

25. Convert 1:10,000 to a percent strength.

    a. 0.0001%
    b. 0.001%
    c. 0.01%
    d. 0.1%

26. Convert 325 mg to grains.

    a. 4
    b. 5
    c. 6.2
    d. 7

27. Convert 5% to a ratio strength.

    a. 1:2
    b. 1:5
    c. 1:20
    d. 1:50

28. How many milliliters would be given for a 50-mg dose if the available drug has a concentration of 10 mg/5 ml?

    a. 5 ml
    b. 10 ml
    c. 20 ml
    d. 25 ml

29. Rx: Zovirax 400-mg tabs, i po, 5 × daily. Disp: 100 tabs. What is the day's supply for the prescription?

    a. 10
    b. 20
    c. 30
    d. 50

30. You need to compound sorbitol 25% 500 ml by mixing sorbitol 70% with sterile water. How much of each will you need?

    a. 321.4 ml of 70% sorbitol and 178.6 ml of sterile water
    b. 250 ml of 70% sorbitol and 250 ml of sterile water
    c. 325 ml of 70% sorbitol and 175 ml of sterile water
    d. 178.6 ml of 70% sorbitol and 321.4 ml of sterile water

chapter 19

Math Practice Test II

Complete this test to review pharmacy calculations.

1. Rx: Diphenhydramine 10-mg/5-ml solution, 500 ml. How much diphenhydramine 12.5-mg/5-ml solution will be needed to prepare the prescription?
   a. 100 ml
   b. 200 ml
   c. 350 ml
   d. 400 ml

2. You need to compound 500 ml of sorbitol 10% by mixing 70% sorbitol with sterile water. How much of each will be needed?
   a. 428.6 ml of 70% sorbitol and 71.4 ml of sterile water
   b. 200 ml of 70% sorbitol and 300 ml of sterile water
   c. 325 ml of 70% sorbitol and 175 ml of sterile water
   d. 71.4 ml of 70% sorbitol and 428.6 ml of sterile water

3. Rx: Allopurinol 300-mg tabs, 450 mg po daily. Disp: 60 tabs. What is the day's supply for the prescription?
   a. 10
   b. 20
   c. 30
   d. 40

4. Rx: Albuterol oral solution 0.5 mg po tid. Disp: 30-day supply. If the pharmacy dispenses albuterol 2-mg/5-ml solution, how much is needed to fill the prescription?
   a. 1.25 ml
   b. 112.5 ml
   c. 120 ml
   d. 140 ml

5. Rx: Hydrocortisone 0.25% ointment, 120 g. How many grams of hydrocortisone 2.5% should be mixed with ointment base to prepare the prescription?
   a. 5 g
   b. 10 g
   c. 12 g
   d. 60 g

6. Furosemide 40-mg tabs cost $23.80/100 tabs and the pharmacy applies a 40% markup on cost plus a $6.50 dispensing fee. What will the patient be charged for 30 tabs?
   a. $16.50
   b. $13.64
   c. $10.00
   d. $7.14

7. How much sorbitol 70% must be mixed with sterile water to prepare 500 ml of sorbitol 10% solution?
   a. 71 ml
   b. 429 ml
   c. 350 ml
   d. 150 ml

8. If the recommended dose of a drug is 500 mg/m^2 per day in two divided doses, how much drug will a patient take in each dose? The patient's BSA = 1.3 m^2.
   a. 125 mg
   b. 250 mg
   c. 325 mg
   d. 650 mg

9. Convert 5 mg to mcg.
   a. 0.005 mcg
   b. 5000 mcg
   c. 50 mcg
   d. 0.05 mcg

10. Tetracycline 250-mg caps cost $3.40/100 caps and the pharmacy applies a 36% markup on cost + $8.00 dispensing fee. What will a patient be charged for 30 caps?
    a. $1.02
    b. $1.36
    c. $9.02
    d. $9.39

11. What is the percent strength of a 480-ml of solution containing 30 g of active ingredient?
    a. 144%
    b. 62.5%
    c. 14.4%
    d. 6.25%

12. How many teaspoons are in 25 ml?
    a. 1½
    b. 2
    c. 3
    d. 5

13. Order: NS 1 L with 35,000 units of heparin infusing @ 10 ml/hr. Calculate the hourly dosage of heparin.
    a. 350 units/hr
    b. 700 units/hr

c. 1400 units/hr
d. 3500 units/hr

14. Rx: Cimetidine 300 mg po qid. Disp: 1-month supply. How many Cimetidine 150-mg tabs are needed to fill the prescription?
    a. 120
    b. 180
    c. 240
    d. 360

15. Rx: Fluoxetine 20 mg po bid. Disp: 90 × 20-mg caps. What is the prescription's days' supply?
    a. 10
    b. 20
    c. 30
    d. 45

16. If the adult dose is 200 mg, what is an appropriate dose for a child weighing 22 kg? (Use Clark's rule.)
    a. 29.3 mg
    b. 64.5 mg
    c. 46.5 mg
    d. 93.2 mg

17. If the adult dose is 250 mg, what is the appropriate dose for a child who weighs 35 lb, using Clark's Rule?
    a. 43.75 mg
    b. 58 mg
    c. 60 mg
    d. 75 mg

18. How many grams of NaCl are there in two 500-ml bags of D5 NS?
    a. 7.5 g
    b. 4.5 g
    c. 2.5 g
    d. 9 g

19. Rx: Cefazolin 1.5 g IVPB q8h. The 2-g vial states that after reconstitution with 9.5 ml of sterile water, the concentration of the resulting solution is 2 g/10 ml. What is the powder volume of the vial?
    a. 1.5 ml
    b. 0.5
    c. 10 ml
    d. 2 ml

20. Rx: Heparin IV @ 2100 units/hr. The IV bag contains NS 1 L with 30,000 units of heparin. Calculate the rate in ml/hr.
    a. 35 ml/hr
    b. 50 ml/hr
    c. 60 ml/hr
    d. 70 ml/hr

21. If 2500 ml of D5W is infused, how many grams of dextrose will the patient receive?
    a. 100 g
    b. 120 g
    c. 125 g
    d. 130 g

22. Rx: Cefazolin 2 g IVPB BID. How many cefazolin 10-g vials will the technician need to reconstitute to prepare a 7-day supply?
    a. 2
    b. 3
    c. 4
    d. 5

23. A 100-ml IV bag has a strength of 70%. How many grams of solute does this represent?
    a. 3 g
    b. 7 g
    c. 30 g
    d. 70 g

24. How many grams of active ingredient will you need to prepare 500 ml of a 20% solution?
    a. 10 g
    b. 15 g
    c. 100 g
    d. 150 g

25. Rx: Penicillin 250,000 units IVPB q6h. The 20,000,000-unit vial states that the concentration after reconstitution is "500,000 units/ml." How many milliliters will need to be withdrawn to prepare one dose?
    a. 0.25 ml
    b. 0.5 ml
    c. 1 ml
    d. 1.5 ml

26. If you are using 30 ml of acetic acid to prepare a total volume 120 ml, what is the percentage of acetic acid?
    a. 2.5%
    b. 25%
    c. 40%
    d. 50%

27. Rx: Heparin IV @ 2500 units/hr. The IV bag contains NS 1 L with 20,000 units of heparin. The IV set delivers 10 gtt/ml. Calculate the rate in gtt/min.
    a. 20 gtt/min
    b. 21 gtt/min
    c. 25 gtt/min
    d. 30 gtt/min

28. Convert 2:20,000 to a percent strength.
    a. 0.0001%
    b. 0.001%
    c. 0.01%
    d. 0.1%

29. A 20,000,000-unit penicillin vial states that the concentration after reconstitution is "500,000 units/ml." How many milliliters are there in the vial after it is reconstituted by the technician?
    a. 10
    b. 20
    c. 40
    d. 50

30. How many milliliters should be given for a 35 mg dose if the available drug has a concentration of 10 mg/ml?
    a. 0.35 ml
    b. 3.5 ml
    c. 7 ml
    d. 8 ml

20 Math Practice Test III

C omplete this test to review pharmacy calculations.

1. Rx: Ampicillin 250-mg caps, 500 mg po q8h × 10 days. How many capsules are needed to fill the prescription?
   a. 30
   b. 60
   c. 50
   d. 40

2. Rx: Docusate sodium oral solution 30 mg po tid. Disp: 30-day supply. If the pharmacy dispenses docusate sodium 50-mg/5-ml solution, how much will the patient take for each dose?
   a. 1.25 ml
   b. 2.5 ml
   c. 3 ml
   d. 3.5 ml

3. Rx: Naproxen 500 mg ii po bid. Disp: 60 tabs. What is the prescription's days' supply?
   a. 10
   b. 12
   c. 15
   d. 30

4. Rx: Triamcinolone 0.025% ointment, 120 g. How many grams of triamcinolone 0.5% will be mixed with an ointment base to prepare the prescription?
   a. 5 g
   b. 6 g
   c. 8 g
   d. 60 g

5. Amitriptyline 100-mg tabs cost $142.50/1000 tabs and the pharmacy applies a 40% markup on cost plus a $10.50 dispensing fee. What will the patient be charged for 90 tabs?
   a. $190.05
   b. $12.83
   c. $23.33
   d. $28.46

6. Order: Diphenhydramine 75 mg IV q6h. How many diphenhydramine 50 mg/ml, 2 ml mdv, will be needed for a 24-hr supply?
   a. 1
   b. 2
   c. 3
   d. 4

7. What is the selling price for a prescription for 30 tablets, if 100 tablets cost $65.30 and the pharmacy applies a 30% markup on cost?
   a. $5.86
   b. $19.59
   c. $24.75
   d. $25.47

8. How many tablespoons are there in 450 ml?
   a. 10½
   b. 20
   c. 30
   d. 50

9. How much dextrose 50% must be mixed with sterile water to prepare 2 L of dextrose 10% solution?
   a. 200 mL
   b. 400 mL
   c. 500 mL
   d. 650 mL

10. Order: NS 500 with 40,000 units of heparin infusing @16 ml/hr. Calculate the hourly dosage of heparin.
    a. 350 units/hr
    b. 600 units/hr
    c. 640 units/hr
    d. 1280 units/hr

11. Rx: Ranitidine 150 mg po q12h. Disp: 3-month supply. How many ranitidine 150-mg tabs will be needed to fill the prescription?
    a. 120
    b. 180
    c. 240
    d. 360

12. If the adult dose is 250 mg, what is an appropriate dose for a six-year-old child? (Use Young's rule.)
    a. 12.5 mg
    b. 38.3 mg
    c. 125 mg
    d. 83.3 mg

13. How many grams of NaCl are there in two 1-L bags of D5 ½ NS?
    a. 7.5 g
    b. 4.5 g

c. 2.5 g
d. 9 g

14. Rx: Heparin IV @1400 units/hr. The IV bag contains NS 1 L with 20,000 units of heparin. Calculate the rate in ml/hr.
    a. 35 ml/hr
    b. 50 ml/hr
    c. 60 ml/hr
    d. 70 ml/hr

15. If the adult dose is 50 mg, what is the appropriate dose for a child who weighs 20 kg?
    a. 14.7 mg
    b. 15.6 mg
    c. 6.7 mg
    d. 6.6 mg

16. If 1000 ml of NS is infused, how many grams of sodium chloride will the patient receive?
    a. 0.45 g
    b. 0.5 g
    c. 4.5 g
    d. 9 g

17. A 100-ml IV bag has a strength of 20%. How many grams of solute does this represent?
    a. 20 g
    b. 0.2 g
    c. 30 g
    d. 70 g

18. How many grams of active ingredient will you need to prepare 2 L of a 25% solution?
    a. 1500 g
    b. 1000 g
    c. 500 g
    d. 250 g

19. Ampicillin 250-mg caps cost $69.87/500 caps and the pharmacy applies a 16.2% markup on cost + $15.30 dispensing fee. What will a patient be charged for 40 caps?
    a. $47.77
    b. $21.80
    c. $15.30
    d. $5.59

20. Rx: Penicillin 750,000 units IVPB q6h. The 1,000,000-unit vial states that the concentration after reconstitution is "500,000 units/ml." How many milliliters will need to be withdrawn to prepare one dose?
    a. 0.25 ml
    b. 0.5 ml
    c. 1 ml
    d. 1.5 ml

21. Rx: Cefazolin 500 mg IVPB q8h. How many cefazolin 10-g vials will the technician need to reconstitute to batch 100 doses?
    a. 10
    b. 30
    c. 3.3
    d. 5

22. If you are using 90 ml of acetic acid to prepare a total volume of 16 oz, what is the percentage of acetic acid?
    a. 1.87%
    b. 5.3%
    c. 18.8%
    d. 53.3%

23. Rx.: D5W @120 ml/hr. The IV set delivers 10 gtt/ml. Calculate the rate in gtt/min.
    a. 20 gtt/min
    b. 21 gtt/min
    c. 25 gtt/min
    d. 30 gtt/min

24. Convert 1:15,000 to a percent strength (round your answer).
    a. 0.006%
    b. 0.007%
    c. 0.07%
    d. 0.6%

25. Convert 10,000 mcg to mg.
    a. 0.1 mg
    b. 1 mg
    c. 10 mg
    d. 100 mg

26. Rx: Ceftriaxone 0.5 g IVPB q12h. The 1-g vial states that after reconstitution with 8.5 ml of sterile water, the concentration of the resulting solution is 100 mg/ml. What is the powder volume of the vial?
    a. 1.5 ml
    b. 0.5

c. 10 ml
d. 2 ml

27. A 1,000,000-unit penicillin vial states that the concentration after reconstitution is "250,000 units/ml." How many milliliters of penicillin are there in the vial after it is reconstituted?
    a. 1
    b. 2
    c. 4
    d. 5

28. What is the percent strength of 480 ml of solution containing 69.12 g of active ingredient?
    a. 144%
    b. 62.5%
    c. 14.4%
    d. 6.25%

29. How many milliliters should be given for a 35-mg dose if the available drug has a concentration of 5 mg/ml?
    a. 0.35 ml
    b. 3.5 ml
    c. 7 ml
    d. 8 ml

30. You need to compound 2 L of 15% dextrose by mixing 5% dextrose and 20% dextrose. How much of each solution will you need?
    a. 250 ml of 5% dextrose and 750 ml of 20% dextrose
    b. 667 ml of 5% dextrose and 1333 ml of 20% dextrose
    c. 1333 ml of 5% dextrose and 667 ml of 20% dextrose
    d. 750 ml of 5% dextrose and 250 ml of 20% dextrose

Trade/Generic/ Classification Practice Test I

Complete this test to review drug trade name, generic name, and classification knowledge.

1. The trade name for dexamethasone is:
   a. Desyrel
   b. Dexasone
   c. Diflucan
   d. Deltasone

2. Fosinopril sodium is the generic name for:
   a. Minocin
   b. Mirapex
   c. Mobic
   d. Monopril

3. Which of the following is used to treat dry eyes?
   a. fluticasone propionate
   b. hydrocortisone
   c. cyclosporine emulsion
   d. gentamicin

4. Lexapro is the trade name for:
   a. dutasteride
   b. escitalopram
   c. ezetimibe
   d. omeprazole

5. Which of the following is used to treat major depressive disorder?
   a. Effexor
   b. Elavil
   c. Elocon
   d. Estrace

6. Tamsulosin is the generic name for:
   a. Flovent
   b. Flomax
   c. Flonase
   d. Tamiflu

7. Which of the following drugs is indicated for the treatment of bipolar disorder?
   a. monteleukast sodium
   b. quetiapine fumerate
   c. atomoxetine
   d. rosuvastatin calcium

8. Which of the following drugs is used to treat hypothyroidism?

   a. levalbuterol
   b. levetiracetam
   c. levonorgestrel
   d. levothyroxine

9. Which of the following is used to treat rheumatoid arthritis?

   a. Lodine
   b. Zetia
   c. Vytorin
   d. Tricor

10. The generic name for Abilify is:

    a. acyclovir
    b. allopurinol
    c. aripiprazole
    d. azithromycin

11. Which of the following is not an ACE inhibitor?

    a. Monopril
    b. Vasotec
    c. Tenoric
    d. Capoten

12. The generic name for Prevacid is:

    a. losartan
    b. lansoprazole
    c. lovastatin
    d. lisinopril

13. Which of the following drugs is used to treat salt and water retention associated with congestive heart failure?

    a. ibandronate sodium
    b. ibuprofen
    c. indapamide
    d. indomethacin

14. The trade name for nifedipine is:

    a. Pamelor
    b. Paxil
    c. Pepcid
    d. Procardia

15. Which of the following is not an opioid analgesic?

    a. oxycodone
    b. phenobarbital
    c. propoxyphene napsylate
    d. morphine

16. The generic name for Cialis is:

    a. travoprost
    b. torsemide
    c. terazosin
    d. tadalafil

17. Which of the following is used to treat patients with type II diabetes mellitus?

    a. simvastatin
    b. sitagliptin phosphate
    c. solifenacin succinate
    d. sumatriptan succinate

18. Which of the following is not used to treat psychotic disorders?

    a. ziprasidone
    b. aripiprazole
    c. irbesartan
    d. olanzapine

19. Which of the following drugs is used to treat ulcerative colitis?

    a. ibandronate sodium
    b. methotrexate
    c. indapamide
    d. mesalamine

20. Norelgestromin and ethinyl estradiol are the generic names for:

    a. Ortho Novum 1/35
    b. Loestrin
    c. Ortho-Cyclen
    d. Ortho Evra

21. Byetta is the trade name for:

    a. eszopiclone
    b. etodolac
    c. exenatide
    d. ezetimibe

22. Which of the following drugs is not a calcium channel blocker?

    a. amlodipide
    b. diltiazem
    c. verapamil
    d. bumetanide

23. Which of the following drugs is not used to treat hyperlipidemia?

    a. ezetimibe
    b. gemfibrozil
    c. felodipine
    d. fenofibrate

24. Fentanyl is the generic name for:

    a. Dolophine
    b. Duoneb
    c. Duragesic
    d. Dyazide

25. Which of the following drugs is not an SSRI antidepressant?

    a. Lexapro
    b. Zoloft
    c. Celexa
    d. Chantix

26. Cephalexin is the generic name for:
    a. Keflex
    b. Keppra
    c. Klonopin
    d. Lamictal

27. Which of the following is used to treat bipolar disorder?
    a. lisinopril
    b. lithium carbonate
    c. lorazepam
    d. losartan

28. Which of the following is not an insulin product?
    a. Humalog
    b. Novolin
    c. Lantus
    d. Glycolax

29. Telmisartan is the generic name for:
    a. Mevacor
    b. Micardis
    c. Micronase
    d. Mirapex

30. Which of the following is not a macrolide antibiotic?
    a. Zmax
    b. Biaxin
    c. Minocin
    d. Erythrocin

31. Pamelor is the trade name for:
    a. nortriptyline
    b. minocycline
    c. glyburide
    d. nystatin

32. Atomoxetine is the generic name for:
    a. Singulair
    b. Spiriva
    c. Strattera
    d. Synthroid

33. Which of the following drugs is used in the treatment of bronchospasms associated with COPD?
    a. Diovan
    b. Demadex
    c. Duoneb
    d. Dilantin

34. Clarinex is the trade name for:
    a. desloratadine
    b. loratadine
    c. diphenydramine
    d. dicyclomine

35. Which of the following is not an oral contraceptive?

36. Verapamil is the generic name for:
    a. Inderal
    b. Indomethacin
    c. Isoptin
    d. Imitrex

37. Which of the following is used to treat diarrhea?
    a. desloratadine
    b. diphenoxylate and atropine
    c. divalproex sodium
    d. docusate sodium

38. Which of the following is not a proton pump inhibitor?
    a. Aciphex
    b. Prilosec
    c. Provigil
    d. Nexium

39. Valium is the trade name for:
    a. diltiazem
    b. digoxin
    c. diclofenac sodium
    d. diazepam

40. Eszopiclone is the generic name for:
    a. Lovaza
    b. Lozol
    c. Lumigan
    d. Lunesta

41. Voltaren is the trade name for:
    a. diazepam
    b. diclofenac sodium
    c. dicyclomine
    d. diltiazem

42. Cefdinir is the generic name for:
    a. Keflex
    b. Cefzil
    c. Omnicef
    d. Ceftin

43. Which of the following drugs is used to treat hypertension and symptomatic heart failure?
    a. Vesicare
    b. Voltaren
    c. Viagra
    d. Vasotec

44. Doxycycline is the generic name for:
    a. E-mycin
    b. Vibramycin
    c. Zithromax
    d. Sumycin

The options for question 35:
a. Loestrin 24 FE
b. Kariva
c. Darvocet-N
d. Yaz

45. Skelaxin is the trade name for:
    a. mesalamine
    b. metaxalone
    c. methadone
    d. methocarbamol

46. Azelastine HCl is the generic name for:
    a. Atarax
    b. Atacand
    c. Astelin
    d. Asacol

47. Which of the following is a CNS stimulant?
    a. metolazone
    b. metoclopramide
    c. methylprednisolone
    d. methylphenidate

48. Metoprolol succinate is the generic name for:
    a. Lopressor
    b. Tenormin
    c. Toprol-XL
    d. Lunesta

49. Which of the following drugs is used to treat recurrent ventricular fibrillation?
    a. alendronate sodium
    b. allopurinol
    c. alprazolam
    d. amiodarone

50. Which of the following drugs is used to treat UTI?
    a. phenytoin
    b. niacin
    c. nifedipine
    d. nitrofurantoin

51. Which of the following is used in the treatment of seizures?
    a. Diflucan
    b. Trileptal
    c. Motrin
    d. Mirapex

52. Adipex-P is the trade name for:
    a. phenytoin sodium
    b. phentermine
    c. phenobarbital
    d. phenazopyridine

53. Oxybutynin chloride is the generic name for:
    a. Ditropan
    b. Dolophine
    c. Drisdol
    d. Duoneb

54. Glucophage is the trade name for:
    a. glyburide
    b. metformin
    c. glyburide and metformin
    d. glipizide

55. Which of the following is used to treat bacterial conjunctivitis?
    a. Zocor
    b. Zymar
    c. Zyprexa
    d. Zyrtec

56. Which of the following is not used to treat erectile dysfunction?
    a. sildenafil citrate
    b. tadalafil
    c. enalapril
    d. vardenafil

57. Combivent is the trade name for:
    a. ipratropium bromide and metaproterenol
    b. ipratropium bromide
    c. salmeterol
    d. ipratropium bromide and albuterol

58. Which of the following is not a skeletal-muscle relaxant?
    a. methocarbamol
    b. metaxalone
    c. atomoxetine
    d. carisoprodol

59. Zocor is the trade name for:
    a. sertraline
    b. sildenafil
    c. simvastatin
    d. sitagliptin

60. Which of the following is used to treat spasticity resulting from multiple sclerosis?
    a. Strattera
    b. Lioresal
    c. Zoloft
    d. Imitrex

61. Montelukast sodium is the generic name for:
    a. Spiriva
    b. Sinequam
    c. Singulair
    d. Seroquel

62. Which of the following drugs is used as a topical analgesic?
    a. Westcort
    b. Nizoral
    c. Lidoderm
    d. Mycolog II

60. Amaryl is the trade name for:
    a. glimepiride
    b. gemfibrozil
    c. glyburide
    d. glipizide

64. Which of the following is used to treat glaucoma?
    a. Alphagan
    b. Namenda
    c. Cozaar
    d. Imdur

65. Lisinopril and HCTZ are the generic name a for:
    a. Zestril
    b. Prinzide
    c. Hytrin
    d. Hyzaar

66. Tegretol is the trade name for:
    a. carvedilol
    b. carisoprodol
    c. carbidopa
    d. carbamazepine

67. Plaquenil is used in the treatment/prevention of:
    a. inflammation
    b. hypertension
    c. high cholesterol
    d. malaria

68. Apresoline is the trade name for:
    a. hydroxyzine pamoate
    b. hydralazine
    c. hydroxyzine HCl
    d. hydrocortisone

69. The generic name for Caduet is:
    a. aripiprazole
    b. amlodipine besylate
    c. amlodipine besylate and atorvastatin
    d. amlodipine besylate and benazepril

70. Demadex belongs to which of the following drug classifications?
    a. loop diuretic
    b. analgesic
    c. antihyperlipidemic
    d. skeletal-muscle relaxant

71. The generic name for Hyzaar is:
    a. losartan
    b. losartan with HCTZ
    c. lovastatin
    d. lisinopril

72. The generic name for Zyrtec is:
    a. cephalexin
    b. cetirizine
    c. citalopram
    d. clarithromycin

73. Which of the following is classified as an antibiotic?
    a. Tussionex
    b. Allegra
    c. Altace
    d. Cipro

74. Which of the following drugs is used to treat hypercholesterolemia?
    a. Zocor
    b. Zofran
    c. Zoloft
    d. Zovirax

75. Which of the following is not used to treat duodenal ulcers?
    a. Pepcid
    b. Zantac
    c. Axid
    d. Vesicare

76. Which of the following drugs is used to treat ADHD?
    a. Flovent
    b. Focalin
    c. Folate
    d. Fosamax

77. Cyclosporine is the generic name for:
    a. Biaxin
    b. Restasis
    c. Bumex
    d. Namenda

78. Triamcinolone acetonide is a:
    a. CNS stimulant
    b. corticosteroid
    c. muscle relaxant
    d. water-soluble vitamin

79. Prempro is the trade name for:
    a. estradiol
    b. conjugated estrogens
    c. medroxyprogesterone
    d. conjugated estrogens and medroxyprogesterone

80. Which of the following is used to treat ADHD?
    a. Aricept
    b. Adderall
    c. Ultracet
    d. Atacand

81. Which of the following drugs is used to treat metastatic breast cancer?
    a. Nizoral
    b. Nolvadex
    c. Norvasc
    d. Novolog

82. Prilosec is the trade name for:
    a. olanzapine
    b. olmesartan
    c. olopatadine
    d. omeprazole

83. Which of the following drugs is used to treat seizures?
    a. Ditropan
    b. Diovan
    c. Dilantin
    d. Diflucan

84. Colace is the trade name for:
    a. divalproex sodium
    b. docusate sodium
    c. docusate calcium
    d. donepezil

85. Which of the following is not a penicillin antibiotic?
    a. Trimox
    b. Augmentin
    c. Veetids
    d. Cipro

86. Which of the following is the trade name for insulin glargine, rDNA origin?
    a. Lamictal
    b. Lanoxin
    c. Lantus
    d. Lasix

87. Which of the following drugs is used to treat symptomatic trichomoniasis?
    a. Bentyl
    b. Cogentin
    c. TobraDex
    d. Flagyl

88. Atacand is the trade name for:
    a. carisoprodol
    b. carbidopa
    c. carbamazepine
    d. candesartan cilexetil

89. Which of the following is an antifungal drug?
    a. Zyloprim
    b. Allegra
    c. Lotrisone
    d. Reglan

90. Benicar is the trade name for:
    a. olmesartan
    b. olanzapine
    c. omeprazole
    d. olopatadine

Trade/Generic/ Classification Practice Test II

Complete this test to review drug trade name, generic name, and classification knowledge.

1. Which of the following drugs is used to treat hypertension and hyperlipidemia?
   a. atenolol and chlorthalidone
   b. amoxicillin and clavulanate potassium
   c. amlodipine besylate and atorvastatin
   d. amlodipine besylate and benazepril

2. Zetia belongs to which of the following drug classifications?
   a. loop diuretic
   b. analgesic
   c. antihyperlipidemic
   d. skeletal-muscle relaxant

3. Which of the following is used to treat gout?
   a. acyclovir
   b. allopurinol
   c. aripiprazole
   d. azithromycin

4. The generic name for Celexa is:
   a. cephalexin
   b. cetirizine
   c. citalopram
   d. clarithromycin

5. The generic name for Prevacid is:
   a. losartan
   b. lansoprazole
   c. lovastatin
   d. lisinopril

6. Which of the following is used to stop coughing?
   a. Tussionex
   b. Allegra
   c. Altace
   d. Cipro

7. The trade name for bimatoprost is:
   a. Lovaza
   b. Lozol
   c. Lumigen
   d. Lyrica

8. Which of the following is used to treat seizures?
   a. oxycodone
   b. phenobarbital
   c. propoxyphene napsylate
   d. morphine

9. The generic name for Demadex is:
   a. travoprost
   b. torsemide
   c. terazosin
   d. tadalafil

10. Which of the following is used to treat active duodenal ulcers?
    a. Pepcid
    b. Levsin
    c. Altace
    d. Vesicare

11. Which of the following is used to treat osteoporosis?
    a. Flovent
    b. Focalin
    c. Folate
    d. Fosamax

12. Which of the following drugs is used to treat glaucoma?
    a. glipizide
    b. aripiprazole
    c. irbesartan
    d. latanoprost

13. Methocarbamol is a:
    a. CNS stimulant
    b. corticosteroid
    c. muscle relaxant
    d. water-soluble vitamin

14. Norgestrel and ethinyl estradiol are the generic names for:
    a. Ortho Novum 1/35
    b. Loestrin
    c. Ovral
    d. Ortho Evra

15. Which of the following is used to treat osteoarthritis?
    a. eszopiclone
    b. etodolac
    c. exenatide
    d. ezetimibe

16. Plendil is the trade name for:
    a. ezetimibe
    b. famotidine
    c. felodipine
    d. fenofibrate

17. Which of the following is used to treat severe pain?
    a. Dolophine
    b. Duoneb
    c. Duragesic
    d. Dyazide

18. Provera is the trade name for:
    a. estradiol
    b. conjugated estrogens
    c. medroxyprogesterone
    d. conjugated estrogens and medroxyprogesterone

19. Which of the following is used to treat Alzheimer's disease?
    a. Aricept
    b. Adderall
    c. Ultracet
    d. Atacand

20. Mevacor is the trade name for:
    a. lisinopril
    b. lithium carbonate
    c. lovastatin
    d. losartan

21. Which of the following is used to treat fungal infections?
    a. Nizoral
    b. Nolvadex
    c. Norvasc
    d. Novolog

22. Which of the following is used in the treatment of allergic conjunctivitis?
    a. olanzapine
    b. olmesartan
    c. olopatadine
    d. omeprazole

23. Pramipexole dihydrochloride is the generic name for:
    a. Mevacor
    b. Micardis
    c. Micronase
    d. Mirapex

24. Which of the following is an anticholinergic?
    a. Levbid
    b. Lantus
    c. Levitra
    d. Lamictal

25. Which of the following is indicated for prophylaxis and chronic treatment of asthma?
    a. Singulair
    b. Spiriva
    c. Strattera
    d. Synthroid

26. Which of the following is used to treat hypertension?
    a. Diovan
    b. Demadex
    c. Duoneb
    d. Dilantin

27. Which of the following drugs is used to treat bladder instability associated with voiding in patients with uninhibited neurogenic or reflex neurogenic bladder?
    a. Ditropan
    b. Diovan
    c. Dilantin
    d. Diflucan

28. Which of the following drug is an oral contraceptive?
    a. Benicar
    b. Kariva
    c. Byetta
    d. Imitrex

29. Aricept is the trade name for:
    a. divalproex sodium
    b. docusate sodium
    c. docusate calcium
    d. donepezil

30. Propranolol is the generic name for:
    a. Inderal
    b. Indomethacin
    c. Isoptin
    d. Imitrex

31. Which of the following drugs is used to treat manic episodes associated with bipolar disorder?
    a. atropine
    b. diphenoxylate and atropine
    c. divalproex sodium
    d. docusate sodium

32. Which of the following drugs is used to treat mild-to-moderate heart failure?
    a. Lamictal
    b. Lanoxin
    c. Lantus
    d. Lasix

33. Which of the following is used to treat arrhythmias?
    a. Cordarone
    b. Prilosec
    c. Capoten
    d. Lanoxin

34. Cardizem is the trade name for:
    a. diltiazem
    b. digoxin
    c. diclofenac sodium
    d. diazepam

35. Bentyl is the trade name for:
    a. diazepam
    b. diclofenac sodium
    c. dicyclomine
    d. diltiazem

36. Cefuroxime is the generic name for:
    a. Keflex
    b. Cefzil
    c. Omnicef
    d. Ceftin

37. Which of the following drugs is used to treat erectile dysfunction?
    a. Sertraline
    b. Sildenafil citrate
    c. Simvastatin
    d. Sitagliptin phosphate

38. Tetracycline is the generic name for:
    a. E-mycin
    b. Vibramycin
    c. Zithromax
    d. Sumycin

39. Which of the following drugs is used to treat seasonal allergic rhinitis?
    a. Zyloprim
    b. Allegra
    c. Nizoral
    d. Reglan

40. Which of the following is a corticosteroid?
    a. metolazone
    b. metoclopramide
    c. methylprednisolone
    d. methylphenidate

41. Benicar is the trade name for:
    a. olmesartan
    b. olanzapine
    c. omeprazole
    d. olopatadine

42. Metoprolol tartrate is the generic name for:
    a. Lopressor
    b. Tenormin
    c. Toprol-XL
    d. Lunesta

43. Procardia is the trade name for:
    a. phenytoin
    b. niacin
    c. nifedipine
    d. nitrofurantoin

44. Meloxicam is the generic name for:
    a. Minocin
    b. Mirapex
    c. Mobic
    d. Monopril

45. Which of the following drugs is indicated for vaginal candidiasis?
    a. Diflucan
    b. Trileptal
    c. Motrin
    d. Mirapex

46. Vitamin D is the generic name for:
    a. Ditropan
    b. Dolophine
    c. Drisdol
    d. Duoneb

47. Which of the following drugs is used in the prophylactic treatment of asthma?
    a. hydrocortisone
    b. fluticasone propionate
    c. cyclosporine emulsion
    d. gentamicin

48. Olanzapine is the generic name for:
    a. Zocor
    b. Zymar
    c. Zyprexa
    d. Zyrtec

49. Which of the following drugs is used to reduce very high triglyceride levels in adults?
    a. olmesartan medexomil
    b. ipratropium bromide
    c. omega-E-acid ethyl esters
    d. ipratropium bromide and albuterol

50. Which of the following is used to treat ADHD?
    a. benazepril
    b. metaxalone
    c. atomoxetine
    d. carisoprodol

51. Januvia is the trade name for:
    a. sertraline
    b. sildenafil
    c. simvastatin
    d. sitagliptin

52. Oseltamivir phosphate is the generic name for:
    a. Osmivir
    b. Flomax
    c. Flonase
    d. Tamiflu

53. Doxepin is the generic name for:
    a. Spiriva
    b. Sinequan

    c. Singulair
    d. Seroquel

54. Crestor is the trade name for:
    a. monteleukast sodium
    b. quetapine fumerate
    c. atomoxetine
    d. rosuvastatin calcium

55. Biaxin is classified as a:
    a. macrolide antibiotic
    b. narcotic analgesic
    c. penicillin antibiotic
    d. tetracycline antibiotic

56. Xopenex is the trade name for:
    a. levothyroxine
    b. levetiracetam
    c. levonorgestrel
    d. levalbuterol

57. Which of the following is used to treat Alzheimer's disease?
    a. Alphagan
    b. Namenda
    c. Cozaar
    d. Imdur

58. Hyoscyamine sulfate is the generic name for:
    a. Hytrin
    b. Levsin
    c. Zestril
    d. Hyzaar

59. Which of the following is used to treat mild-to-severe heart failure?
    a. carvedilol
    b. carisoprodol
    c. carbidopa
    d. carbamazepine

60. Which of the following is used to treat high cholesterol levels?
    a. Lodine
    b. Ziac
    c. Vytorin
    d. Tricor

61. Indocin is used in the treatment of:
    a. inflammation
    b. hypertension
    c. high cholesterol
    d. malaria

62. Which of the following drugs is indicated for the treatment of hypertension?
    a. hydroxyzine pamoate
    b. hydralazine
    c. hydroxyzine HCl
    d. hyoscyamine sulfate

63. The trade name for trazodone is:
    a. Desyrel
    b. Dexasone
    c. Diflucan
    d. Deltasone

64. The generic name for Cozaar is:
    a. losartan
    b. losartan with HCTZ
    c. lovastatin
    d. lisinopril

65. Which of the following is an ACE inhibitor?
    a. Avodart
    b. Zestril
    c. Coreg
    d. Aricept

66. The generic name for Motrin is:
    a. ibandronate sodium
    b. ibuprofen
    c. indapamide
    d. indomethacin

67. The trade name for ondansetron is:
    a. Zocor
    b. Zofran
    c. Zoloft
    d. Zovirax

68. Requip is the trade name for:
    a. simvastatin
    b. ropinirole
    c. solifenacin succinate
    d. rosuvastatin

69. Which of the following is used in the treatment of short-term anxiety?
    a. Biaxin
    b. Boniva
    c. Bumex
    d. BuSpar

70. Lozol is the trade name for:
    a. ibandronate sodium
    b. ibuprofen
    c. indapamide
    d. indomethacin

71. Which of the following drugs is used to treat edema associated with CHF?
    a. amlodipine
    b. bumetanide
    c. doxazosin
    d. capoten

72. Which of the following drugs is used to stop smoking?
    a. Lexapro
    b. Chantix

    c. Celexa
    d. Coumadin

73. Which of the following is not used as adjunctive treatment for seizures associated with epilepsy?
    a. Levsinex
    b. Keppra
    c. Klonopin
    d. Lamictal

74. Which of the following is not used to treat diabetes?
    a. Glucovance
    b. Remeron
    c. Januvia
    d. Byetta

75. Which of the following is used to treat oral candidiasis?
    a. nortryptyline
    b. minocycline
    c. glyburide
    d. nystatin

76. Which of the following drugs is used to treat irritable bowel syndrome?
    a. desloratadine
    b. loratadine
    c. diphenhydramine
    d. dicyclomine

77. Which of the following is a penicillin antibiotic?
    a. Keflex
    b. Augmentin
    c. Minocin
    d. Cipro

78. Eszopiclone is the generic name for:
    a. Lovaza
    b. Lozol
    c. Lumigan
    d. Lunesta

79. Which of the following drugs is used to treat Parkinsonism?
    a. Bentyl
    b. Cogentin
    c. TobraDex
    d. Flagyl

80. Which of the following drugs is used to treat musculoskeletal conditions in adults?
    a. carisoprodol
    b. carbidopa
    c. carbamazepine
    d. candesartan cilexetil

81. Asacol is the trade name for:
    a. mesalamine
    b. metaxalone
    c. methadone
    d. methocarbamol

82. Which of the following drugs is used for in the treatment of heart failure in patients with left ventricular systolic dysfunction?
    a. Atarax
    b. Atacand
    c. Astelin
    d. Asacol

83. Which of the following drugs is used in the management of anxiety disorders?
    a. amiodarone
    b. allopurinol
    c. alprazolam
    d. alendronate sodium

84. Which of the following is used in the treatment of the pain and irritation associated with UTI?
    a. phenytoin sodium
    b. phentermine
    c. phenobarbital
    d. phenazopyridine

85. Glucovance is the trade name for:
    a. glyburide
    b. metformin
    c. glyburide and metformin
    d. glipizide

86. Which of the following is not used in the treatment of hypertension?
    a. proglitazone
    b. olmesartan medoxomil
    c. fosinopril
    d. candesartan cilexetil

87. Which of the following is used to treat overactive bladder?
    a. tolterodine tartrate
    b. sertraline
    c. enalapril
    d. vardenafil

88. Amitriptyline is the generic name for:
    a. Effexor
    b. Elavil
    c. Elocon
    d. Estrace

89. Which of the following drugs is used in the treatment of acute migraine attacks?
    a. Strattera
    b. Lioresal
    c. Zoloft
    d. Imitrex

90. Which of the following is not used to improve glycemic control in adults with type II diabetes mellitus?
    a. glimepiride
    b. gemfibrozil
    c. glyburide
    d. glipizide

Appendix A
Review of Abbreviations and Terminology

A major part of being a successful pharmacy technician is knowing the abbreviations that are commonly used in pharmacy. Although it is not all-inclusive, the following table does list the most common abbreviations you will need to know as a pharmacy technician. Note that as a working pharmacy technician, you may see abbreviations written in a variety of different ways. For example, some abbreviations may be written in all uppercase or in all lowercase letters, with or without periods. In most cases the abbreviations mean the same.

(BID = bid = B.I.D. = b.i.d.)

ABBREVIATION	MEANING
Routes of Administration	
AAA	Apply to affected area
ad	Right ear
AS	Left ear
AU	Both ears
ID	Intradermal
IM	Intramuscular
IPPB	Intermittent positive-pressure breathing (inhalation)
IV	Intravenous or Roman numeral 4
IVP	Intravenous push
IVPB	Intravenous piggyback
NPO	Nothing by mouth
OD	Right eye
OS	Left eye
OU	Each or both eyes
po	By mouth, orally
pr	Rectally
SL	Sublingual
sq, SQ, sc, subq	Subcutaneous
S&S or S/S	Swish and swallow or swish and spit
Schedules	
ā, á	Before
ac	Before meals
ad lib	At liberty, at pleasure
a.m.	Morning
ASAP	As soon as possible
ATC	Around the clock
bid	Twice daily
c̄, ć	With
crm	Cream
d	Day
hr, h	Hour
hs	Bedtime
KVO	Keep vein open
MR	May repeat
MRx1	May repeat 1 time
Noc, N, n	Night
NR, non rep	No refills, no repeat
p	After
pc	After meals
p.m.	Evening
prn	As needed
q	Every
qAM	Every morning
qh, q	Every hour
qhs	Every night at bedtime
qid	Four times daily
qPM	Every evening
qshift	Every shift
q4h	Every 4 hours
q6h	Every 6 hours
q8h	Every 8 hours
q12h	Every 12 hours
q24h	Every 24 hours
s	Without
stat	At once, immediately, now
tid	Three times daily

(*continued*)

ABBREVIATION	MEANING
TKO	To keep vein open
ud	As directed
wa	While awake
Dosage Forms	
amp	Ampule
cap(s)	Capsule(s)
CR	Controlled release
DA	Delayed action
DR	Delayed release
DS	Double strength
EC	Enteric-coated
gtt, gtts	Drop, drops
inh	Inhalation or inhaler
inj	Injection
liq	Liquid
MDI	Metered-dose inhaler
ophth	Ophthalmic
otic	Ear
pwd	Powder
SA	Sustained action
soln, sol	Solution
SR	Sustained release
supp	Suppository
susp	Suspension
tab(s)	Tablet(s)
TPN	Total parenteral nutrition
ung, oint	Ointment
IV Solutions	
½ NS	Sodium chloride 0.45%
¼ NS	Sodium chloride 0.2% or 0.225%
D5W	Dextrose 5% water
D10W	Dextrose 10% water
D20W	Dextrose 20% water
D30W	Dextrose 30% water
D40W	Dextrose 40% water
D50W	Dextrose 50% water
D70W	Dextrose 70% water

ABBREVIATION	MEANING
D5 ¼ NS	Dextrose 5% water 0.2% sodium chloride *(D5W 0.2% NaCl)*
D5 ½ NS	Dextrose 5% water 0.45% sodium chloride *(D5W 0.45% NaCl)*
D5NS	Dextrose 5% water 0.9% sodium chloride *(D5W 0.9% NaCl)*
D5LR	Dextrose 5% water and lactated Ringer's *(D5WLR)*
LR	Lactated Ringer's
NS	Sodium chloride 0.9% (normal saline)
Miscellaneous	
@*	At
&	And
ABX	Antibiotic
ad	To, up to
ASO	Automatic stop order
bm	Bowel movement
BP	Blood pressure
CI	Controlled substance—Schedule I
CII	Controlled substance—Schedule II
CIII	Controlled substance—Schedule III
CIV	Controlled substance—Schedule IV
CV	Controlled substance—Schedule V
cc*	Cubic centimeters
Cath	Catheter
Cont	Continue, continuous
CP	Chest pain
CS	Controlled substance
DBP	Diastolic blood pressure
DC, D/C, DC'd	Discontinue, discontinued or discharge, discharged
disp	Dispense
fs, FS	Floor stock or finger stick
gm	Gram

ABBREVIATION	MEANING
gr	Grain
HA	Headache
H.O.	House officer
HR	Heart rate
~~I.U.~~	~~International units~~
IVF	Intravenous fluids
L	Liter
LOC	Laxative of choice or loss of consciousness
mcg	Micrograms
meds	Medications
mEq	Milliequivalent
mg	Milligram
ml	Milliliter
mM	Millimole
narc	Narcotic
NGT, Ng tube	Nasogastric tube
NKDA, nka	No known drug allergies, no known allergies
no., #	Number
NTE	Not to exceed
N/V, N&V	Nausea and vomiting
PCA	Patient-controlled analgesic
pt	Patient
qs	Sufficient quantity
qs ad	Sufficient quantity up to
R	Right
Rx	Prescription, take, take thou, recipe
SBP	Systolic blood pressure
Sig	Directions
SOB	Shortness of breath
ss	Half
SZ	Seizure
T, temp	Temperature
T>	Temperature greater than
T<	Temperature less than
tbsp	Tablespoon

ABBREVIATION	MEANING
tsp	Teaspoon
TO	Telephone order
~~U~~	~~Units~~
USP	United States Pharmacopeia
VO	Verbal order
VS	Vital signs
x	Times or for
µg*	Micrograms
'	Hour
"	Minutes
/	Per, or, and, with
>*	Greater than
<*	Less than
≥	Greater than or equal to
≤	Less than or equal to
↑	Increase
↓	Decrease
Δ	Change
°	hour or degree (24° = 24 hour or 24 degrees)

Chemical Elements

Ag	Silver
Au	Gold
Ca	Calcium
Cl	Chloride
Cu	Copper
Fe	Iron
H	Hydrogen
Hg	Mercury
I	Iodine
K	Potassium
Li	Lithium
Mg	Magnesium
N	Nitrogen
Na	Sodium
O	Oxygen
P	Phosphorus
Zn	Zinc

(*continued*)

ABBREVIATION	MEANING
Chemical Compounds	
ACTH	Adrenocorticotropic hormone (corticotrophin)
$AgNO_3$	Silver nitrate
APAP	Acetaminophen
ASA	Aspirin
ASA EC	Aspirin, enteric-coated
B_1	Thiamine
B_6	Pyridoxine
B_{12}	Cyanocobalamin
BSS	Balanced salt solution
CaCl	Calcium chloride
$CaCO_3$	Calcium carbonate
D5W	Dextrose 5% in water
DES	Diethylstilbestrol
dig	Digoxin
DPT	Diphtheria, pertussis, tetanus
epi	Epinephrine
ETOH	Ethyl alcohol
$FeSO_4$	Ferrous sulfate
gent	Gentamicin
HBIG	Hepatitis immune globulin
HC	Hydrocortisone
HCl	Hydrochloride
HCTZ	Hydrochlorothiazide
Hep-lock	Heparin lock flush
H_2O	Water
H_2O_2	Hydrogen peroxide
INH	Isoniazid
IVIG	Intravenous immune globulin
KCl	Potassium chloride
KI	Potassium iodine
KPO_4	Potassium phosphate
L-Dopa	Levodopa
$LiCO_3$	Lithium carbonate
mag cit	Magnesium citrate
MMR	Measles, mumps, rubella
MOM	Milk of magnesia
MVI	Multiple vitamins
NaCl	Sodium chloride
$NAHCO_3$, NaBicarb	Sodium bicarbonate
$NaPO_4$	Sodium phosphate
NS	Normal saline
NTG	Nitroglycerin
Pb, Phenobarb	Phenobarbital
PCN	Penicillin
PCN G	Penicillin G
Penicillin VK	Penicillin VK
PO_4	Phosphate
PPD	Purified protein derivative
PTU	Propylthiouracil
SO_4	Sulfate
SSKI	Saturated solution of potassium iodide
tobra	Tobramycin
vit C	Ascorbic acid
vit K	Phytonadione
ZnO	Zinc oxide
$ZnSO_4$	Zinc sulfate

Abbreviations with ~~strikethrough~~ are included in the Joint Commission "DO NOT USE" list and are not supposed to be used in an institutional setting. Also included in the list are the use of a trailing zero (X.0 mg) and lack of a leading zero (.X mg).

Abbreviations followed by an asterisk (*) are being considered for possible inclusion in the "DO NOT USE" list. Also being considered are abbreviations for apothecary units and any abbreviations for drug names.

Pharmaceutical Terminology

Knowledge of terminology is necessary for basic understanding of any language. Review the following terms and definitions as they apply to the pharmacy and medical settings.

A

absorption the time it takes for a drug to work after it has been administered; the rate at which the drug passes from the intestines into the bloodstream

active ingredient the chemical in a medication that is known or believed to have a therapeutic effect *acute* refers to a disease or illness with a sudden onset and a short duration

additive a substance added to a liquid solution that is intended for IV use

admixtures a substance that is produced from mixing two or more substances

adverse reaction an unwanted or unexpected side effect or reaction to a medication; may also result from an interaction among two or more medications

aerosol a medication dosage form that contains a gaseous substance consisting of fine liquid or solid particles

alcoholic solution solution that contains only alcohol as the dissolving agent

allergic reaction sensitivity to a specific substance that is contacted through the skin, inhaled into the lungs, swallowed, or injected

allergy a sensitivity of the immune system to a chemical or drug; causes symptoms from rashes to more severe symptoms such as irregular breathing

amphetamines substances that are frequently abused as a stimulant medication; used to treat narcolepsy and eating disorders

analeptic a substance that stimulates the central nervous system

analgesic a substance used to relieve acute or chronic pain

anaphylactic shock a hypersensitivity reaction to another substance

anesthetic a substance that relieves pain by interfering with the nerve transmission that alerts the brain of pain

angiotensin-converting enzyme (ACE) inhibitors used to treat hypertension (high blood pressure) and heart failure by blocking the enzyme that activates angiotensin—a natural substance that narrows the blood vessels, causing high blood pressure

anorectic a substance that suppresses the appetite

antacid a substance that relieves high acid levels in the gastric (stomach) area

antagonist a substance that opposes the action of another drug or substance

antianxiety refers to substances that reduce or relieve anxiety

antibiotic a substance that is used to kill or stop the growth of bacteria in the body

antibody a protein produced by the immune system to respond to foreign substances in the body

anticholinergic a substance that inhibits hypersecretion and gastrointestinal motility

anticoagulant a substance that stops blood clotting (also known as a blood thinner)

anticonvulsant a substance that stops brain nerve firing in order to suppress convulsive seizures

antidepressant a substance that helps maintain proper hormone balance levels to decrease depressive moods

antidiarrheal a substance that relieves and decreases gastrointestinal activity that produces diarrhea

antidote a substance that counteracts the effects of a poisoning agent

antiemetic a substance that relieves nausea and vomiting

antiflatulent a substance that relieves the pressure of excess intestinal gas

antifungal a substance that kills fungus growing in or on the body

antihistamine a substance that stops the effects of histamine release, which cause sneezing, watery eyes, and congestion

antihypertensive a substance that works to lower blood pressure

anti-inflammatory a substance that reduces and relieves inflammation

antineoplastic a substance that is used to kill cancer cells

antioxidant a chemical produced by the body in response to a foreign organism, bacteria, or virus

antiplatelets substances that reduce the ability of platelets to stick together and form a clot

antipruritic a substance that relieves itching

antipsychotics substances that block and inhibit the stimulatory actions of dopamine

antipyretic a substance that relieves and lowers high fever

antispasmodic a substance that relieves stomach-muscle spasms

antitussive a substance that relieves severe cough

antiviral refers to drugs that fight viral infections in the body

aqueous containing water

aseptic techniques techniques that are used to eliminate and protect against bacteria and other microorganisms

astringent a substance that stops secretions or controls bleeding

auxiliary labels labels that are placed on a medication package to provide information and instructions for use

B

beta-blockers substances used in the treatment of hypertension, angina, arrhythmia, and cardiomypathy; may also be used to minimize the possibility of sudden death after a heart attack

binding agent a substance that holds all of the ingredients in a tablet together

bioequivalence refers to a substance that acts on the body with the same strength and similar bioavailability as the same dosage of a sample of a given substance

blood sugar level the measure of glucose (sugar) level in the bloodstream

brand name the proprietary name of a drug, exclusive to a manufacturer for selling and distributive purposes

bronchodilator a substance that relaxes the bronchial smooth muscles in the respiratory system

buccal tablet a tablet that is dissolved in the lining of the cheek rather than swallowed whole

bulk compounding the process of compounding large quantities of a substance for dispensing or distribution

bulk manufacturing the process of manufacturing large quantities of a substance for selling or distribution

bulking agent a chemical substance that is required to produce the desired result

C

calcium channel blockers substances used to treat and reduce hypertension (high blood pressure) and disorders that affect the blood supply to the heart; also used in the treatment of irregular heartbeats

capsule a solid dosage form of a medication that is usually made of gelatin, which holds fine particles of a solid or liquid particle

chewable tablets tablets that are chewed rather than swallowed whole

chronic refers to a disease or illness that has a long duration (such as for a lifetime)

clinical trial a scientific experiment that tests the effect of a drug in human test patients; required by the FDA for approval of a new medication

communicable refers to a disease or illness that can be transmitted to another person

compound a substance made from a combination of two or more substances

contagious the time period during which an infectious person can transmit the disease to another person through direct or indirect contact

contraindication part of a patient's condition that does not agree with the treatment

controlled-release medications medications that are released and metabolized in the body over a period of time

controlled substance a drug with a high abuse potential; manufacturing and distribution are regulated by the federal government to limit abuse and harm

corticosteroids substances used to prevent minor asthma attacks or to treat severe attacks

cream a dosage form of a medication that is a semisolid preparation, usually applied externally to soothe, lubricate, or protect

cure the effective treatment of a disease or illness, leading to elimination of all symptoms

D

decongestant a substance that shrinks the mucous membranes that cause congestion

dehydration excessive loss of water from the body

diagnosis a process by which a health-care professional (doctor, nurse, or technician) determines the patient's condition or disease following tests and examinations

disease a physical process in which the body or specific organs are being destroyed, causing harm and characteristic symptoms to the patient

distribution the process following absorption by which a drug is passed to the cells of various organs

diuretic a substance that increases the water output in the kidneys and reduces water retention in the body

dopamine a neurotransmitter associated with the regulation of movement, emotions, pain, and pleasure

drops a liquid dosage form of medication that is placed in the eye or ear

drug a chemical compound intended for the use in diagnosis, treatment, or prevention of a disease in human or animals; any substance that is intended to produce an alteration to the chemistry and/or functioning in the body

E

effervescent tablet a tablet that is dissolved into a liquid before administration

electrolytes salts that the body requires in its fluids and that are essential in nerve, muscle, and heart functions

elimination the process following distribution by which a drug is broken down and the excess is excreted through the urine

elixir a liquid dosage form that contains flavored water and alcohol mixtures

emulsion a liquid dosage form consisting of a mixture of two products that normally do not mix together

enema a process by which a medicated fluid is injected into the rectum

estrogens hormones that are produced in the ovaries and are responsible for the development and maintenance of female secondary sex characteristics

excretion the process by which the body eliminates waste after metabolism and distribution

expectorant a substance that removes mucus from the upper respiratory system

F

Food and Drug Administration (FDA) the federal agency responsible for the approval, review, and regulation of drugs and dietary supplements

formulary a preferred list of medications that insurance plans allow members to get at a lower out-of-pocket expense

fungicide a substance that kills fungi

G

generic name the nonproprietary name of a drug; also known as the chemical name of the drug

genetically engineered drugs substances that have had foreign genes inserted into their genetic codes artificially

glucagon a hormone produced in the pancreas that causes the automatic release of glucose

glucose the primary energy source and sugar found in the bloodstream

glycogen the principal substance for storing carbohydrates in the body; it is stored in the liver, turned into glucose, and released into the bloodstream when the blood sugar level gets low

H

half-life the amount of time it takes for half of a substance to be broken down in the body and excreted

hazardous waste any substance that is potentially dangerous and toxic to living organisms; must be disposed of properly

health the physical, emotional, or mental well-being of a person

health care procedures, techniques, tests, and examinations that are used to prevent or treat health problems, and maintain a patient's health and well-being

histamine H_2 blockers substances that reduce acid secretion by blocking histamine from reaching the H_2 receptors

hydroalcoholic solution a solution that contains water and alcohol

hypersensitivity an exaggerated response to a given stimulus

hypnotic a substance that relaxes the central nervous system to produce sleep

I

immediate-release medications medications that are released and metabolized immediately following administration

immunosuppressant a substance that is used to prevent the body from rejecting an organ transplant (also known as an antirejection drug) *inactive ingredients* the remaining ingredients other than the active ingredient that are found in a drug; used to flavor, digest, color, and bind the whole substance

infusion a slow injection of solution or emulsion into a vein or subcutaneous tissue

inhalation the administration of a medication directly into the lungs by the mouth or nose

inhaler a dosage form that uses a gaseous substance to force fine solid or liquid particles into the respiratory system through the nose or mouth

insulin a hormone secreted by the pancreas that helps the body digest sugars and starches; manufactured insulin is available for use when the pancreas does not produce enough on its own

intolerance an extreme sensitivity to a drug or other substance

intracardiac refers to administration of a medication by injection directly into the heart

intradermal refers to administration of a medication by injection into the skin

intramuscular refers to administration of a medication within or into a muscle

intravenous refers to administration of a medication within or into a vein

inventory the supplies of medications that the pharmacy stocks for dispensing

L

labeling the process of identifying a particular medication with the patient's and physician's information for dispensing

laxative a substance that increases defecation

legend drug a medication that requires a prescription written by a physician before it can be dispensed to a patient

local refers to a small area or single part of the body (for example, a local anesthetic)

lotion a liquid dosage form that contains a powdered substance in a suspension, used externally to soothe, cool, dry, and protect

M

medical devices devices or products used for medical procedures or diagnostic tests

medication order a prescription, usually given in a hospital or other institutional setting

migraine a severe headache caused by extreme changes in the blood vessels in the brain

muscle relaxants substances used to treat involuntary, painful contraction of muscles by slowing the passage to the muscles of nerve signals that cause pain

N

narcotic a drug that is potentially highly abused as a pain reliever, causing dependency and tolerance

narrow therapeutic range the bioequivalence range of a brand drug and its generic counterpart in which very small changes in dosage level could result in toxicity

nonaqueous containing no water

nonlegend drug a medication that does not require a prescription before dispensing; more commonly referred to as an over-the-counter medication

nonsteroidal anti-inflammatory agent a substance that inhibits production of the enzymes that are necessary for the synthesis of prostaglandins, reducing pain and inflammation

O

Occupational Safety and Health Administration (OSHA) the federal agency that is responsible for safety guidelines in the workplace

ointment a semisolid (mixture of a liquid and solid) dosage form that is applied externally to deliver medication, lubricate, and protect

ophthalmic refers to administration of a medication through the eye

opiate a drug that originates from the opium poppy, such as morphine or codeine

opioid a drug, hormone, or other substance that has sedative or narcotic effects similar to substances containing opium or its derivatives

oral refers to administration of a medication by mouth

otic refers to administration of a medication in the ear

overdose an action resulting from ingesting too much of a substance or drug; may result from one dose or multiple doses over the course of time

P

package insert a supplement provided by the manufacturer giving specific details, instructions, and warnings regarding the medication

parenteral refers to administration of medication by any other route than oral; administration by injection

patch a dosage form in which the medication is delivered through a solid application applied to the skin and absorbed into the bloodstream

patent a federally granted, exclusive right to create and sell a product for a specific period of time before other manufacturers can create and sell the identical product

pharmacist a licensed health-care professional who is skilled and trained to dispense medications as ordered by a physician and counsel patients on their drug therapies

pharmacokinetics the study of the rates at which drugs are metabolized, distributed, and excreted from the body after consumption

pharmacology the study of drugs and their effects on the body

placebo a pill-like preparation that contains no active or chemical ingredient, usually given for its psychological effects (commonly referred to as a sugar pill)

prescription a direction given by a physician for the preparation and use of a medication for a specific patient to be dispensed by a pharmacist

progestin a female reproductive hormone that causes menstruation as it triggers the shedding of the uterine lining

proton pump inhibitor a substance that reduces gastric acid buildup by blocking the release of protons by proton pumps

psychotherapeutic drugs substances that are used to relieve the symptoms of mental and psychiatric illnesses, such as depression, psychosis, and anxiety

psychotropic a substance that affects a person's ability to distinguish reality from imagination

R

recreational drugs drugs (usually illegal) that are often used in a social setting for their pleasurable effects rather than medicinal value

rectally refers to administration of a solid or liquid medication through the rectum

S

Schedule I drugs drugs classified by the Drug Enforcement Agency as having high abuse potential and with no FDA approval for medicinal use (illegal drugs)

Schedule II drugs drugs classified by the Drug Enforcement Agency as having high abuse potential with severe dependence liability (narcotics, amphetamines, stimulants)

Schedule III drugs drugs classified by the Drug Enforcement Agency as having less abuse potential than Schedule II drugs and moderate dependence liability (non-narcotic stimulants, nonbarbituate sedatives, anabolic steroids)

Schedule IV drugs drugs classified by the Drug Enforcement Agency as having less abuse potential than Schedule III drugs and limited dependence liability (sedatives, antianxiety agents, non-narcotic analgesics)

Schedule V drugs drugs that have limited abuse potential; available as prescription or over-the-counter drugs (cough syrups with small amounts of codeine, antitussives, antidiarrheals)

sedative a substance that relieves anxiety and tension; calms and relaxes

side effect a predicted, unwanted reaction to a substance or combination of substances

slow-release medication a medication that is released and metabolized in the body over a period of time

solution a liquid dosage form in which the medication is completely dissolved in a liquid

sterilize to cleanse objects, wounds, burns, and so on, of microorganisms such as bacteria

stimulants a class of medications that are intended to increase alertness and physical activity

subcutaneous refers to administration of a medication under the skin

sublingual tablet a tablet that is dissolved under the tongue rather than swallowed whole

suppository a solid medication given through the vagina or rectum

suspension a liquid dosage form in which the solid particles are not completely dissolved

symptom a condition that usually comes before the onset of a disease or illness; an abnormality that indicates the existence of a disease or illness

syrup a liquid dosage form that consists of water and sugar mixed with the medication

T

tablet a solid dosage form in which the ingredients are compacted into a small, formed shape

tolerance the condition in which the body has become unresponsive to a substance after prolonged exposure

topical refers to a substance used externally for relief of swelling, itching, or infection

transdermal refers to administration of a medication through the skin (for example, patches)

U

U.S. Pharmacopeia (USP) a nonprofit organization, recognized by the FDA, that publishes standards on prescription drugs, over-the-counter medications, dietary supplements, and health-care products

V

vaginal tablet a tablet that is dissolved in the mucous lining of the vagina

vaginally refers to administration of a solid or liquid medication through the vagina

vasodilator a substance that causes the blood vessels to widen

W

withdrawal symptom an effect that occurs with sudden stopping of the use of a substance after prolonged use

Medical Terminology

A

acne vulgaris a skin condition that occurs as a result of the overproduction of oil by the oil glands of the skin and results in pimples, blackheads, and whiteheads on the surface of the skin

addiction physical or psychological dependence on a chemical substance such as alcohol; refers to any habit that cannot easily be given up

amnesia loss of memory (may be short- or long-term)

anatomy the study of the structures in living things

anemia a condition in which there are very few red blood cells in the bloodstream that can carry oxygen to the tissues

anesthesiologist a physician who specializes in administering drugs to anesthetize or sedate patients before a surgical procedure and who monitors a patient's vital signs while under anesthesia

angina pectoris a condition characterized by an attack of chest pain caused by an insufficient supply of oxygen to the heart

anorexia an eating disorder characterized by a refusal to maintain body weight in a healthy range, low self-esteem, and an intense fear of gaining weight

arrhythmia an irregular heartbeat

arteriosclerosis a condition characterized by thickening and hardening of the arteries

arthritis a condition characterized by inflammation of the joints

asthma a condition that affects the breathing of a patient by restricting the airway and oxygen supply as a result of inflammation, swelling, and irritation

attention-deficit disorder (ADD) a mental disorder characterized by developmentally inappropriate levels of attention, concentration, activity, distractibility, and impulsivity

attention-deficit hyperactivity disorder (ADHD) a mental disorder characterized by impulsive behavior, difficulty concentrating, and hyperactivity that affects social, academic, or occupational functioning

autoimmune disorder a disorder characterized by an immune response against the body's own tissues

B

bacteria single-celled microorganisms that are abundant in most living things; may be beneficial or cause harm to a person

benign refers to a condition or abnormal growth that is not cancerous (such as a tumor or cyst)

blood pressure the force exerted by blood against the walls of the arteries; measured when the heart contracts and relaxes

bloodstream the area in which the blood flows through the capillaries, veins, and arteries

body mass index (BMI) a measurement of body fat based on the patient's height and weight

bronchitis acute inflammation of the bronchial tubes in the lungs

C

carcinogen any agent capable of causing cancer

cardiologist a physician who specializes in the treatment of cardiac (heart) disorders and illnesses

cardiovascular disease conditions of the heart and circulation system

catalyst a substance that speeds up a chemical reaction without being changed or destroyed by the reaction

cavity a hollow space in a structure

cerebral refers to the brain

chemotherapy prevention or treatment of cancerous disease by using toxic chemical agents

cholesterol a substance produced in the liver and necessary for normal functioning of the body, including production of hormones, bile, and vitamin D

clinical refers to diagnostic tests, labs, and procedures that require close observation of patients

congestive heart failure a potentially fatal condition of the cardiovascular system in which the heart has lost its ability to pump blood in and out

contraceptives drugs and devices used for the prevention of pregnancy; can also be used for hormone regulation

cranial refers to the skull or head

cystitis inflammation of the urinary bladder

D

dementia a disease characterized by progressive memory loss and by learning and thinking disorders; often leads to Alzheimer's disease

dependency physical and/or psychological reliance on a chemical substance or habit

depression a mental disorder in which the person feels sad and helpless; characterized by personality changes and a loss of socialization, communication, and energy

dermatologist a physician who specializes in the treatment of skin disorders and illnesses

detoxification a process in which a patient is medically supervised during withdrawal from alcohol or drug dependency

diabetes a condition characterized by lack of insulin production in the pancreas, which is essential for digesting and retrieving energy from food

distal refers to a body part that is farthest from the point of attachment

E

edema abnormal swelling caused by a buildup of fluids in tissues and organs

emergency medicine specialist a physician who specializes in the treatment of emergency situations and trauma

emphysema an irreversible disease caused usually by long-term smoking, in which there has been severe damage to the alveoli (tiny air sacs) in the lungs, resulting in a decrease in the exchange of gases; results in wheezing, coughing, and shortness/difficulty of breath

endorphin a chemical or ingredient produced by the body that relieves pain and stress

erythrocyte a red blood cell

esophagitis inflammation of the esophagus as a result of acid buildup

euphoria a feeling of great happiness and well-being

excretion the process by which waste is eliminated from the body

external refers to the outer or outside part of a structure

G

gastric ulcer a tear in the normal tissue lining of the stomach wall

gastritis inflammation of the normal tissue lining of the stomach wall

gastroenterologist a physician who specializes in the treatment of digestive disorders and illnesses

gastroesophageal reflux disease (GERD) a condition that occurs when incompletely digested food is forced back up the esophagus; the food is very acidic and irritates the esophagus, causing heartburn and other symptoms

gastrointestinal tract the part of the digestive system that includes the mouth, esophagus, stomach, and intestines; aids in digesting and processing food in the body

geriatric refers to the care and treatment of elderly patients

glaucoma an eye condition caused by a buildup of pressure caused by reduced drainage of fluid from the eye, possibly resulting in loss of vision

gynecologist a physician who specializes in the treatment of disorders of the female reproductive organs

H

heartburn a painful burning sensation in the esophagus, just below the breastbone

hemorrhage severe, uncontrollable bleeding (may be external or internal)

hepatitis inflammation of the liver

herpes simplex an acute viral disease characterized by watery blisters on the skin and mucous membranes; commonly known as cold sores

hormone a chemical substance that stimulates and regulates certain bodily functions

hormone replacement therapy (HRT) a therapy developed for women to help increase the declining amounts of estrogen caused by menopause

hyperglycemia high blood glucose (sugar)

hyperlipidemia high cholesterol

hypertension long-term high blood pressure

hypoglycemia low blood glucose (sugar)

I

immunity the body's ability to fight off infections from bacteria and viruses

impotence the inability to achieve and maintain penile erection

inflammation redness, swelling, pain, and heat in a body tissue(s) caused by physical injury, infection, or irritation

influenza a contagious viral infection of the nose, throat, and lungs that often occurs in the winter season

inpatient a person who has been admitted to a hospital or other medical facility to receive treatment for a disease

internal refers to the inner or inside part of a structure

L

leukemia a condition characterized by high white blood cell counts

leukocyte a white blood cell

lipids organic compounds consisting of fats and other substances; used to measure cholesterol

M

malignant refers to an abnormal condition or growth in which a group of cells causes harm and destruction to other cells and tissues (for example, cancerous cells)

metabolism the physical and chemical processes of the body that convert consumed food into energy for use by the tissues and organs

metastasis the spreading of a disease from one organ to another organ or part of the body

N

narcolepsy a rare, chronic sleep disorder characterized by constant daytime fatigue and sudden attacks of sleep

nausea a feeling of sickness in the stomach, usually accompanied by the urge to vomit

neurologist a physician who specializes in the treatment of disorders and illnesses of the brain and central nervous system

neuropathic refers to a disease of the nerves

neurotransmitter a substance released by one nerve cell that activates or inhibits a neighboring nerve cell

O

obstetrician a physician who specializes in the care of pregnant women before and during the birth of babies

oncologist a physician who specializes in the treatment of cancer

ophthalmologist a physician who specializes in the treatment of poor vision and eye disorders with medication, corrective lenses, and surgery

organ a part of the body made up of tissues that performs a specialized function; part of an organ system

orthopedist a physician who specializes in the treatment of injuries and structural disorders of the bones and joints

osteoporosis a loss in total bone density that may result from calcium deficiency, menopause, certain endocrine diseases, advanced age, medications, or other risk factors

otolaryngologist a physician who specializes in the treatment of disorders and illnesses of the ear, nose, and throat

outpatient refers to patients who receive treatment from a hospital or other medical facility on a scheduled basis without being admitted for overnight or continuous stay

P

pain a feeling of slight or severe discomfort caused by an injury or illness

panic attack a sudden, repeated episode of extreme fear, panic, and anxiety

parietal refers to the wall of a structure

pathogen a microorganism that causes a disease (bacteria or virus)

pathologist a physician who studies the history, causes, and progress of diseases by examining specimens of body tissues, blood, fluids, and secretions

pathology the study of the nature of disease

peripheral at or toward the surface of the body or its parts

physiology the study of the function of living things

prevention taking steps before a health condition or other abnormality occurs or worsens

primary care the medical care a person receives from a general practitioner or family physician

primary care physician usually an internal medicine or family physician who can treat a variety of illnesses; refers a patient to a specialist if further specialized care or treatment is necessary

prognosis medical assessment of the expected outcome and course of a particular disease

proximal refers to a body part that is nearest to the point of attachment

psychiatrist a physician who specializes in the treatment of mental, emotional, and behavioral disorders; uses medications and psychotherapy

psychotherapy nondrug treatment of psychological disorders performed as behavioral or cognitive therapy

pulmonary refers to the lungs and respiratory system

R

radiologist a physician who uses technologies such as X-rays, radiation therapy, and ultrasound machines to view, analyze, and treat medical problems

receptor part of the nerve cell that recognizes a neurotransmitter and communicates with other nerve cells

respiration the process by which gases are passed through the lungs and distributed throughout the body

S

seasonal affective disorder (SAD) a type of depression that occurs during the fall and winter months only

secondary care the medical care a person receives from a specialist after being referred by his or her primary physician

serotonin a neurotransmitter in the brain that functions to regulate moods, appetite, sensory perception, and other central nervous system functions

spasm an involuntary muscle contraction

specialist a physician who is experienced in a certain area of study for treatment and prevention

surgeon a physician who is trained to perform surgical procedures and operations on patients in order to provide treatment or cure for an illness

syndrome a set of symptoms that are characteristic of a particular disease

systemic refers to the whole body

T

terminally ill the condition of having an illness or disease for which there is no treatment or cure available; expected result of the disease is death

testosterone a hormone produced in high amounts in males that regulates certain characteristics of muscle building, sexual organs, hair growth, and the deepening of the voice during puberty

toxic refers to a poisonous substance

U

urinary incontinence the inability to control the holding of urine in the bladder

urologist a physician who specializes in the treatment of disorders of the urinary tract, as well as problems in the male reproductive organs

V

vaccine a preparation that contains killed or weakened viruses or bacteria, which is administered to a person to provide active immunity against a disease

vascular refers to the blood vessels and circulatory system

vertigo a condition characterized by dizziness

virus very small infectious organisms that require a living cell to reproduce

visceral refers to the structures inside the body

Appendix B
Professional Resources

Reference Books

Clinical Books

- *American Hospital Formulary Service Drug Information (AHFS)*
- *Drug Facts and Comparisons*
- *Drug Handbook for the Allied Health Professional*
- *Martindale's*
- *Physician's Drug Reference* (paid for by drug manufacturers)

Product Information

American Drug Index
First Data Bank

Pharmaceutical Management

Applied Therapeutics: The Clinical Use of Drugs
Manual of Therapeutics
Merck Manual

Certification/Accreditation/ Regulations

ACPE—Accreditation Council for Pharmacy Education

www.acpe-accredit.org
312-664-3575 (phone)
312-664-4652 (fax)
135 S. LaSalle Street, Suite 4100
Chicago, IL 60603-4810

ExCPT—Exam for the Certification of Pharmacy Technicians

www.nhanow.com
800-499-9092
11161 Overbrook Road
Leawood, KS 66211

NABP—National Association of Boards of Pharmacy

www.nabp.net
847-391-4406 (phone)
847-391-4502 (fax)

1600 Feehanville Drive
Mount Prospect, IL 60056

PTCB—Pharmacy Technician Certification Board

www.ptcb.org
800-363-8012 (phone)
202-888-1699 (fax)
2200 C Street NW
Suite 101
Washington, DC 20037

National Associations

AAPT—American Association of Pharmacy Technicians

www.pharmacytechnician.com

APhA—American Pharmacists Association

www.pharmacist.com
202-628-4410 / 800-237-2742 (phone)
202-783-2351 (fax)
2215 Constitution Avenue, NW
Washington, DC 22037

ASHP—American Society of Health-System Pharmacists

www.ashp.org
301-657-3000 / 866-279-0681 (phone)
7272 Wisconsin Avenue
Bethesda, MD 20814

CAPT—Canadian Association of Pharmacy Technicians

www.capt.ca
416-410-1142 (phone)
9-6975 Meadowvale Town Centre Circle, Suite #164
Mississauga, Ontario L5N 2V7

NACDS—National Association of Chain Drug Stores

www.nacds.org
703-549-3001 (phone)

703-836-4869 (fax)

1776 Wilson Blvd., Suite 200

Arlington, VA 22209

NACP—National Community Pharmacists Association

www.ncpanet.org

703-683-8200 / 800-544-7447 (phone)

703-683-3619 (fax)

100 Daingerfield Road

Alexandria, VA 22314

NPTA—National Pharmacy Technician Association

www.pharmacytechnician.org

888-247-8700 (phone)

888-247-8706 (fax)

PO Box 683148

Houston, TX 77268

PTEC—Pharmacy Technician Educators Council

www.rxptec.org

Other

APHA—American Public Health Association

www.apha.org

CDC—Centers for Disease Control

www.cdc.gov

DEA—U.S. Drug Enforcement Administration

www.dea.gov

FDA—U.S. Food & Drug Administration

www.fda.gov

RxList

www.rxlist.com

USP—United States Pharmacopeia

www.usp.gov

WebMD

www.webmd.com

Appendix C
Answers

Chapter 1 Review Questions

1. d	2. c	3. c	4. b	5. a
6. b	7. b	8. c	9. d	10. b

Chapter 2 Review Questions

1. a	2. c	3. b	4. a	5. b
6. b	7. c	8. a	9. c	10. b

Chapter 3 Review Questions

1. a	2. d	3. b	4. c	5. d
6. b	7. a	8. a	9. b	10. c

Chapter 4 Review Questions

1. d	2. b	3. a	4. c	5. b
6. d	7. a	8. c	9. a	10. b

Chapter 5 Review Questions

1. d	2. b	3. c	4. a	5. d
6. c	7. b	8. a	9. d	10. b

Chapter 6 Review Questions

1. c	2. d	3. a	4. c	5. b
6. d	7. b	8. a	9. d	10. b

Chapter 7 Review Questions

1. d	2. d	3. a	4. b	5. d
6. b	7. d	8. b	9. d	10. c

Chapter 8 Review Questions

1. c	2. a	3. b	4. c	5. d
6. c	7. b	8. d	9. d	10. b

Chapter 9 Review Questions

1. c	2. a	3. c	4. d	5. a
6. a	7. d	8. c	9. b	10. d

Chapter 10 Review Questions

1. c	2. b	3. d	4. a	5. d
6. c	7. b	8. d	9. d	10. d

Chapter 11 Review Questions

1. a	2. b	3. d	4. d	5. c
6. b	7. e	8. a	9. d	10. c

Chapter 12 Review Questions

n/a

Chapter 13 Review Questions

1. c. Pepcid and Zantac are both H_2 antagonists.
2. b. Enalapril is an ACE inhibitor.
3. a.
$$\frac{76.78}{100} = \frac{x}{30}$$
$$100x = 76.78 \times 30$$
$$100x = 2303.4$$
$$x = 23.03 \,(\text{AWP for 30 tabs})$$
$$\underline{+7.75} \,\,(\text{Dispensing fee})$$
$$\$30.78 \,\text{Total for 30 tabs}$$

4. c. Because methylphenidate is a Schedule II drug, it cannot be written with refills.
5. b. A technician should always forward questions of this nature to the pharmacist, because technicians cannot legally counsel patients.
6. b.

2.5		0.5	Total parts 1.5
	1.5		
1		1	

$$\frac{0.5}{1.5} \times 60 = 20\text{g of } 2.5\%$$
$$\frac{1}{1.5} \times 60 = 40\text{g of } 1\%$$

The correct answer is 40 g of 1% and 20 g of 2.5%.

7. d. Whenever an investigational drug is used, a physician must initiate the order for the drug.

$$\frac{3}{100} = \frac{x}{150}$$
$$100x = 450$$
$$x = 4.5 \text{ g}$$
$$4.5 \text{ g} \times 1000 \text{ mg/g} = 4500 \text{ mg}$$
$$\frac{500 \text{ mg}}{\text{tab}} = \frac{4500 \text{ mg}}{x}$$
$$500x = 4500 \text{ mg}$$
$$x = 9 \text{ tablets}$$

8. b.
9. d. An antipyretic is indicated to reduce fever.
10. b. medication name and strength, lot number, and expiration date.

11. c.
$$\frac{250 \text{ mg}}{5 \text{ mL}} = \frac{400 \text{ mg}}{x \text{ mL}}$$
$$250 \times x = 5 \times 400$$
$$250x = 2000$$
$$x = 8 \text{ mL}$$

Each dose will be 8 mL. 8 mL tid for 10 days equals 240 mL total volume needed.

12. b. A Luer lock syringe should always be used when mixing hazardous medications

13. c.
$$\frac{1400 \text{ mL}}{12 \text{ hr}} \bigg| \frac{40 \text{ gtt}}{1 \text{ mL}} \bigg| \frac{1 \text{ hr}}{60 \text{ min}} = \frac{56,000 \text{ gtt}}{720 \text{ min}}$$
$$= 77.7 \text{ gtt/min}$$

Round up to 78 gtt/min.

14. d. Inventory turnover refers to how often medications are used and reordered.

15. b. The co-payment is the portion of the retail price that the patient must pay.

16. d. 42 capsules will be needed to give a patient 1 capsule tid for 14 days.

17. c. Federal law requires records to be kept for a minimum of 2 years.

18. b. Prescription medications are also called legend drugs.

19. c. Stock rotation consists of always keeping the shortest expiration dates to the front of the shelf, to ensure that they are dispensed first.

20. c. The drug propranolol is classed as a beta-blocker.

21. b.
$$\frac{2 \text{ mEq}}{\text{ml}} = \frac{8 \text{ mEq}}{x \text{ mL}}$$
$$2x = 8$$
$$x = 4 \text{ ml}$$

22. b. An invoice is the wholesaler's bill to the pharmacy, and it is used by the pharmacy when paying for the drug order.

23. a. Diphenhydramine is the generic name for Benadryl.

24. c.

10		3	Total parts 8
	5		
2		5	

$$\frac{3}{8} \times 120 = 45 \text{ grams of } 10\%$$
$$\frac{5}{8} \times 120 = 75 \text{ grams of } 2\%$$

25. a. 2–8°C equals 36–46°F, which is the required temperature for storage under refrigeration.

26. b.
$$\frac{5}{100} = \frac{x}{300}$$
$$x = 15$$

27. d. Confidentiality protects identity and health information of patients from those who are not authorized to have such information.

28. c. Any controlled substance in Schedule III, IV, or V may be refilled up to five times within 6 months after the prescription is written.

29. b. The four-digit group in an NDC number signifies the drug product.

30. d. Lortab is classified as a Schedule III controlled substance.

31. d. Glucotrol is the trade name for glipizide.

32. a. 125 ml/hr × 24 hr = 3000 ml

33. c. 164 lb/2.2 = 74.5 kg
74.5 kg × 5 mg = 372.5/day
372.5 mg/3 doses = 124.2 mg/dose
This will round down to 124 mg/dose.

34. b. Ranitidine is classed as an H_2 antagonist.

35. d. Lisinopril and glyburide are the generic names for Prinivil and Diabeta, respectively.

36. c.
$$\frac{0.5}{100} = \frac{x}{60}$$
$$100x = 30$$
$$x = 0.3 \text{ g}$$
$$0.3 \text{ g} \times 1000 \text{ mg/g} = 300 \text{ mg}$$

37. b. 2 tabs po q4–6h prn coincides with the directions given.

38. a.

15%		5
	10%	
5%		5

The ratio 5:5 can be reduced to a 1:1 ratio.

39. c. Doxycycline, a tetracycline derivative, can make the skin especially sensitive to the sun. This condition is known as photosensitivity.

40. d. First convert 2 g to milligrams by multiplying by 1000 (1 g = 1000 mg). Then 2000 mg ÷ 250 mg (each dose) = 8 doses.

41. d. Nitroglycerin should always be stored in its original container, which is air-tight and light-resistant. Exposure to light will decrease the potency of the nitroglycerin over a period of time.

42. c. The blower on the laminar airflow workbench should run for at least 30 minutes before use to ensure that the air within the hood meets the standards of ISO5.

43. a. The 18-gauge needle has the largest bore. (Hint: The smaller the number, the bigger the needle.)

44. a. A "No alcohol" auxiliary label should always be placed on the container when dispensing metronidazole to a patient. Consuming alcohol while using this drug will cause an antabuse-type reaction, including severe nausea and profuse vomiting.

45. b. 500 mL × 15% = 1500 mL × x%

$$500 × 0.15 = 1500 × x$$
$$75 = 1500x$$
$$0.05 = x$$
$$5\% = x$$

46. d. Because furosemide is a non–potassium-sparing diuretic, it causes loss of potassium along with the fluid that is lost. Potassium supplements are usually given in conjunction with a drug of this nature.

47. b. Instill 3 drops in the left ear three times daily as needed for pain.

48. c. A patient who is allergic to penicillin has a 1-in-10 chance of being allergic to a cephalosporin. This is known as cross-sensitivity.

49. b. $\frac{1}{2}$ gr = 30 mg

50. b. $\dfrac{1000 \text{ mL}}{12 \text{ hr}} \bigg| \dfrac{15 \text{ gtt}}{1 \text{ mL}} \bigg| \dfrac{1 \text{ hr}}{60 \text{ min}}$

$$= \frac{15{,}000 \text{ gtt}}{720 \text{ min}} = 20.83 \text{ gtt/min}$$

Round up to 21 gtt/min.

51. c. Zovirax and Epivir are both antiviral agents. (Hint: *vir* is in both drug names.)

52. b. $\dfrac{40 \text{ mEq}}{1000 \text{ mL}} = \dfrac{x \text{ mEq}}{80 \text{ mL}}$

(Hint: 1 L = 1000 mL.)

$$40 × 80 = 1000 × x$$
$$3200 = 1000x$$
$$3.2 \text{ mEq} = x$$

There are 3.2 mEq in 80 mL, and the patient will receive 80 mL/hr. Therefore, the patient will receive 3.2 mEq of KCl per hour.

53. a. Na is the chemical symbol for sodium.

54. d. A 5-micron filter needle will be sufficient to filter out tiny glass fragments from an opened ampoule.

55. b. Rifampin is used to treat tuberculosis.

56. d. The volume of liquid is always read at the bottom of the meniscus.

57. b. $\dfrac{2}{100} = \dfrac{1}{x}$

$$2x = 100$$
$$x = 50$$

58. b. The Poison Prevention Packaging Act of 1970 states that child-resistant caps should be used on all dispensing containers unless the drug is exempt or the patient requests otherwise.

59. c. 180 mL = 6 oz (Hint: 30 mL = 1 oz)

60. a. Inspections every six months are required to ensure that the laminar airflow workbench is working properly.

61. b. 142 lb ÷ 2.2 (2.2 lb = 1 kg) = 64.5 kg

15 mg × 64.5 kg = 968.1 mg/day

968.1 ÷ 3 (number of equal doses) Round up to 323 mg.

62. b. The FDA's MedWatch form is used to report any adverse drug reactions.

63. c. $4.50 × 30% = $1.35

$4.50 + $1.35 = $5.85

64. b. Tetracycline and tetracycline-derivative drugs should never be administered with antacids or dairy products. This medication will bind to the antacids or dairy products and simply pass through without being absorbed systemically.

65. c. Temazepam is classed as a Schedule IV drug, as are most sedatives and hypnotics.

66. d. 15–30°C is equivalent to 59–86°F. This is the correct temperature for room-temperature storage.

67. b. A formulary is a list of accepted medications from which a physician may prescribe. This formulary is standardized and approved by the pharmacy and therapeutics (P&T) committee.

68. d. Any information that could identify a patient is considered protected health information under HIPAA.

69. d. Vinblastine is a chemotherapeutic agent and therefore should be handled as a hazardous medication. A spill kit should be used to clean the area if a spill/breakage occurs.

70. c. When cleaning the laminar airflow workbench, always clean the hanging bar and sides first. When cleaning the sides, clean from top to bottom, working outward from the filter. Always clean the work surface last. Never spray anything directly onto the HEPA filter, because doing so could weaken or damage it.

71. b. 120 mL × 0.05% = x mL × 5%

$$120 × 0.0005 = x × 0.05$$
$$0.05 = 0.05x$$
$$1.2 = x$$

72. b. 60 ml/hr × 20 = 1200 hr total volume needed. Therefore, two bags will be sufficient to complete the 20-hr infusion.

73. a. The packing slip is used by the wholesaler to pull the drug order in the warehouse. The packing slip accompanies the drug order to the pharmacy.

74. d. 200 mL × $\dfrac{1}{200}$ = 500 mL × x%

$$200 × 0.0005 = 500 × x$$
$$0.1 = 500x$$
$$0.0002 = x$$
$$0.02\% = x$$

75. c. A secondary infusion attached to a main IV line is called a piggyback.

76. a. The 000 is the largest size empty gelatin capsule used in extemporaneous compounding. (Hint: The smaller the number, the larger the capsule.)

77. b. When working in the laminar airflow workbench, all manipulations should be at least 6 inches within the hood.

78. d. A phone call is not considered a direct copy. A nurse or a pharmacist may receive a telephoned order from a physician, but a nurse cannot simply call an initial order to the pharmacy. The written documentation of the order must be reviewed by a pharmacist before it can be filled.

79. a. Amlodipine is classed as a calcium channel blocker.

80. c. A want book is a list of items that need to be ordered when using a manual inventory system.

81. c. The second letter corresponds to the first letter of the prescriber's last name.

    Add $1 + 5 + 6 = 12$

    Add $3 + 5 + 7 = 15 \times 2 = 30$

    Add $12 + 30 = 42$

    2 is the check digit, so this is the only number that could be a valid DEA number.

82. c. A Class III drug recall is the least severe of all recall classes. This type of recall is not likely to cause harm to the patient.

83. b. A DEA Form 222c is used to order Schedule II controlled substances.

84. d. Controlled substances, investigational drugs, and chemotherapy drugs all require special handling. Check your pharmacy P&P for specifics.

85. a. The Orange Book is most often used to find generic equivalent drugs.

86. d. Nursing station inspections are a responsibility of the pharmacy technician and are performed to ensure that drugs are being stored and used correctly in patient-care areas.

87. b. Warfarin and aspirin used together without a doctor's approval and appropriate monitoring could result in hemorrhage, since both of these drugs are anticoagulants. This could be a major drug–drug interaction.

88. b. 35 units + 15 units = 50 units/day

    50 units $\times$ 30 days = 1500 units/30 days

    Since each vial of insulin holds 1000 units, the patient will need two vials.

89. d. Nitroglycerin tablets and injections should always be dispensed in the original glass container. If it is dispensed in a plastic container, the medication may adhere to the plastic.

90. b. Ampicillin injection should always be diluted with normal saline for best stability. If it is mixed with dextrose, stability is greatly diminished.

Chapter 14 Review Questions

1. c. compounding

2. b. The Automix is used for TPN compounding, the PhaSeal for chemotherapy preparation, and the Pyxis and MedCarousel for medication dispensing.

3. b. A tablet can be prepared by either compression or molding.

4. c. Employee performance appraisal

5. a. Mixing calcium gluconate and sodium phosphate together in a syringe will cause an insoluble precipitate of calcium phosphate.

6. d. A suspension contains undissolved drug particles.

7. d. A POS system is a point-of-sale system that deducts products from inventory when they are sold.

8. d. Aspirin is contraindicated for a patient on warfarin, because it can increase bleeding of the stomach lining, thin the blood, and decrease coagulation.

9. d. The trade name for ramipril is Altace.

10. d. all of the above

11. b. The Omnibus Budget Reconciliation Act of 1990 required pharmacists to perform drug utilization reviews, keep proper records, and counsel Medicaid patients.

12. a. Most capsules are available in either hard or soft-shell gelatin or some other form of soluble material.

13. b. Venlafaxine

14. d. Methyldopa is approved to treat HTN during pregnancy.

15. b. Of the available answers, clonidine is the only one used to treat hypertension and available in a patch.

16. a. Total parts = 100. Therefore, 12.5 parts/100 parts $\times$ 454 grams = 56.75 grams.

17. a. Lidocaine is used to treat arrhythmias.

18. a. Of the choices, digitalis is the only drug used for atrial flutter and fibrillation.

19. b. A disintegrator is added to facilitate dissolution of the drug.

20. b. Phytonadione produces the opposite effect as warfarin.

21. a. Safe Medical Devices Act

22. b. DEA Form 222 is used to order CII drugs.

23. d. angina pectoris

24. c. Total parts = 15.5. 1.5 parts/15.5 parts $\times$ 12 kg = 1.16 kg.

25. d. Non–potassium-sparing diuretics cause loss of potassium along with the fluid that is lost. Potassium supplements are usually given in conjunction with a drug of this nature.

26. d. A sig code is used to facilitate order entry.

27. d. Whenever state and federal guidelines differ, always follow the guideline that is the most strict.

28. d. $\dfrac{100 \text{ mg}}{\text{ml}} = \dfrac{500 \text{ mg}}{x \text{ ml}}$

$100x = 500$

$x = 5 \text{ ml}$

29. c. $1 \text{ g} = 1000 \text{ mg}$

$\dfrac{1000 \text{ mg}}{10 \text{ ml}} = \dfrac{600 \text{ mg}}{x}$

$1000x = 6000$

$x = 6 \text{ ml}$

30. d. Controlled substances can be kept under lock and key or dispersed in the regular stock in a way that deters diversion and theft.

31. b. Survanta is a natural bovine lung extract.

32. a. Consuming alcohol while using this drug will cause an antabuse-type reaction, including severe nausea and profuse vomiting.

33. d. The Kefauver-Harris Amendment was passed because of birth defects due to thalidomide.

34. b. Tetracycline and tetracycline-derivative drugs should never be administered with antacids or dairy products. This medication will bind to the antacids or dairy products and simply pass through without being absorbed systemically.

35. a. Patients should always be advised to drink plenty of water when taking trimethoprim and sulfamethoxazole, to prevent crystalluria and stone formation.

36. d. Tetracycline causes the skin to be more sensitive to sunlight.

37. c. Antibiotics by nature kill or inhibit microorganisms.

38. b. The lot number is needed to identify the recalled drug product.

39. c. Syringes used for oral liquid medications must not be able to accept a needle, to ensure proper administration of the liquid.

40. d. The Drug Enforcement Administration is the federal agency responsible for enforcing the CSA.

41. c. pc means after meals.

42. c. Prescriptions are not the primary records of acquisition by a pharmacy.

43. b.

44. d. Fat-soluble vitamins are A, D, E, and K.

45. c. The maximum amount the patient is prescribed is 2 tabs every 4 hours, which is 12 tabs per day. 12 tabs × 14 days = 168 tablets.

46. d. A gel-cap is the only choice for masking the taste.

47. a. If the patient is to receive 1.5 mg/minute, then he or she will receive 90 mg/hr (1.5 mg × 60). The concentration of the IV is 8 mg/ml (2000 mg/ 250 ml).

$\dfrac{8 \text{ mg}}{\text{ml}} = \dfrac{90 \text{ mg}}{x}$

$8x = 90$

$x = 11.25 \text{ ml}$; round down to 11 ml/hr.

48. b. Type I diabetes is considered insulin-dependent.

49. c. A broad-spectrum drug works against both gram-positive and gram-negative organisms.

50. d.

51. b. $\dfrac{2 \text{ mEq}}{\text{ml}} = \dfrac{30 \text{ mEg}}{x}$

$2x = 30$

$x = 15 \text{ ml}$

52. d. MAC is the maximum allowable cost.

53. d. all of the above

54. d. $\dfrac{x}{100} = \dfrac{150 \text{ g}}{3785}$

$3785x = 15,000$

$x = 3.96$

55. b. Anabolic steroids are Schedule III drugs.

56. a. The Poison Prevention Packaging Act requires drugs to be dispensed in child-resistant containers unless the drug is exempt or the patient/prescriber requests otherwise.

57. c. Fosamax

58. d. Digoxin is a cardiac glycoside.

59. b. Morphine is classified as an opiate.

60. d. Oxytocin is used to induce labor contractions.

61. b. Antihypertensives manage high blood pressure.

62. b. The Prescription Drug Marketing Act prohibits the sale of drug samples.

63. d. After continued use, a patient may build up a tolerance to a drug and may require higher doses.

64. a. Class I drugs are not approved for legal use in the United States.

65. c. Dr. Jones, AJ1234563, follows the format for a valid DEA number.

66. d. The pharmacy's policies and procedures manual is the best choice for inventory procedures specific to your pharmacy.

67. c. Turnover

68. b. Hypoglycemia: hypo = low, glycemia = sugar

69. a. The law does not specifically state that the sale must be made by the pharmacist or a certified pharmacy technician.

70. c. Syrup of ipecac is used to induce vomiting.

71. b. Insulin is not derived from horse.

72. a. The patient's phone number is not required to be written on a prescription.

73. a. Patients with an allergy to penicillin are more likely to have a cross-sensitivity to cephalosporins.

74. c. $100/5000 = 0.02$

75. c. The pharmacy technician should always follow the specific policy of the pharmacy.

76. b. A 5-micron filter is the standard size for filtering particulates.

77. a. employee handbook

78. b. accounts receivable ledger

79. b. managed care

80. c. NDC numbers are divided into three sections, with the first five digits indicating the manufacturer; the next four digits indicating the product name, strength, and dosage form; and the last two digits indicating the package size.

81. b.

82. a. pharmaceutical care

83. a. Class I recall has the possibility of severe complications or death.

84. d. both b and c

85. c. informed consent

86. b. a wholesaler

87. b. Drug samples cannot be sold or distributed by a licensed pharmacy.

88. c. The Durham-Humphrey Amendment first distinguished between OTC and prescription drugs.

89. a. $\dfrac{3}{100} = \dfrac{x}{454}$

$100x = 1362$

$x = 13.62 \text{ g} \times 1000 \text{ mg/g} = 13{,}620 \text{ mg}$

90. a. accounts payable ledger

Chapter 15 Review Questions

1. b. the process by which a nongovernmental agency or association grants recognition to an individual who has met certain predetermined qualifications specified by that agency or association

2. d.

3. a. An interface is a connection between two or more computer systems.

4. c. activities of technicians outside the workplace

5. b. quality assurance

6. a. Sterile product preparation should be performed 6 in. from the front edge of the hood.

7. d. $1.5 \text{ g} = 1500 \text{ mg}$. If the concentration is 250 mg/ml, then the total volume contains 1500 mg.

$\dfrac{250 \text{ mg}}{\text{ml}} = \dfrac{1500 \text{ mg}}{x \text{ ml}}$

$250x = 1500$

$x = 6 \text{ ml}$

8. d. The patient's telephone number is not required on a prescription label.

9. c. as many times as the prescriber indicates on the prescription within a specified time period

10. d. Add $3 + 9 + 4 = 16$. Add $6 + 1 + 5 = 12 \times 2 = 14$. Add sums $16 + 24 = 40$. Therefore, the check digit is 0.

11. a. CI drugs have no accepted medical use in the United States.

12. c. 50 g

13. b. Household cleaners must be packaged in child-proof containers.

14. a. placed under the tongue

15. d. OBRA 90 requires DURs, record keeping, and counseling

16. c. Alprazolam

17. a. Synthroid is measured in micrograms.

18. a. Legend drugs require a prescription.

19. d. 0.9% sodium chloride is considered isotonic.

20. d. Patients do not have to be paid to participate in investigational studies.

21. d. $1.5 \text{ tsp} = 7.5 \text{ ml}$. $7.5 \text{ ml} \times 3 \text{ (TIO)} \times 10 \text{ days} = 225 \text{ mL}$

22. b. Because the prescription does not specify otic or ophthalmic, the pharmacist must contact the prescriber for verification/clarification.

23. d. Tagamet and cimetidine are H2 antagonists indicated for ulcers.

24. d. 750 mg $\times$ 2 doses per day $\times$ 7 days = 10,500 mg/1000 mg per vial = 10.5 vials. Therefore, the technician needs 11 vials to prepare the order.

25. d. Final volume − diluent volume = powder volume. $50 - 34.6 = 15.4 \text{ ml}$.

26. d. Technicians cannot dispense drug information.

27. d. $\dfrac{25}{100} = \dfrac{x}{480}$

$100x = 480 \times 25$

$100x = 12{,}000$

$x = 120$

28. b. This error code means that the patient is not enrolled in the insurance program or that the patient's name is misspelled; check for errors.

29. b. Notify the pharmacist that the patient has orders for two drugs of the same class.

30. c. Only regular insulin can be given IV.

31. c. Deductible amounts must be met before third parties begin coverage.

32. d. Oral ampicillin suspension is not sterile; therefore, it does not need to be prepared using aseptic technique.

33. d. The ADI does not contain specifics regarding parenteral medications; it includes only trade/generic names, indications, and so on.

34. d. all of the above

35. c. Discreetly notify the pharmacist so that the appropriate action may be taken.

36. d. Etoposide is a chemotherapy drug, so it should not be mixed in a horizontal hood, but in a vertical hood or biological safety cabinet.

37. b. Because technicians cannot provide drug information, the technician should inform the pharmacist that the mother would like help choosing a non-prescription product.

38. c. Patient package inserts are required with oral inhalers.

39. c. A technician can answer this question because it does not involve professional judgment or drug information.

40. b. A strength is needed to fill the prescription, so the technician should alert the pharmacist to the problem.

41. d. All the choices could contribute to a medication error. Failure to rotate stock could result in dispensing an expired or short-date drug; preparing more than one prescription at a time could result in the wrong medication going to the wrong patient; and not reading the label could result in the wrong drug or strength being used.

42. a. Notify the pharmacist if the patient is also buying aspirin; there is an interaction between these medications, and the patient should not take the medications together.

43. b. Trailing zeros (7.0 mg) should not be used because if the decimal point is not clear, the amount could be mistaken for 70 mg, not 7 mg.

44. d. all of the above

45. c. Explain the situation to the pharmacist, correct the error, document the error per procedure, and have the patient return to the pharmacy for the correct prescription.

46. c. Diazepam is a CIV drug and is not ordered on Form 222.

47. c. Unit-dose medications are not patient-specific; therefore, patient information is not printed directly on the drug label.

48. d. Refer the question to the pharmacist, because technicians cannot dispense drug information.

49. a. o.u. = both eyes

50. d. 30 cc = 30 ml = 2 tbsp

51. a. Oral polio vaccine is frozen for long-term storage.

52. d. When only a month and year are given in an expiration date, the drug is usable until the last day of that month.

53. b. U-100 means 100 units/ml. Therefore, 35 units = 0.35 ml.

54. a. A technician should never call a prescriber for clarification on an abbreviation.

55. d. Vinblastine is a chemotherapy drug.

56. d. Prescribers can give CIII drugs a maximum of five refills that must be used within six months after date of issuance.

57. b. cyclophosphamide

58. d. aseptic technique

59. c. carbamazepine

60. d. all of the above

61. d. Triazolam is a hypnotic used to induce sleep.

62. a. a.u. = both ears; therefore, an otic suspension should be dispensed.

63. c. $100 \div 1000 = 0.1$

64. b. The full quantity of the original prescription is for a 12-month supply (3 months with 3 refills). Therefore, if 1 month's worth is dispensed, the patient will get 11 refills for a 12-month supply.

65. c. Ask the patient the type of allergic reaction experienced, note the patient's response, and alert the pharmacist so the pharmacist can question the patient regarding the reaction.

66. b. If a prescription is marked (according to state law) that no substitutions are allowed, then a trade name must be dispensed unless the prescriber is contacted to okay a substitution.

67. c. 1 tbsp = 15 ml; 360 ml/15 ml per tbsp = 24 tbsp

68. b. 1 fluid ounce = 30 ml; $3 \times 30 = 90$

69. d. 2000 ml $\div$ 10 hr = 200 ml/hr

70. d. 1 mg = 1000 mcg; a 950-mcg dose = 0.95 mg.

71. b. If the patient wants the insurance to pay the maximum amount, then the generic drug must be dispensed.

72. d. The last step in filling a new prescription is RPh counseling.

73. d. All drug interaction messaging should be directed to the pharmacist.

74. a. $$\frac{125 \text{ mg}}{5 \text{ml}} = \frac{250 \text{ mg}}{x \text{ ml}}$$
$$125x = 1250$$
$$x = 10 \text{ ml}$$

75. d. Alert the pharmacist about any drug interaction messages.

76. c. Cefazolin is an antibiotic.

77. d. The physician's DEA number is required on all controlled-substance prescriptions, but not on the prescription container labels.

78. b. The tip and plunger must remain sterile.

79. d. Vertical flow hoods provide the best preparer protection, because contaminated air is not blown at the operator.

80. a. Amphotericin B must be protected from light. IV bags are covered with amber bags.

81. d. 500 mg × 4 (qid) × 7 = 14,000 mg; 14,000 mg/ 250-mg tablets = 56 tablets.

82. c. Tobramycin injection does not have to be refrigerated. IVs compounded with the injection should be refrigerated.

83. a. Sepsis is a severe infection in the body and is not normally treated at home.

84. d. Pancrease is not a laxative.

85. a. Tobramycin is available as an injection, topical cream, and ophthalmic solution.

86. d. Ibuprofen is available only in oral dosage forms.

$$\frac{80 \text{ mg}}{2 \text{ ml}} = \frac{130 \text{ mg}}{x \text{ ml}}$$

$$80x = 130$$

$$x = 3.25 \text{ ml}$$

87. b.

88. b. $\dfrac{1000 \text{ ml}}{480 \text{ min}} = \dfrac{10 \text{ gtt}}{\text{ml}} = 20.8 \text{ gtt/min}$

Round up to 21 gtt/min.

89. c. Federal law does not allow refills on CII drugs.

90. c. Cefotaxime is a cephalosporin antibiotic, not chemotherapy or hazardous.

Chapter 16 Review Questions

1. d. Any person (pharmacist or tech) who signs a DEA Form 222 must have the power to do so.

2. b. At a minimum, compounding equipment must be cleaned at least once daily, usually before use. Equipment should also be cleaned after it is used and anytime it is contaminated.

3. d. Suspensions and emulsions contain particles that are not dissolved, so they are considered suspensions.

4. d. The DEA Form 222 has 10 lines; therefore, a maximum of 10 different drugs could be ordered on one form.

5. d.

6. c. Patient profiles should always be updated with correct information.

7. b. The FDA regulates GMPs.

8. a. Hiring practices for the organization may not be found in the pharmacy's P&P manual, but in the organization's P&P manual.

9. d. 0.75 g = 750 mg; therefore, the patient needs 15 ml or 1 tablespoon.

10. d. Vitamin B-1 is thiamine.

11. c. 1000 mcg = 1 mg; therefore, the patient is to receive 1 mg per minute. 1 mg × 60 minutes = 60 mg per hour. The concentration of the IV is 2 mg/ml (500 mg/250 ml), so the IV rate is 30 mg/ml.

12. b. A patient's insurance coverage should not affect the drug dosage that the physician prescribes.

13. c. Because the active ingredients in a liquid are already dissolved, they will deteriorate faster than those that have to dissolve in the body.

14. b. Batch repackaging involves repackaging large amounts for general use in the pharmacy. Extemporaneous repackaging is repackaging a drug for a specific patient or order.

15. b. A compounding slab is used to mix topical medications.

16. c. A "refill too soon" message indicates that the days' supply entered in the computer does not match how the patient is using the drug. Either the patient is using the drug incorrectly or the pharmacy entered the days' supply incorrectly.

17. c. Prn means as needed; therefore, a prn drug is given only under specific circumstances and is not scheduled around the clock.

18. b. Isotretinoin is used to treat acne; if it is taken by a pregnant woman, it can cause birth defects or miscarriage.

19. c. The ScriptPro is used to fill retail prescriptions; the Automix is used to compound TPNs; and the Pyxis and Omnicell are automated medication dispensing devices used in hospital settings.

20. d.

21. c. Technicians must always refer drug information or counseling questions to the pharmacist.

22. b. 4 oz = 120 ml ratio has a total of 4 parts. If you divide 120 ml by 4 parts, you get 30 ml for each part. Therefore, 3 × 30 ml = 90 and 1 × 30 ml = 30 ml.

23. c. 1.5^2 m^2 × 20 mg/m^2 = 30.4 mg per day

$$\frac{50 \text{ mg}}{50 \text{ ml}} = \frac{30.4 \text{ mg}}{x \text{ ml}} = 20.8 \text{ gtt/min}$$

$$50x = 1520$$

$$x = 30.4 \text{ ml}$$

$$\frac{10 \text{ mg}}{\text{ml}} = \frac{40 \text{ mg}}{x \text{ ml}} = 20.8 \text{ gtt/min}$$

24. b. $10x = 40$

$$x = 4 \text{ ml for each dose}$$

4 ml per dose × 3 doses per day (q8h) = 12 ml total. Therefore, you need to send 2 mdv.

25. c. 2000 ml ÷ 24 hr = 83.3 ml/hr. Round down to 83 ml/hr.

26. c. $\dfrac{250 \text{ mg}}{5 \text{ ml}} = \dfrac{373 \text{ mg}}{x \text{ ml}}$

$$250x = 375(5)$$

$$250x = 1875$$

$$x = 7.5 \text{ ml} = 1\frac{1}{2} \text{ tsp}$$

27. b. Rifampin will cause discoloration of the urine and feces.

28. b. U-100 means 100 units per milliliter.

29. d. Percodan contains aspirin, so it should not be taken because of the interaction between warfarin and aspirin.

30. a. The IV route has the fastest onset of action, because the drug is injected directly into the bloodstream.

31. b. Unit-dose drug packages are not specific to any one patient. Therefore, the patient's name is not printed on the drug label.

32. c. Drugs that require patient package inserts (PPIs) must include them with each prescription or refill.

33. d. $42.10 ÷ 100 = $0.421 for each tablet
$0.421 × 60 tablets = $25.26 for 60 tabs
$25.25 + (25.25 × 0.25) = $31.575; rounded to the nearest penny.

34. d

35. a. 0.5% means 0.5 g per 100 g.
$$\frac{0.5\text{ g}}{100\text{ mg}} = \frac{x\text{ mg}}{120\text{ g}}$$
$$100x = 60$$
$$x = 0.6\text{ g}$$

36. b. $\dfrac{30\text{ mg}}{5\text{ ml}} = \dfrac{38.4\text{ mg}}{x\text{ ml}}$
$$30x = 192$$
$$x = 6.4\text{ ml}$$

37. d. 40 lb ÷ 2.2 kg/lb = 18.18 kg
18.18 kg × 30 mg/kg/day = 545.4 mg/day 545.4 mg/day ÷ 2 divided doses = 272.7 mg/dose; round up to 273 mg.

38. d. 10 g = 10,000 mg
10,000 mg ÷ 125 mg/dose = 80 doses

39. a. The gauge refers to the diameter of the needle's shaft. The lumen refers to the inner diameter of the needle.

40. d. The IDC-9 code is the code set for diagnosis required by HIPAA standards.

41. c. 20 mg × 2 caps per dose × 2 doses per day = 80 mg per day

42. c. $\dfrac{1\text{ mg}}{\text{ml}} = \dfrac{x\text{ mg}}{100\text{ ml}}$
$x = 100$; therefore, 100 mg is needed to prepare 100 ml of a 1-mg/ml solution.

43. c. Cyclosphosphamide is a chemotherapy drug, and a chemo spill kit is required to be near anyone who prepares or administers chemo drugs.

44. d.

45. b. Nitroglycerin is required to be dispensed in its original glass container to maintain its potency.

46. d. % strength = # of grams of active ingredient per 100 g of product. 250 mg = 0.25 g; therefore,
$$\frac{0.25\text{ g}}{30\text{ g}} = \frac{x\text{ g}}{100\text{ g}}$$
$$30x = 25$$
$$x = 0.8333\text{ ml}$$
$x = 0.8333$ g are in 100 g of product; therefore, the percent strength is 0.83%.

47. d. All unused investigational drugs should be returned to the manufacturer per guidelines.

48. c. The generic name for Pamelor is nortriptyline.

49. a. Perpetual inventory maintains a running total of all inventory. Therefore, the pharmacy must document all sales and purchases as they occur.

50. b. NDC numbers are divided into three sections, with the first five digits indicating the manufacturer; the next four digits indicating the product name, strength, and dosage form; and the last two digits indicating the package size.

51. c. As drugs are ordered and placed into inventory, the drugs with the shortest expiration date should be moved to the front of the shelf to ensure that those drugs are used first.

52. b. A hospital formulary is a listing of all approved drugs used in the institution.

53. c. Acetaminophen with codeine is a Schedule III drug.

54. d. A purchase order shows the technician what drugs have been ordered.

55. c. Inventory turnover indicates how often the pharmacy uses its inventory.

56. c. When only a month and year are indicated on an expiration date, the drug is usable until the last day of that month.

57. c. Meperidine is a CII drug, and all CIIs are ordered on a DEA Form 222.

58. b. Actos is an oral antidiabetic drug.

59. b. A PAR level indicates the minimum level to be kept on the shelf. If the level falls below the PAR level, then the technician orders enough drugs to bring the quantity up to the PAR level.

60. c. The *Physician's Desk Reference* contains a compilation of manufacturers' package inserts.

61. b. Paxil is indicated for the treatment of major depressive episode.

62. b. $\dfrac{2\text{ mEq}}{\text{ml}} = \dfrac{8\text{ mEq}}{x\text{ mL}}$
$$2x = 8$$
$$x = 4\text{ ml}$$

63. b. An invoice is the wholesaler's bill to the pharmacy, and it is used by the pharmacy when paying for the drug order.

64. c.

10		3	Total parts 8
	5		
2		5	

$$\frac{3}{8} \times 120 = 45 \text{ grams of } 10\%$$

$$\frac{5}{8} \times 120 = 75 \text{ grams of } 2\%$$

65. a. 2–8°C equals 36–46°F, which is the required temperature for storage under refrigeration.

66. d. $200 \text{ mL} \times \frac{1}{200} = 500 \text{ mL} \times x\%$

$$200 \times 0.0005 = 500 \times x$$

$$0.1 = 500x$$

$$0.0002 = x$$

$$0.02\% = x$$

67. d. Antibiotics are often considered an "automatic stop order," which means that the pharmacy will automatically stop filling the order after a predetermined period of time unless the doctor renews or reorders the medication. This will prevent patients from taking antibiotics for extended periods of time, which in turn could cause drug resistance.

68. c. $100 \div 10,000 = 0.01$

69. d. During medication delivery rounds, or simply "rounds," the technician picks up new orders and drops off orders that have been filled.

70. c. Insurance claim errors decrease the payments received by the pharmacy.

71. b. Refrigeration temperature range is between 2 and 8°C.

72. c. If possible, always document any damage or missing boxes before the delivery person leaves the pharmacy.

73. a. Class I recalls have the potential for serious harm or death to the patient.

74. d. The Occupational Safety and Health Administration requires MSDSs.

75. d. Diazepam is not exempt. Oral inhalers, nitroglycerin sl tabs, and all hospital unit dose medications are exempt.

76. b. If a refill section is left blank, then the pharmacy must not give any refills.

77. c. The Omnibus Budget Reconciliation Act requires pharmacists to counsel Medicaid patients.

78. c. Always follow the return policies of your pharmacy.

79. a. Remington's Pharmaceutical Sciences is the go-to source for information on compounding medications.

80. d. When patients take their medication as directed, they are complying with the prescription.

81. d. The five rights of medication administration are the right route, the right dose, the right medication, the right patient, and the right time.

82. c. Pharmaceutical scales and balances should be certified for accuracy at least yearly.

83. d. All health-care providers (doctors, pharmacists, pharmacy technicians), health plans (insurance company), and health-care clearing houses are considered covered entities.

84. c. ScriptPro is used in retail Pharmacies; Pyxis, Omnicell, and AcuDose are used in institutional settings.

85. d. Policies and procedures manuals contain all the pharmacy's best practices.

86. c.

87. b. Zovirax

88. d. In clinical pharmacy, the pharmacist uses his or her drug information expertise to enhance and optimize patient care and outcomes.

89. d. Each state has its own state board of pharmacy, which creates and enforces all pharmacy licensing and laws in that state.

90. d. The active ingredient causes the desired effect.

Chapter 17 Review Questions

1. a. Co-payment is a set amount that the patient pays for each prescription.

2. b. Line 2 has the first error. The balance should be 45 not 44.

3. b. Only a signature can prove that a patient picked up a prescription.

4. c. Drugs are not necessarily used for life-sustaining or supporting efforts.

5. c. A five-drawer filing system is not allowed.

6. a. There is no particular pH level that an IV should have, although infusion of isotonic IVs is easier on the patient and causes fewer complications.

7. c. The patient's phone number is not required on the prescription label. All other information is required.

8. a. Sterilizing filters are 0.2 microns or smaller in size.

9. d. $150 \text{ ml} \div 50 \text{ ml/hr} = 3 \text{ hr}$

10. a. Laminar airflow hoods are designed to provide an ultraclean, almost sterile environment for IV preparation.

11. b. Unlike a side effect, an adverse effect is usually severe in nature and is not expected.

12. b. Prescriptions in the institutional setting are called medication orders, physician's orders, doctor's orders, drug orders, or orders.

13. b. MSDSs contain information on what to do if you have an accident with the substance on the sheet.

14. a. $0.5 \text{ kg} \times 1000 \text{ g/kg} = 500 \text{ g}$

    $25 \text{ mg} \times 1 \text{ g}/1000 \text{ g} = 0.025 \text{ g}$

    $10 \text{ g} + 500 \text{ g} + 0.025 \text{ g} = 510.025 \text{ g}$

15. d. The Joint Commission requires the separation of dosage forms for safety reasons.

16. b. Controlled substances usually have an automatic stop order, which means the pharmacy will stop filling the order after a predetermined period of time unless the doctor renews the order.

17. c. Drugs destroyed in the liver during the first-pass effect are not absorbed into the body.

18. c. The CSA classified controlled substances into one of five schedules based on abuse potential.

19. c. PR stands for per rectum or rectally.

20. c. Only one item may be ordered per line on DEA Form 222.

21. c. U&C stands for usual and customary.

22. b. Continuous infusions run at a slow constant rate over a long period of time.

23. a. DEA Form 222 is used to order CII medications.

24. c. Intermittent infusions are small volumes given over short periods of time. IVPBs are a type of intermittent infusion.

25. d. Pastilles are sucked in the mouth.

26. b. Extended-release medications are designed to release medication over longer periods of time, therefore reducing the frequency of doses.

27. b. PR = rectally

28. d. $1.17 \text{ kg} \times 1000 \text{ g/kg} = 1170 \text{ g}$

    $260 \text{ mg} \times 1 \text{ g}/1000 \text{ mg} = 0.26 \text{ g}$

    $1170 + 1.59 + 0.26 = 1171.85 \text{ g}$

29. d. All of these containers are considered for one-time usage.

30. d. Patient confidentiality is mandated by the federal law HIPAA.

31. c. Sig means directions for use.

32. c. Phosphate should be added first, then all other additives should be added; the TPN should be mixed in between additions. Add any calcium last, before any drug with color.

33. b. A point-of-sale (POS) system maintains a continuous record of all inventory items purchased and sold.

34. b. 2 kg = 2000 g = 2,000,000 mg. Therefore, 2,000,000 mg ÷ 325 mg = 6153.8 tablets can be made from the acetaminophen. 5 g = 5000 mg.

    Therefore, 5000 mg, 2 mg = 2500 tablets can be made from the chlorpheniramine.

35. b. Normal saline (0.9% sodium chloride) is isotonic.

36. d. Size 1 capsules are the smallest in size. The larger the capsule number, the smaller the capsule size.

37. d. GERD is gastroesophogeal reflux disease, and esomeprazole is used to tread GERD.

38. d. Nitroglycerin is good for only approximately six months after the glass bottle is opened, even if the medication is still within the manufacturer's expiration date.

39. c. Expiration dates with the month and year indicate that the drug is good until the last day of the month.

40. d. Because the patient is administering the IV at home, the directions must be transcribed out for the patient.

41. c. Sedatives and hypnotics are Schedule IV controlled substances.

42. a.

43. a. 3500 ml of Dextrose 10% can be made from 500 ml of Dextrose 70%.

44. a. The *Handbook of Injectable Drugs* is the go-to guide for parenteral medications.

45. d. Pharmacy techs are involved in all of the processes.

46. d. all of the above

47. a. No drugs can be dispensed by a pharmacy technician without a pharmacist's approval.

48. d. It is within a technician's scope of duty to retrieve lab data for the pharmacist to use in making clinical judgments on patient care, as long as the technician is not making any judgments on the patient's care.

49. a. If a generic substitution is made, the drugs must have the same active ingredient and cause the same effect on the body.

50. d. USP 797 requires that sterile alcohol and sterile water be used.

51. c. Fluorouracil is a chemotherapy drug.

52. d. 25,000 units ÷ 500 ml = 50 units/ml

53. d. All the statements are true.

54. d. Technicians should not call a doctor to discuss drug therapy.

55. d. Technicians cannot counsel, but they can instruct someone to call poison control.

56. d. A package insert is prepared by the manufacturer and is intended for the clinician.

57. a. Always notify the pharmacist if you see a potential drug interaction such as between cisapride and fluconazole.

58. d. ADI provides all the above information.

59. b. MSDSs do not give specific antidote dosing.

60. d. Oral inhalers usually are not taken with food.

61. b. $6.80 − (6.80 ÷ 40\%) = $4.08

62. c. The oral route is the easiest and least complicated ROA.

63. b. A troche is also called a lozenge.

64. d. Hydromorphone is a CII drug.

65. d. $\dfrac{24 \text{ mEq}}{x \text{ ml}} = \dfrac{08 \text{ mEq}}{\text{ml}}$

$$0.8x = 24$$
$$x = 30 \text{ ml}$$

66. d. Vitamin K is necessary for proper blood coagulation.

67. d. Technicians are responsible for all the duties in home care.

68. c. This type of reimbursement is called capitation.

69. d. All the above types of data can be collected by the technician at the prescription drop off window.

70. c. 32.5 ml of a 10 mg/5 ml drug will deliver a dose of 65 mg.

71. d. All the above are examples of quality control.

72. b. A patient's deductable must be met before an insurance company will begin to pay additional benefits or expenses.

73. d. Gowns, gloves, and masks should be worn when preparing chemotherapy or hazardous drugs.

74. b. 1 tab × 2 doses per day × 10 days = 20 tabs

75. d. Techs are only allowed to fill med carts and are generally not allowed to perform any of the other duties.

76. c. 1 tbsp = 15 ml
    15 ml × 32 = 480 ml

77. d. For extended stability, amphotericin should be mixed in D5W.

78. d. Baxa is a pharmaceutical company, not an automated dispensing system.

79. c. Never recap needles before disposal.

80. a. Phentermine is indicated for the short-term use in weight reduction along with exercise and diet.

81. c. The prescriber's signature is required on the original prescription, but it is not on the prescription label.

82. b. Proper aseptic technique minimizes the chance of contaminating sterile products.

83. a. Reorder points indicate the maximum and minimum amounts of inventory to be kept.

84. a. Erythromycin 2% solution is a topical solution.

85. b. Cimetidine is an H_2 antagonist and is not generally found on a crash cart.

86. d. 1 L = 1000 mL
    1000 mL ÷ 125 mL/hr = 8 hr
    Each 1-L bag will last 8 hr, so three 1-L bags are needed for a 24-hr supply.

87. b. Proper hand washing is the most basic and effective way for a technician to prevent contamination.

88. d. Etodolac is indicated for osteoarthritis and rheumatoid arthritis.

89. b. 4 tabs daily × 2 days = 8 tabs
    3 tabs daily × 2 days = 6 tabs
    1 tab BID × 2 days = 4 tabs
    1/2 tab BID × 2 days = 2 tabs
    1/2 tab BID × 2 days = 1 tabs
             Total = 21 tabs

90. a. 1000 ml 480 min × 20 gtt/ml = 41.6; round up to 42 gtt/min.

Chapter 18 Review Questions

1. b. $0.25\% \times x \text{ ml} = 0.1\% \times 500 \text{ ml}$
   $$0.25x = 50$$
   $$x = 200 \text{ ml}$$

2. d. $\dfrac{2 \text{ mg}}{5 \text{ ml}} = \dfrac{3 \text{ mg}}{x \text{ ml}}$

   $$2x = 15$$
   $$x = 7.5 \text{ ml per dose}$$

   7.5 ml per dose × 3 doses per day (TID) × 14 days = 315 m

3. c. $1\% \times x \text{ g} = 0.5\% \times 60 \text{ g}$
   $$x = 30 \text{ g}$$

4. b. $70\% \times x \text{ ml} = 25\% \times 1000 \text{ ml}$
   $$70x = 25,000$$
   $$x = 357.14; \text{ round down to 357 ml.}$$

5. d. 1 tbsp = 15 ml
   4350 ÷ 15 = 290

6. d. 1 tsp = 5 ml
   12.5 ÷ 5 = 2.5

7. d. 1 tab × 4 doses per day × 90 days = 360 tabs

8. c. 100 caps ÷ 4 caps per day = 25-day supply

9. b. 26.4 lb ÷ 2.2 lb/kg = 12 kg
   12 kg × 30 mg per day = 360 mg per day
   360 mg ÷ 3 doses per day = 120 mg per dose
   $\dfrac{125 \text{ mg}}{5 \text{ ml}} = \dfrac{120 \text{ mg}}{x \text{ ml}}$
   $$125x = 600$$
   $$x = 4.8 \text{ ml}$$

10. a. Powder volume = final volume − diluent volume. After reconstitution, if 10 ml has 1 g of drug, then the total volume of the vial is 20 ml, because it is a 2-g vial.
    $$x = 20 \text{ ml} - 15.5$$
    $$x = 4.5 \text{ ml}$$

11. c. If the patient is receiving 1400 units per hour, then you need to calculate how many milliliters contain 1400 units.

Concentration: 40,000 units ÷ 1000 ml
$$= 40 \text{ units/ml}$$
$$\frac{40 \text{ units}}{\text{ml}} = \frac{1400 \text{ units}}{x \text{ ml}}$$
$$40x = 1400$$
$$x = 35 \text{ ml}$$
the IV will run at 35 ml/hr.

12. c. 48 lb ÷ 2.2 lb/kg = 21.82 kg
21.82 kg × 20 mg/kg = 436.4 mg per day
436.4 mg ÷ 3 doses per day = 145.47 mg
$$\frac{187 \text{ mg}}{5 \text{ ml}} = \frac{145.47 \text{ mg}}{x \text{ ml}}$$
$$187x = 727.35$$
$$x = 3.88; \text{ round up to } 3.9 \text{ ml}$$

13. d. $$\frac{70 \text{ g}}{100 \text{ ml}} = \frac{x \text{ g}}{80 \text{ ml}}$$
$$100x = 5600$$
$$x = 56 \text{ g} \times 1000 = 56,000 \text{ mg}$$

14. b. 3 g × 9 doses = 27 g are needed. 27 g ÷ 10 g/vial = 2.7 vials, which means you need three vials.

15. c. Percent strength = gram per 100. Therefore, if you have 100 ml of 30%, you have 30 g of active drug.

16. b. 3785 ml/gal × 2.5 gal = 9462.5 ml
$$\frac{45.6 \text{ g}}{100 \text{ ml}} = \frac{x \text{ g}}{9462.5 \text{ ml}}$$
$$10x = 431,490$$
$$x = 4314.9 \text{ g}$$

17. d. 1/2 NS = 0.45% sodium chloride
Percent strength = # grams per 100 ml
$$\frac{0.45 \text{ g}}{100 \text{ ml}} = \frac{x \text{ g}}{500 \text{ ml}}$$
$$100x = 225$$
$$x = 2.25 \text{ g}$$

18. c. $23.40 ÷ 100 = 0.234 per cap × 60 caps
$$= \$14.04$$

19. c. −0.5 g = 500 mg
$$\frac{250 \text{ g}}{5 \text{ ml}} = \frac{500 \text{ mg}}{x \text{ ml}}$$
$$250x = 2500$$
$$x = 10 \text{ ml}$$

20. c. $$\frac{258 \text{ ml}}{946 \text{ ml}} = \frac{x \text{ ml}}{100 \text{ ml}}$$
$$946x = 25,800$$
$$x = 27.3 \text{ ml}$$
If there are 27.27 ml of drug in 100 ml, then the percentage is 27.3%.

21. b. 35,000 units/1000 ml = 35 units/ml
5 units/ml × 20 ml/hr = 700 units/hr

22. d. $$\frac{56 \text{ g}}{473 \text{ ml}} = \frac{x \text{ g}}{100 \text{ ml}}$$
$$473x = 5600$$
$$x = 11.8 \text{ g}$$
If there are 11.8 g of drug in 100 ml, then the percentage is 11.8%.

23. c. IV conc = 40,000 units/1000 ml = 40 units/ml
$$\frac{40 \text{ units}}{\text{ml}} = \frac{2000 \text{ units}}{x \text{ ml}}$$
$$40x = 2000$$
$$x = 50 \text{ ml}$$
Therefore, the IV rate is 50 ml/hr. Now 50 ml/60 min × 15 gtt/ml = 12.5; round up to 13 gtt/min.

24. a. $10.23 ÷ 100 tabs = $0.1023 per tab
$0.1023 × 90 tabs = $9.207
$9.207 + (9.207 × 32%) = $12.15324 + 4.50
= 16.65324; round down to $16.65.

25. c. 100 ÷ 10,000 = 0.01

26. b. 1 gr = 65 mg
325 mg ÷ 65 mg/gr = 5 gr

27. c. 100 ÷ 5 = 20; therefore, the ratio is 1:20.

28. d. $$\frac{10 \text{ mg}}{5 \text{ ml}} = \frac{50 \text{ mg}}{x \text{ ml}}$$
$$10x = 250$$
$$x = 25 \text{ ml}$$

29. b. 100 tabs ÷ 5 tabs per day = 20-day supply

30. d. Sterile water contains 0% of sorbitol.

70		25	Total parts 70
	25		
0		45	

$$\frac{25}{70} \times 500 \text{ ml} = 178.57 \text{ ml of } 70\%$$
$$\frac{45}{70} \times 500 \text{ ml} = 321.4 \text{ ml of sterile water}$$

Chapter 19 Review Questions
Math Practice Test II

1. d. 12.5 × x ml = 10 × 500 ml
$$12.5x = 50,000$$
$$x = 400 \text{ ml}$$

2. Sterile water contains 0% sorbitol.

70		10	Total parts 70
	10		
0		60	

$$\frac{10}{70} \times 500 \text{ ml} = 71.4 \text{ ml of } 70\%$$

$$\frac{60}{70} \times 500 \text{ ml} = 428.6 \text{ ml of sterile water}$$

3. d. 60 tabs ÷ 1.5 tabs per day = 40-day supply

4. b. $\dfrac{2 \text{ mg}}{5 \text{ ml}} = \dfrac{0.5 \text{ mg}}{x \text{ ml}}$

   $2x = 2.5$

   $x = 1.25$ ml per dose

   1.25 ml per dose × 3 doses per day (TID) × 30 days = 112.5 ml

5. c. $2.5\% \times x \text{ g} = 0.25\% \times 120 \text{ g}$

   $x = 12$ g

6. a. $23.80 ÷ 100 tabs = $0.238 per tab

   $0.238 × 30 tabs = $7.14

   $7.14 + (7.14 × 40%) = 9.996 + 6.50 = 16.496; round up to $16.50.

7. a. $70\% \times x \text{ ml} = 10\% \times 500 \text{ ml}$

   $70x = 5000$

   $x = 71.428$; round down to 71 ml.

8. c. 500 mg × 1.3 m2 = 650 mg per day

   650 mg ÷ 2 doses per day = 325 mg per dose

9. b. 1 mg = 1000 mcg

   5 mg × 1000 mcg/mg = 5000 mcg

10. d. $3.40 ÷ 100 = 0.034 per cap × 30 caps = $1.02

    $1.02 + (1.02 × 36%) = 1.3872 + $8.00 = 9.3872 = $9.39

11. d. $\dfrac{30 \text{ g}}{480 \text{ ml}} = \dfrac{x \text{ g}}{100 \text{ ml}}$

    $480x = 3000$

    $x = 6.25$ g

12. d. 1 tsp = 5 ml

    $25 ÷ 5 = 5$

13. a. 35,000 units/1000 ml = 35 units/ml

    35 units/ml × 10 ml/hr = 350 units/hr

14. c. 2 tabs × 4 doses per day × 30 days = 240 tabs

15. d. 90 caps ÷ 2 caps per day = 45-day supply

16. b. 22 kg = 48.4 lbs

    (48.4 lbs × 200 mg)/ 150 = 64.5 mg

17. b. $\dfrac{35 \times 250}{150} = 58.3$

18. d. NS = 0.9% sodium chloride. Percent strength = # grams per 100 ml.

19. b. Powder volume = final volume − diluent volume

    $x = 10$ ml − 9.5

    $x = 0.5$ ml

20. d. If the patient is receiving 2100 units per hour, you need to calculate how many milliliters contain 2100 units.

    Concentration = 30,000 units ÷ 1000 ml = 30 units/ml

    Therefore, the IV will run at 70 ml/hr.

21. c. $\dfrac{5 \text{ g}}{100 \text{ ml}} = \dfrac{x \text{ g}}{2500 \text{ ml}}$

    $100x = 12,500$

    $x = 125$ g

22. b. 2 g × 2 doses per day × 7 days = 28 g needed

    28 g ÷ 10 g/vial = 2.8 vials. Therefore, you need three vials.

23. d. Percent strength = gram per 100. Therefore, if you have 100 ml of 70%, you have 70 g of active drug.

24. c. $\dfrac{20 \text{ g}}{100 \text{ ml}} = \dfrac{x \text{ g}}{500 \text{ ml}}$

    $100x = 10,000$

    $x = 100$ g

25. b. $\dfrac{500,000 \text{ units}}{\text{ml}} = \dfrac{250,000 \text{ units}}{x \text{ ml}}$

    $500,000x = 250,000$

    $x = 0.5$ ml

26. b. $\dfrac{30 \text{ ml}}{120 \text{ ml}} = \dfrac{x \text{ ml}}{100 \text{ ml}}$

    $120x = 3000$

    $x = 25$ ml

    If there are 25 ml of drug in 100 ml, the percentage is 25%.

27. b. IV concentration = 20,000 units1000 ml = 20 units/ml

    $\dfrac{20 \text{ units}}{\text{ml}} = \dfrac{2500 \text{ units}}{x \text{ ml}}$

    $20x = 2500$

    $x = 125$ ml

    Therefore, the IV rate is 125 ml/hr.

    125 ml/60 min × 10 gtt/ml = 20.8; round up to 21 gtt/min

28. c. 200 ÷ 20,000 = 0.01

29. c. $\dfrac{500,000 \text{ units}}{\text{ml}} = \dfrac{20,000,000 \text{ units}}{x \text{ ml}}$

    $500,000x = 20,000,000$

    $x = 40$ ml

    $500,000x = 20,000,000$

    $x = 40$ ml

30. b. $\dfrac{10 \text{ mg}}{\text{ml}} = \dfrac{35 \text{ mg}}{x \text{ ml}}$

    $10x = 35$

    $x = 3.5$ ml

Chapter 20 Review Questions

Math Practice Test III

1. b. 2 caps per dose × 3 doses per day × 10 days = 60 caps

2. c. $\dfrac{50 \text{ mg}}{5 \text{ ml}} = \dfrac{30 \text{ mg}}{x \text{ ml}}$

   $50x = 150$

   $x = 3$ ml per dose

3. c. 60 tabs ÷ 4 tabs per day = 15-day supply

4. b. $0.5\% \times x \text{ g} = 0.0.25\% \times 120 \text{ g}$

   $x = 6$ g

5. d. \$142.50 ÷ 1000 tabs = \$0.1425 per tab

   \$0.1425 × 90 tabs = \$12.825

   \$12.825 + (12.825 × 40%) = 17.955 + 10.50 = 28.455; round up to \$28.46.

6. c. 75 mg × 4 doses per day = 300 mg

   $\dfrac{50 \text{ mg}}{\text{ml}} = \dfrac{300 \text{ mg}}{x \text{ ml}}$

   $50x = 300$

   $x = 6$ ml

   Therefore, 6 ml are needed for the day; if each vial contains 2 ml, you need 3 vials.

7. d. \$65.30 ÷ 100 caps = 0.653 per cap

   0.653 × 30 caps = \$19.59 (cost for 30 caps)

   \$19.59 (cost) + \$5.88 (markup) = \$25.47 (selling price)

8. c. 1 tbsp = 15 ml

   450 ÷ 15 = 30

9. b. $50\% \times x \text{ ml} = 10\% \times 2000 \text{ ml}$

   $50x = 20,000$

   $x = 400$ ml

10. d. 40,000 units/500 ml = 80 units/ml

    80 units/ml × 16 ml/hr = 1280 units/hr

11. b. 1 tab × 2 doses per day × 90 days = 180 tabs

12. d. (6 × 250 mg)/(6 + 12) = 83.3 mg

13. d. 1/2 NS = 0.45% sodium chloride. Percent strength = # grams per 100 ml; therefore,

    $\dfrac{0.45 \text{ mg}}{100 \text{ ml}} = \dfrac{x \text{ g}}{2000 \text{ ml}}$

    $100x = 900$

    $x = 9$ g

14. d. If the patient is receiving 1400 units per hour, you need to calculate how many milliliters contain 1400 units.

    Concentration = 20,000 units ÷ 1000 ml = 20 units/ml

    $\dfrac{20 \text{ units}}{\text{ml}} = \dfrac{1400 \text{ units}}{x \text{ ml}}$

    $20x = 1400$

    $x = 70$ ml

    The IV will run at 70 ml/hr.

15. a. 20 kg × 2.2 lb/kg = 44 lb

    $\dfrac{44 \times 50}{150} = 14.666$; round up to 14.7

16. d. $\dfrac{0.45 \text{ g}}{100 \text{ ml}} = \dfrac{x \text{ g}}{1000 \text{ ml}}$

    $100x = 450$

    $x = 9$ g

17. a. Percent strength = g per 100. Therefore, if you have 100 ml of 20%, you have 20 g of active drug.

18. c. $\dfrac{25 \text{ g}}{100 \text{ ml}} = \dfrac{x \text{ g}}{2000 \text{ ml}}$

    $100x = 50,000$

    $x = 500$ g

19. b. \$69.87 ÷ 500 = 0.13974 per cap × 40 caps = \$5.5896

    \$5.5896 + (5.5896 × 16.2%) = 6.4951 + \$15.30 = 21.7951 = \$21.80

20. d. $\dfrac{500,000 \text{ units}}{\text{ml}} = \dfrac{750,000 \text{ units}}{x \text{ ml}}$

    $500,000x = 750,000$

    $x = 1.5$ ml

21. d. 500 mg × 100 doses = 50,000 mg

    500 mg ÷ 1000 mg/g = 50 g needed

    50 g ÷ 10 g/vial = 5 vials

22. c. 16 oz = 480 ml

    $\dfrac{90 \text{ ml}}{480 \text{ ml}} = \dfrac{x \text{ ml}}{100 \text{ ml}}$

    $480x = 9000$

    $x = 18.75$ ml

    If there are 18.75 ml of drug in 100 ml, the percentage is 18.75 or 18.8%.

    If there are 14.4 g of drug in 100 ml, the percentage is 14.4%.

23. a. 120 ml/60 min × 10 gtt/ml = 20 gtt/min

24. b. 100 ÷ 15,000 = 0.00666 = 0.007%

25. c. 1 mg = 1000 mcg

    10,000 mcg × 1 mg/1000 mcg = 10 mg

26. a. Powder volume = final volume – diluent volume

    $\dfrac{100 \text{ mg}}{\text{ml}} = \dfrac{1000 \text{ mg}}{\text{ml}}$

    $100x = 1000$

    $x = 10$ ml

    If the concentration is 100 mg/ml and you have a vial of 1 g (1000 mg), the final volume is 10 ml.

    $x = 10 \text{ ml} - 8.5$

    $x = 1.5$ ml

27. c.
$$\frac{\dfrac{250{,}000 \text{ units}}{\text{ml}} = \dfrac{1{,}000{,}000 \text{ units}}{x \text{ ml}}}{250{,}000x = 1{,}000{,}000}$$
$$x = 4 \text{ ml}$$

28. c.
$$\frac{69.12 \text{ g}}{480 \text{ ml}} = \frac{x \text{ g}}{100 \text{ ml}}$$
$$480x = 6912$$
$$x = 14.4 \text{ ml}$$

If there are 14.4 g of drug in 100 ml, the percentage is 14.4%.

29. c.
$$\frac{5 \text{ mg}}{\text{ml}} = \frac{35 \text{ mg}}{x \text{ ml}}$$
$$5x = 35$$
$$x = 7 \text{ ml}$$

30. b.

20		10
	15	
5		5

Total parts 15

$$\frac{10}{15} \times 2000 \text{ ml} = 1333 \text{ ml of } 20\%$$

$$\frac{5}{15} \times 2000 \text{ ml} = 667 \text{ ml } 5\%$$

Chapter 21 Review Questions

1. d	2. d	3. c	4. b	5. a
6. b	7. b	8. d	9. a	10. c
11. c	12. b	13. c	14. d	15. b
16. d	17. b	18. c	19. d	20. d
21. c	22. d	23. c	24. c	25. d
26. a	27. b	28. d	29. b	30. c
31. a	32. c	33. c	34. a	35. c
36. c	37. b	38. c	39. d	40. d
41. b	42. c	43. d	44. b	45. b
46. c	47. d	48. c	49. d	50. d
51. b	52. b	53. a	54. b	55. b
56. c	57. d	58. c	59. c	60. b
61. c	62. c	63. a	64. a	65. b
66. d	67. d	68. b	69. c	70. a
71. b	72. b	73. d	74. a	75. d
76. b	77. b	78. b	79. d	80. b
81. b	82. d	83. c	84. b	85. d
86. c	87. d	88. d	89. c	90. a

Chapter 22 Review Questions

1. c	2. c	3. b	4. c	5. b
6. a	7. c	8. b	9. b	10. a
11. d	12. d	13. c	14. c	15. b
16. c	17. c	18. c	19. a	20. c
21. a	22. b	23. d	24. a	25. a
26. a	27. a	28. b	29. d	30. a
31. c	32. b	33. a	34. a	35. c
36. d	37. b	38. d	39. b	40. c
41. a	42. a	43. c	44. c	45. a
46. c	47. b	48. c	49. c	50. c
51. d	52. d	53. b	54. d	55. a
56. d	57. b	58. b	59. a	60. c
61. a	62. b	63. a	64. a	65. b
66. b	67. b	68. b	69. d	70. c
71. b	72. b	73. a	74. b	75. d
76. d	77. b	78. d	79. b	80. a
81. a	82. b	83. c	84. d	85. c
86. a	87. a	88. b	89. d	90. b

Index

A

AAPT. *See* American Association of Pharmacy Technicians (AAPT)

AAS in Pharmacy Technology. *See* Associates of Applied Science (AAS) in Pharmacy Technology

Abbreviations
  metric system, 119
  sig code, 84–86

Abilify, 137

Abraxane, 142

Accreditation Council on Pharmacy Education (ACPE), 6, 14

Acetaminophen, 22–23, 27, 66, 67

Aciphex, 139

ACPE. *See* Accreditation Council on Pharmacy Education (ACPE)

Activase, 142

Active ingredient, determining percent strength of, 126

Actonel, 141

Actos, 138

ADA. *See* Americans with Disabilities Act of 1990 (ADA)

Adacel, 142

ADC. *See* Automated Dispensing Cabinets (ADC)

Adderall XR, 139

ADE. *See* Adverse Drug Events (ADE)

Administration, routes of, 22, 24, 49–50, 80. *See also specific administrations*

Advair Diskus, 137

Advair HFA, 142

Adverse Drug Events (ADE), 11, 17, 44, 68

Adverse Events Reporting System 1998, 44

AERS. *See* Adverse Events Reporting System 1998

Afinitor, 141

Aggrenox, 141

Alimta, 138

Alligations, 133

Aloxi, 141

Ambulatory pharmacies, 3–4

American Association of Pharmacy Technicians (AAPT), 19, 45

American Pharmacists Association (APhA), 2, 7, 19

American Society of Health System Pharmacist (ASHP), 6–7, 19, 73, 103

Americans with Disabilities Act of 1990 (ADA), 7, 16

Aminoglycosides, 25

Amphetamine Salts, 140, 142

Analgesics, 22

Anaphylactic reactions, 30

AndroGel, 138

Angiomax, 141

Antibiotics, 22, 23, 25, 51

Antidepressants, 27, 32, 66, 98

Antihistamines, 27, 32, 38–39

Anti-Tampering Act of 1983, 42

APhA. *See* American Pharmacists Association (APhA)

Apothecary system, 118
  apothecary-to-metric conversions, 120–122

Aranesp, 139

Asacol, 140

Asclepius (god of medicine), 1

Aseptic technique, 48–51, 54–55

ASHP. *See* American Society of Health System Pharmacist (ASHP)

Aspirin, 32, 66, 82

Associates of Applied Science (AAS) in Pharmacy Technology, 5

Atorvastatin Calcium, 138, 139

Atripla, 137

Automated Dispensing Cabinets (ADC), 104, 114–115

Auxiliary warning labels, 66–67, 81

Avastin, 137

Avodart, 140

Avonex, 138

B

Back orders, 100

Balance's readability, 57

Bar code scanning, 76, 113–114

Batch compounding (batching), 56

Benicar, 139

Benicar HCT, 139

Betaseron, 139

Biologics Control Act (1902), 2

Black box warning, 65

BNDD. *See* Bureau of Narcotics and Dangerous Drugs (BNDD)

Boats, 58

Boxed warnings. *See* black box warning

Brand name drugs with generic equivalents practice tests, 189–200

Brand names, 25–27

Budesonide, 138

Bulwer-Lytton, Edward, 2

Bureau of Narcotics and Dangerous Drugs (BNDD), 35

Business math, 134–135

Byetta, 141

Bystolic, 140